HORMONES AND BREAST CANCER

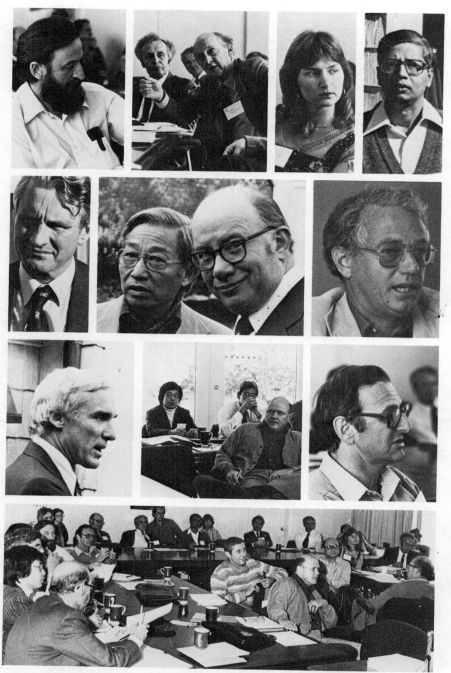

Row 1: M. C. Pike; J. B. Brown, R. Bulbrook; R. Ottman; Y. N. Sinha.
Row 2: F. de Waard; T. Dao, J. Meites; B. Henderson.
Row 3: C. Welsch; R. Shiu, J. Rosen, R. Moon; S. Korenman.
Row 4: Participants at an afternoon session.

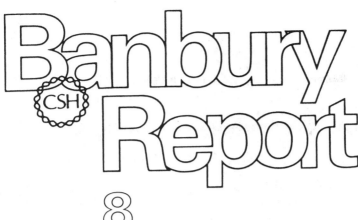

8

HORMONES AND BREAST CANCER

Edited by

MALCOLM C. PIKE
University of Southern California

PENTTI K. SIITERI
University of California School of Medicine

CLIFFORD W. WELSCH
Michigan State University

COLD SPRING HARBOR LABORATORY
1981

BANBURY REPORT SERIES

Banbury Report 8
Hormones and Breast Cancer

Printed in the United States of America

Cover and book design by Emily Harste

Library of Congress Cataloging in Publication Data

Main entry, under title:

Hormones and breast cancer.
    (Banbury report ; 8)
    Includes index.
    1. Breast—Cancer—Etiology—Congresses. 2. Endo-
crine gynecology—Congresses. 3. Hormones, Sex—
Physiological effect—Congresses. I. Pike, Malcolm C.,
1935-   . II. Siiteri, Pentti K., 1926-
III. Welsch, Clifford W., 1935-   . IV. Series:
Banbury Center. Banbury report ; 8.
RC280.B8H65   616.99'449071   80-28015
ISBN 0-87969-206-5
ISSN 0198-0068

Participants

James B. Brown, Department of Obstetrics and Gynecology, University of Melbourne, Australia

Richard D. Bulbrook, Department of Clinical Endocrinology, Imperial Cancer Research Fund, London

Philip Cole, Epidemiology Program of the Comprehensive Cancer Center, University of Alabama, Birmingham

Thomas L. Dao, Department of Breast Surgery and Breast Cancer Research Unit, Roswell Park Memorial Institute

Frits de Waard, Department of Epidemiology, University of Utrecht, The Netherlands

Brian E. Henderson, Department of Family and Preventive Medicine, University of Southern California Medical School, Los Angeles

Russell Hilf, Department of Biochemistry and University of Rochester Cancer Center

Peter Hill, American Health Foundation

Jennifer L. Kelsey, Department of Epidemiology and Public Health, Yale University School of Medicine

Stanley G. Korenman, Department of Medicine, UCLA-San Fernando Valley Program, VA Medical Center

Marc Lippman, Medicine Branch, National Cancer Institute

Victor K. McElheny, Banbury Center, Cold Spring Harbor Laboratory

Joseph Meites, Department of Physiology, Michigan State University, East Lansing

Richard C. Moon, Life Sciences Division, IIT Research Institute

Satyabrata Nandi, Department of Zoology and Cancer Research Laboratory, University of California, Berkeley

Ruth Ottman, Department of Genetics, University of California, Berkeley

Nicholas L. Petrakis, Department of Epidemiology and International Health, University of California, San Francisco

Malcolm C. Pike, Department of Family and Preventive Medicine, University of Southern California School of Medicine, Los Angeles

Jeffrey M. Rosen, Department of Cell Biology, Baylor College of Medicine

Albert Segaloff, Department of Medicine, Alton Ochsner Medical Foundation

Claire J. Shellabarger, Medical Department, Brookhaven National Laboratory

Robert P. C. Shiu, Department of Physiology, University of Manitoba, Winnipeg

Pentti K. Siiteri, Department of Obstetrics, Gynecology and Reproductive Sciences, University of California, San Francisco

Yagya N. Sinha, Scripps Clinic and Research Foundation

David A. Sirbasku, Department of Biochemistry and Molecular Biology, The University of Texas Medical School, Houston

William Topp, Cold Spring Harbor Laboratory

Reijo Vihko, Department of Clinical Chemistry, University of Oulu, Finland

James D. Watson, Cold Spring Harbor Laboratory

Clifford W. Welsch, Department of Anatomy, Michigan State University, East Lansing

Barnett Zumoff, Institute for Steroid Research and the Department of Oncology, Montefiore Hospital and Medical Center

Preface

Breast cancer, which tragically accounted for 19% of the 183,000 female cancer deaths recorded in the United States in 1978, presents some of the most tangled puzzles faced by researchers attempting to sort out the influences of genetic endowment and the environment in cancer causation.

Wide variation in overall breast cancer rates between such countries as Japan and the United States, or between women in Japan and women of Japanese ancestry in the United States, point to still-unidentified environmental factors as major influences on breast cancer. But the very slow change in breast cancer rates in the United States in 1953-78, as tabulated by Richard Doll and Richard Peto in their study for the U.S. Office of Technology Assessment, indicates that such environmental influences have varied little over a long period in which such factors as fat in the diet may have changed substantially.

The importance of duration of exposure to estrogen as an influence on breast cancer rates has been underlined not only by experimental work on rodents but also by the discovery by epidemiologists of the enhancement of breast cancer risk by such factors as early age at menarche, late age at menopause, or late age of first full-term pregnancy. Other studies, such as those of women exposed to radiation from the Hiroshima and Nagasaki atomic bombs in the ages near menarche, indicate a developmental period of special vulnerability from exposure to environmental factors.

The Banbury conference on hormones and breast cancer, held from 26 to 29 October 1980, brought together three groups of researchers who have been tackling the puzzles of breast cancer—epidemiologists, animal oncologists and endocrinologists, and human endocrinologists—to report recent findings, explore what remains poorly understood, and suggest new studies to both epidemiologists and endocrinologists. Participants found the conference stimulating, and we at Banbury Center and Cold Spring Harbor Laboratory hope that this promptly published account will prove equally stimulating to a wider technical audience.

As is usual in such a cooperative intellectual enterprise, thanks are owed widely. We are grateful to each of our participants for the effort involved in attendance, preparation of presentations and manuscripts, and thoughtful discussion. We were fortunate to have Malcolm Pike, Pentti Siiteri, and Clifford Welsch as our organizers and volume editors, recruiting our distinguished participants, and overseeing the publication of the papers and lively discussions.

Making possible the 2-year effort of organizing the conference and publishing its results as part of the Banbury program on environmental health risks was support from such generous organizations as the Esther A. and Joseph Klingenstein Fund, the Alfred P. Sloan Foundation, the National Cancer Institute, and the board of trustees of Cold Spring Harbor Laboratory.

Contributing advice and enthusiasm at every step was James Watson, director of Cold Spring Harbor Laboratory, who had the original idea of dedicating the magnificent Banbury estate, given to the Laboratory in 1976 by Charles S. Robertson, to such public-service uses as a program of assessing environmental health problems.

It is a pleasure once again to acknowledge the indispensable contributions to this, the eighth Banbury Report, of Lynda Moran and Judith Cuddihy, editors, Kathleen Kennedy, editorial assistant, Barbara Cowley-Durst, our free-lance editor, and Beatrice Toliver, administrative assistant.

Victor K. McElheny

Contents

SESSION 1:
Review of Epidemiology of Breast Cancer

The Epidemiology of Breast Cancer As It Relates to Menarche, Pregnancy, and Menopause

MALCOLM C. PIKE, BRIAN E. HENDERSON,
AND JOHN T. CASAGRANDE
Department of Family and Preventive Medicine
University of Southern California School of Medicine
Los Angeles, California 90033

Experimental work over the last 20 years has greatly increased our knowledge of breast cancer in a number of animal species, and this work, plus the development of sensitive assays for steroid and peptide hormones, has, we believe, provided the epidemiologist with the basic tools required for the understanding of human breast cancer. Epidemiologists need knowledge of the most recent thinking of animal experimentalists and human endocrinologists if they are to contribute significantly to the understanding of the etiology of breast cancer. Experimentalists and endocrinologists, likewise, need knowledge of the epidemiologic facts of breast cancer if they are to continue to contribute their best efforts to the solution of the human problem.

Because it is the human problem that is to be the focus of this meeting and we continually will be checking the relevance of any theory, wherever derived, by comparing it to human experience, it seemed most sensible to begin this meeting by reviewing the epidemiology of breast cancer. In this brief review, we will ignore the possible effects of drugs, including oral contraceptives and menopausal estrogens, and concentrate rather on the "natural" risk factors of age at menarche, first birth, and menopause. These three factors may be built into a simple mathematical model, which we will use to ask such questions as, "Do we need a Japanese factor to explain the very low breast cancer rates in Japan, or do they simply reflect the Japanese pattern of menarche, pregnancy, and menopause."

INTERNATIONAL VARIATION

There is remarkable variation in breast cancer rates among different countries (Waterhouse et al. 1976). In Table 1, it is shown that, as of 1970, rates were some 6.6 times higher in the United States and Canada than in Japan. Rates nearly as high as those of North America are seen in Switzerland, whereas rates 4.5 times higher than in Japan are seen in many Western European countries and in New Zealand. The rates in South America, the Caribbean, and Eastern Europe

Table 1

Ratios of Age-standardized Breast Cancer Rates in Different Countries

Country	Rate ratio[a]	Country	Rate ratio[a]
Hawaii (white)	6.64	São Paulo, Brazil	3.91
British Columbia	6.61	Norway (rural)	3.31
San Francisco (white)	6.60	Finland	2.72
Geneva, Switzerland	5.83	Warsaw, Poland	2.60
Hawaii (Hawaiian)	5.47	Cali, Columbia	2.30
San Francisco (black)	4.79	Puerto Rico	2.10
Israel (all Jews)	4.59	Bombay, India	1.66
Oxford, United Kingdom	4.50	Singapore (Chinese)	1.60
New Zealand (white)	4.34	Ibadan, Nigeria	1.26
New Zealand (Maori)	4.31	Miyagi, Japan	1.07
Norway (urban)	4.10	Osaka, Japan	1.00

[a]Ratio relative to age-standardized rate of 12.1 per 100,000 per year in Osaka, Japan. Age standardization is to world population, (see Waterhouse et al. [1976] where all the data is given).

are intermediate. This large variation has provided a particularly strong impetus to epidemiologic studies of many kinds (demographic, dietary, and endocrinologic).

These differences in breast cancer rates are not determined by variation in genetic susceptibility. U.S. black breast cancer rates are very similar to U.S. white rates, not to black African rates (see Table 1). Furthermore, studies of Japanese migrants to Hawaii (Haenszel and Kurihara 1968) and California (Buell 1973) show that Japanese-Americans are likely soon to have the high breast cancer rates of U.S. women. Figure 1, for example, compares the rates of breast cancer in Los Angeles white women to Japanese women in Los Angeles and Osaka. Under age 55, the incidence of breast cancer in Japanese women in Osaka is about one-fifth that of white women in Los Angeles, whereas Japanese women in Los Angeles have rates that are within 20% of the white rates. Over age 55, the Japanese-Osaka rates are one-eighth that of Los Angeles white rates, with Japanese-Los Angeles rates some fourfold higher than the Osaka rates, but still only half the Los Angeles white rates. This latter gap presumably will continue to decrease as more Japanese women born in the United States enter the older age groups.

Figure 1 also illustrates another particularly noteworthy feature of Japanese breast cancer rates, namely, that they remain almost constant after the menopause, whereas U.S. rates and rates for many other countries continue to rise.

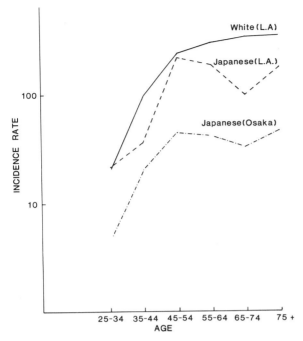

Figure 1

Age-specific breast cancer incidence rates among Los Angeles County whites and Japanese compared to Japanese in Osaka.

SECULAR TRENDS

Before discussing the key risk factors for breast cancer, it is worth pointing out one other facet of U.S. breast cancer rates—the age-adjusted rates have been relatively stable for a long time. The results of the three National Cancer Surveys are shown in Table 2 (Devesa and Silverman 1978). The small increases found by these special surveys are in sharp contrast to the data from the Connecticut Tumor Registry (Connecticut State Department of Health 1967), which show a steady increase in rates since 1935. The Connecticut increases appear as a cohort effect: Compared to the 1900-09 birth cohort, succeeding 10-year birth cohorts have rates that have increased an average of 20%, 38%, and 49%. The reliability of the Connecticut data is, however, open to serious question due to secular changes in the case ascertainment methods used, in particular the decreasing proportion of cases ascertained solely from death certificates. Changes in ascertainment methods and changes in diagnostic criteria (Fox 1979) also cast serious doubt on the recent increases reported from the Surveillance, Epidemiology, and End Results (SEER) program (Pollack and Horm 1980).

Incidence rates usually are considered a much better guide to what is happening than are mortality rates, but this is not necessarily true when in situ

Table 2

Secular Trend in Breast Cancer Incidence Rates, 1938-1970

Years of survey	White	Nonwhite
1937–39	67.1	46.2
1947–48	73.6	50.4
1969–71	73.3	53.7

From Devesa and Silverman (1978).

carcinomas are being diagnosed as cancer and biopsy rates are increasing. These problems are discussed at length by Fox (1979). It is clear that both incidence and mortality rates need to be considered when discussing secular trends.

We conclude that there is no great recent increase in breast cancer rates, and searching for an important cause of breast cancer in some aspect of the modern environment that has been introduced since, say, 1940 is unlikely to be fruitful.

The probable artefactual increases in rates in Connecticut are a clear warning that some fraction of the differences shown in Table 1 are also arte-factual. The major differences are, however, confirmed by mortality statistics.

KEY RISK FACTORS

Age at Menarche

A significantly higher risk of developing breast cancer has been found among women with an earlier age at menarche in many case-control studies (Staszewski 1971). In the United States, the average age at menarche of breast cancer cases has been found to be only a few months younger than that of controls (Henderson et al. 1974); however, Table 3 shows that this translates into a twofold increased risk of breast cancer at young ages when the effect is most evident for menarche before age 12 as compared with menarche at 13 or older.

Table 3

Relative Risk of Breast Cancer by Age at Menarche in Women Aged 32 and Younger

	Age at menarche		
	>11	12	13+
Cases	49	52	62
Controls	61	67	142
Relative risk	1.00	0.90	0.50

From Pike et al. (1981).

Age At First Full-term Pregnancy

Two of the earliest known and most reproducible features of breast cancer epidemiology are the decreased risk associated with increased parity and the increased risk of single women.

MacMahon et al. (1970) made a major advance in our understanding of the role of pregnancy in altering breast cancer risk in their analysis of their international collaborative case-control study. Single and nulliparous married women were found to have the same increased risk of breast cancer, approximately 1.4 times that of married women. Among married women in each country, parous cases had fewer children than parous controls. MacMahon and his colleagues clearly demonstrated, however, that this protective effect of parity was due to a protective effect of early age at first full-term pregnancy (FFTP). Those women with a FFTP under age 20 had about one-half the risk of nulliparous women (Table 4). Controlling for age at FFTP, the number of subsequent births had no influence on the risk of developing breast cancer (Table 5); i.e., the entire protective effect was limited to the first birth and

Table 4
Relative Risk of Breast Cancer by Age at FFTP

Age at FFTP	Relative risk
–19	1.00
20–24	1.20
25–29	1.56
30–34	1.88
35+	2.44
Never	2.00

From MacMahon et al. (1970).

Table 5
Relative Risk of Breast Cancer by Number of Full-term Pregnancies (FTP) after the First FTP (Adjusting for Age at First FTP)

Number of FTPs after the first	Relative risk
0	1.0
1	1.2
2	1.0
3	1.0
4–8	0.9
9+	0.9

From MacMahon et al. (1970).

subsequent births did not lower the risk further. Early abortions before the first full-term pregnancy did not have any protective effect.

Table 4 also shows that nulliparous women did not have quite as high a risk as women whose FFTP was delayed to their late 30s. It is not clear whether this peculiar finding is due to some "abnormality" in the nulliparous women or in the women with late first deliveries.

If it is the women with a late first birth who are "abnormal," then one possible explanation is that they are a group of subfertile women and that the same intrinsic hormonal imbalance, which made them subfertile, is also responsible for their increased risk of breast cancer. An alternative explanation is that the stimulation of breast tissue that accompanies pregnancy promotes previously initiated tumor cells in a woman pregnant at a late age; however, late births other than the first do not have an increased risk associated with them (MacMahon et al. 1970). Yet another possibility was suggested by our recent finding that early abortions (less than 3 months gestation) before the FFTP actually doubled the breast cancer risk in young women (Pike et al. 1981). Women with late FFTP are more likely to fall into this category.

We will see below, however, that the observed relative risk of 2.44 (compared with women with FFTP under 20) associated with late age at FFTP is quite compatible with a reasonable model of breast cancer, and this suggests that the nulliparous may have a slightly lower intrinsic risk of breast cancer.

Age at Menopause

The relationship between menopause and breast cancer risk has been known for some time. Trichopoulos et al. (1972) estimated that women whose natural menopause occurred before age 45 had only one-half the breast cancer risk of those whose menopause occurred after age 55 (see Table 6). Age at menarche is not correlated with age at menopause (Wallace et al. 1978), so that another way of expressing this result is that women with 40 or more years of active menstruation have twice the risk of those with less than 30 years of menstrual activity. Similar results have been obtained in many other studies, and the relationship has been shown to extend beyond age 70.

Table 6
Relative Risk of Breast Cancer by Age at Menopause

	Age at menopause			
	-44	45-49	50-54	55+
Artificial menopause[a]	0.77	1.00	1.34	—
Natural menopause	1.00	1.27	1.47	2.03

Derived from data in Trichopoulos et al. (1972).
[a] Hysterectomy plus bilateral oophorectomy.

Lilienfeld (1956), Feinleib (1968), Trichopoulos et al. (1972), and others have shown that artificial menopause by either bilateral oophorectomy or pelvic irradiation also reduces breast cancer risk (see Table 6). The effect appears to be somewhat greater than that of natural menopause (defined as cessation of periods), and women with artificial menopause induced by hysterectomy and bilateral oophorectomy before age 35 have only 25% the expected breast cancer rate.

Both smoking and weight affect the average age at menopause. Smokers have menopause on average about 2 years before nonsmokers, and a weight increase of between 10 kg and 15 kg increases the average age at menopause by roughly the same amount (Daniell 1978). Although smokers tend to weigh less than nonsmokers, this only accounted for roughly half the smoking effect. Results from a particularly good study in Sweden are shown in Table 7.

The above studies suggest that the average age at menopause should be earlier in Japan by approximately 2 years because Japanese women are at least 15 kg lighter at menopausal ages (Stoudt et al. 1965; Hirayama 1978). We did not observe this in a recent study in Hiroshima (D.G. Hoel et al., in prep.); in fact, we found the median age at natural menopause to be the same as in the United States, and the Japanese had a much lower frequency of artificial menopause.

Weight

There is a strong relationship between weight and breast cancer risk after age 50 that appears not to be due solely to the relation of weight to age at menopause. This relationship is discussed in the accompanying paper by de Waard (this volume). We mention it here because we regard this relationship as almost as fundamental as menarche, FFTP, and menopause in determining breast cancer risk, and we will be referring to it later in discussing Japanese breast cancer rates.

The relationships between smoking and weight and between smoking and age at menopause probably are part of the explanation of the slightly lowered breast cancer rates observed in smokers (Hammond 1966).

Table 7
Smoking Habits, Body Weight, and Menopausal Status of 50-year-old Swedish Women

	Premenopausal		Postmenopausal		
	number	average weight (kg)	number	average weight (kg)	Percent postmenopausal
Smokers	43	66.0	80	62.3	65
Nonsmokers	116	69.8	71	66.7	38

From Lindquist and Bengtsson (1979).

AGE AND THE INCIDENCE OF EPITHELIAL TUMORS

If one considers the incidence, $I(t)$, of cancer at particular sites at age t (i.e., the probability of being diagnosed with the specific cancer within a year at age t) as a function of age, then the different sites fall into one or other of three patterns (Cook et al. 1969). These patterns are: (1) a rapid increase in incidence from childhood to old age, (2) a rapid increase from childhood to middle age with a subsequent slowing down of the rate of increase, and (3) a peak incidence in childhood or early adult life with a subsequent actual decline in the rate. Ignoring tumors in the third category, the most striking feature of the other cancers is their increase with advancing age, and increasing age is undoubtedly the greatest risk factor.

For most tumor sites in the first category, the relationship between incidence and age can be represented by the simple equation

$$I(t) = at^k \tag{1}$$

or

$$\log I(t) = \log a + k \log t. \tag{2}$$

Equation (2) shows that for these tumor sites we will obtain a straight line with slope k if we plot the logarithm of the incidence against the logarithm of age. This linear log-log relationship is illustrated with data for colorectal cancer from the U.S. Third National Cancer Survey (TNCS) in Figure 2 (Cutler and Young 1975). The exponent, k, of age is usually between 4 and 5.

Detailed study of the relationship between lung cancer incidence and cigarette smoking suggests that incidence should be related to duration of smoking rather than age (Peto 1977; Doll and Peto 1978), and a modified form of equation (1),

$$I(t) = a(t - w)^k, \tag{3}$$

provides an excellent description of the lung cancer incidence curve for cigarette smokers, where w is the age at starting to smoke (plus a small minimum latent period). Further studies of lung cancer incidence in ex-smokers show that the incidence remains very nearly constant after smoking ceases, again emphasizing that duration of insult is critical, not age, and suggesting that we write equation (3) as

$$I(t) = a\,[d(t)]^k \tag{4}$$

where $d(t)$ is the relevant age of the tissue. For lung cancer rates at a given cigarette consumption, $d(t)$ is simply duration of smoking to age t.

The incidence rates of tumors in the second category do not fit equations (1) or (3). We showed previously, however, that equation (4) will give a very good description of ovarian cancer rates, which show a marked flattening off at around 50 years of age, if $d(t)$ is defined as follows (Casagrande et al. 1979): $d(t)$ = number of years cycling regularly + 0.3 × number of years since

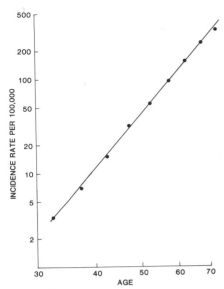

Figure 2

Age-specific incidence rates for colorectal cancer in U.S. white males (TNCS 1969-71 [Cutler and Young 1975])

menarche in which the woman is either pregnant, postmenopausal, or taking oral contraceptives. Time, as measured by $d(t)$, starts at menarche and proceeds regularly with each ovulation, but during periods of anovulation it proceeds at only 30% the pace. This definition of time accommodates the change in the rate of increase in the age incidence at about the time of menopause, as well as the protective effect both of repeated pregnancies and of the use of oral contraceptives (Casagrande et al. 1979).

THE AGE INCIDENCE OF BREAST CANCER

Because equation (4) has been so successful in describing the incidence rates of a variety of epithelial tumors, it is reasonable to assume that it will be able to represent the age-incidence curve for breast cancer with the appropriate definition of $d(t)$. A simple definition incorporating the major breast cancer risk factors of age at menarche, age at FFTP, and age at menopause is:

$$d(t) = f_0 \times \text{(time from menarche to FFTP)}$$
$$+ f_1 \times \text{(time from FFTP to menopause)} \tag{5}$$
$$+ f_2 \times \text{(time from menopause to } t)$$

where $f_0 = 1$ and f_1 and f_2 are both less than 1. Here, $d(t)$ assumes that time starts at menarche, moves regularly (at pace 1) to FFTP, then slows down after

FFTP to pace f_1 until menopause, when it slows down further to pace f_2. Without necessarily believing it, one may think of $f_0 = 1, f_1$, and f_2 as representing the rate of metabolism of breast stem cells in the three periods from menarche to FFTP, FFTP to menopause, and menopause on.

Figure 3 shows the breast cancer incidence rates for U.S. white females for 1969-1971 (Cutler and Young 1975) fitted using equation (4) with the above definition of $d(t)$; k was set at 4.5 in agreement with other epithelial tumors and to agree with the best value of k for lung cancer incidence data (Doll and Peto 1978). Menarche was set at 13 years, roughly in accordance with national figures (MacMahon 1973). To get a good fit to the data, it was necessary to set FFTP at 28 and menopause at 45; i.e., some 4 years later and 3 years earlier than the relevant national figure (MacMahon and Worcester 1966; Heuser 1976). For FFTP, therefore, we consider the beneficial effect starting only 4 years after the event. For menopause, the beneficial effect starts some 3 years before the final menstrual period. The curve shown in the figure was obtained with $f_1 = 0.7$ and $f_2 = 0.115$ and with a minimum latent period of 1 year. Equation (5) has thus become

$$d_A (t) = \text{(time from menarche to FFTP} + 4)$$
$$+ 0.7 \text{ [time from (FFTP} + 4) \text{ to (menopause} - 3)] \qquad (6)$$
$$+ 0.115 \text{ [time from (menopause} - 3) \text{ to } (t - 1)].$$

The fit of equation (6), and equation (4), clearly is pretty good, especially so when one considers the fact that the observed rates are obtained from a cross-sectional survey.

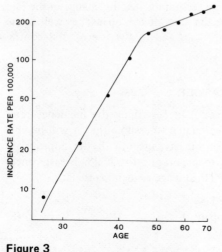

Figure 3
Age-specific incidence rates for breast cancer in U.S. white females (TNCS 1969-71 [Cutler and Young 1975]) and fitted "theoretical" curve from mathematical model

PREDICTED RELATIVE RISKS FOR MENARCHE, FFTP, AND MENOPAUSE

By substituting different ages at menarche, FFTP, and menopause into equation (6), and, hence, into equation (4), we may calculate what the model predicts quantitatively for the effects of age at menarche, FFTP, and menopause.

Age at Menarche

Table 8 shows the predicted relative risks for age at menarche varying from 11 to 14. The effect is most marked at young ages, but it remains significant at all ages. The predictions are in excellent agreement with the observed relative risks shown in Table 3 and with the results of other studies.

Age at FFTP

Table 9 shows the predicted relative risks for age at FFTP. The predicted results are again in excellent agreement with the observed results shown in Table 4.

Age at Menopause

Table 10 shows the predicted relative risks for age at menopause. The predicted results are, of course, in the right direction, but are larger than have been observed in epidemiologic studies. Some of this may be due to our choosing the TNCS as the data to fit (Fig. 3). Other data (e.g., the Second National Cancer Survey) have a less pronounced break in the slope around menopause; this will give a higher value for f_2 and, hence, lower relative risks for different menopausal ages.

Table 8
Predictions from Mathematical Model of Effect of Age at Menarche

Age at menarche	Predicted[a] relative risk at age			
	25-34	35-44	45-54	55-64
11	1.00	1.00	1.00	1.00
12	0.76	0.83	0.85	0.86
13	0.57	0.68	0.72	0.73
14	0.42	0.55	0.61	0.62

Standard conditions: $k = 4.5$, $w = 1$, age at FFTP = 24 with effect delayed 4 yr, $f_1 = 0.7$, menopause = 48 with effect occurring 3 yr earlier, $f_2 = 0.115$, and $a = 5.86845 \times 10^{-10}$.

[a] Predictions calculated at midpoint of age intervals.

Table 9

Predictions from Mathematical Model of Effect of Age at FFTP

Age at FFTP	Predicted[a] relative risk at age		
	35-44	45-54	55-64
15-19	1.00	1.00	1.00
20-24	1.37	1.29	1.28
25-29	1.84	1.65	1.62
30-34	2.42	2.08	2.02
35-39	2.76	2.60	2.50

Standard conditions: $k = 4.5$, $w = 1$, age at menarche = 13, effect of FFTP delayed 4 yr, $f_1 = 0.7$, age at menopause = 48 with effect occurring 3 yr earlier $f_2 = 0.115$, and $a = 5.86845 \times 10^{-10}$.

[a]Predictions calculated at midpoints of age intervals.

Table 10

Predictions from Mathematical Model of Effect of Age at Menopause

Age at menopause	Predicted[a] relative risk at age		
	45-54	55-64	65-74
40-44	1.00	1.00	1.00
45-49	1.67	1.64	1.60
50-54	2.54	2.55	2.45
55-59	–	3.82	3.63

Standard conditions: $k = 4.5$, $w = 1$, age at menarche = 13, age at FFTP = 24 with effect delayed 4 yr, $f_1 = 0.7$, effect of menopause occurs 3 yr earlier, $f_2 = 0.115$, and $a = 5.86845 \times 10^{-10}$.

[a]Predictions calculated at midpoints of age intervals.

PREDICTED BREAST CANCER INCIDENCE IN JAPAN

Equation (6), and equation (4), also may be used to predict the breast cancer incidence in other countries by inserting the relevant median age at menarche, FFTP, and menopause. In particular, we may use this model to predict the breast cancer rate in Japan.

There has been a major decrease in the age at menarche in Japan from 1885 up to the 1955 birth cohort (Kagawa 1978). The Japanese women who have the low breast cancer rates shown in Figure 1 had menarche around 16, i.e., some 3 years later than U.S. women. The relevant age at first full-term pregnancy in Japan may be estimated from the case-control study of MacMahon et al. (1970) at 22, roughly 2 years younger than the U.S. women. (Note: These comparative figures adjust for the much smaller proportion of nulliparous women in Japan.) The median age at menopause in Japan may, however, be a year later than in U.S. women due to a much lower frequency of artificial menopause (D. G. Hoel et al., in prep.).

Whatever three critical ages (menarche, FFTP, menopause) are fitted to the model expressed in equation (6), the fact that f_2 is positive will result in a continually increasing breast cancer rate after the menopause. Figure 1 shows that no such increase occurs in Japan and this implies that $f_2 = 0$ (equation [5]). We believe the reason for this is the weight of postmenopausal Japanese women. The Japanese of Figure 1 were some 10 kg lighter than U.S. women at age 20 (Baldwin 1924; Kagawa 1978) and some 20 kg lighter at age 60 (Stoudt et al. 1965; Hirayama 1978).

With $f_2 = 0$ but keeping $f_1 = 0.7$, as in equation (6), equation (5) becomes

$$d_J(t) = \text{(time from menarche to FFTP} + 4) \tag{7}$$
$$+ 0.7 \text{ [time from (FFTP} + 4) \text{ to (menopause} - 3)].$$

When equation (7) is fitted with the above ages at menarche (16), FFTP (22), and menopause (49), the breast cancer rate at age 50 is 95.4. The observed rate is approximately 40.

The model therefore has reduced the essential or intrinsic difference between the breast cancer rates in the United States and Japan from a factor of 6 to a factor of 2.4 (95.4/40). This is still substantial and suggests that looking for an additional Japanese factor may be rewarding. Equation (7) may be used to estimate the magnitude of such a factor by asking how much further does time have to be slowed down to reduce the breast cancer risk at age 50 from 95.4 to 40. In keeping with the spirit of our derivation of equation (7), we interpret this as follows: What value does F have to take in a modified equation (7):

$$d_J^*(t) = F \times d_J(t) \tag{8}$$

to make equation (8) result in a breast cancer incidence of 40 at age 50? Setting $F = 0.82$ accomplishes this.

DISCUSSION

An early menarche, late age at FFTP, and late age at menopause all increase the risk of breast cancer. These factors may be brought together into a simple mathematical model of breast cancer that assumes different rates of metabolism in the three periods: (1) menarche to FFTP, (2) FFTP to menopause, and (3) menopause on. The possible hormonal basis for these differential rates is discussed in other papers in this volume. This model is shown to predict accurately the known relative risks associated with different ages at menarche and FFTP.

The model overestimates the observed relative risks associated with different ages at menopause. This may be due to using cross-sectional data to estimate the parameters of the model. We currently are attempting a more involved parameter estimation taking differential cohort fertility into account.

The model predicts that nulliparous women should have the highest breast cancer rates. This is known to be untrue. Very little effort has been made to explain why women with a late age at FFTP should have a higher breast cancer rate than nulliparous women—testable hypotheses would be most welcome.

Some two-thirds of the difference in the breast cancer rates between high-risk U.S. women and low-risk Japanese women can be explained by differences in age at menarche and age at FFTP, but we are still left with a Japanese factor. If this Japanese factor is thought of in the same "rate of metabolism" terms, then we estimate that the "rate of metabolism" of breast tissue in the Japanese women born around 1920 was 82% of the equivalent U.S. rate. This small difference may be reflected in similarly small differences in active hormone levels and suggests that studies should be designed with large enough numbers to find such differences statistically significant.

Korenman (1980) has suggested that the perimenopausal period with its associated luteal inadequacy or anovulation is a particularly dangerous period for breast cancer induction due to the exposure of the breast to "unopposed estrogen." Plotting the breast cancer age-incidence curve on a log-log scale as in Figure 3 (which we argued above is the correct scale for such curves), shows, however, that there is no evidence for a period of increased susceptibility to breast cancer induction in the perimenopausal period. Rather, it shows a simple reduction in risk as the perimenopausal period advances.

REFERENCES

Baldwin, B.T. 1924. The use and abuse of height-weight-age tables as indices of health and nutrition. *J. Am. Med. Assoc.* 82:1.

Buell, P. 1973. Changing incidence of breast cancer in Japanese-American women. *J. Natl. Cancer Inst.* 51:147.

Casagrande, J.T., E.W. Louie, M.C. Pike, S. Roy, R.K. Ross, and B.E. Henderson. 1979. "Incessant ovulation" and ovarian cancer. *Lancet* ii:170.

Connecticut State Department of Health. 1967. *Cancer in Connecticut, incidence characteristics 1935-1962.* Connecticut State Department of Health, Hartford, Connecticut.

Cook, P.J., R. Doll, and S.A. Fellingham. 1969. A mathematical model for the age distribution of cancer in man. *Int. J. Cancer* 4:93.

Cutler, S.J. and J.L. Young. 1975. Third National Cancer Survey: Incidence data. *Natl. Cancer Inst. Monogr.* 41.

Daniell, H.W. 1978. Smoking, obesity, and the menopause. *Lancet* ii:373.

Devesa, S. and D. Silverman. 1978. Cancer incidence and mortality trends in the United States: 1935-74. *J. Natl. Cancer Inst.* 60:545.

Doll, R. and R. Peto. 1978. Cigarette smoking and bronchial carcinoma: Dose and time relationships among regular smokers and lifelong non-smokers. *J. Epidemiol. Community Health* 32:303.

Feinleib, M. 1968. Breast cancer and artificial menopause: A cohort study. *J. Natl. Cancer Inst.* 41:315.

Fox, M.S. 1979. On the diagnosis and treatment of breast cancer. *J. Am. Med. Assoc.* 241:489.

Haenszel, W. and M. Kurihara. 1968. Studies of Japanese migrants. I. Mortality from cancer and other diseases among Japanese in the United States. *J. Natl. Cancer Inst.* 51:147.

Hammond, E.C. 1966. Smoking in relation to the death rates of one million men and women. *Natl. Cancer Inst. Monogr.* 19:127.

Henderson, B.E., D. Powell, I. Rosario, C. Keys, R. Hanisch, M. Young, J. Casagrande, V. Gerkins, and M.C. Pike. 1974. An epidemiologic study of breast cancer. *J. Natl. Cancer Inst.* 53:609.

Heuser, R.L. 1976. *Fertility tables for birth cohorts by color: United States, 1917-1973.* Government Printing Office, Washington, D.C.

Hirayama, T. 1978. Epidemiology of breast cancer with special reference to the role of diet. *Prev. Med.* 7:173.

Kagawa, Y. 1978. Impact of westernization on the nutrition of Japanese: Changes in physique, cancer, longevity and centenarians. *Prev. Med.* 7:205.

Korenman, S.G. 1980. Oestrogen window hypothesis of the aetiology of breast cancer. *Lancet* i:700.

Lilienfeld, A.M. 1956. The relationship of cancer of the female breast to artificial menopause and marital status. *Cancer* 9:927.

Lindquist, O. and C. Bengtsson. 1979. Menopausal age in relation to smoking. *Acta Med. Scand.* 205:73.

MacMahon, B. 1973. *Age at menarche.* Vital Health Statistics, series 11, no. 133. DHEW publication number (HRA) 74-1615. National Center for Health Statistics, Rockville, Maryland.

MacMahon, B. and J. Worcester. 1966. *Age at menopause, United States, 1960-1962.* Vital Health Statistics, series 11, no. 19. DHEW, Washington, D.C.

MacMahon, B., P. Cole, T.M. Lin, C.R. Lowe, A.P. Mirra, B. Ravnihar, E.J. Salber, V.G. Valaoras, and S. Yuasa. 1970. Age at first birth and breast cancer risk. *Bull. W.H.O.* 43:209.

Peto, R. 1977. Epidemiology, multistage models and short-term mutagenicity tests. *Cold Spring Harbor Conf. Cell Proliferation* 4:1473.

Pike, M.C., B.E. Henderson, J.T. Casagrande, I. Rosario, and G.E. Gray. 1981. Oral contraceptive use and early abortion as risk factors for breast cancer in young women. *Br. J. Cancer* 43.

Pollack, E. and J. Horm. 1980. Trends in cancer incidence and mortality in the United States, 1969-76. *J. Natl. Cancer Inst.* 64:1091.

Staszewski, J. 1971. Age at menarche and breast cancer. *J. Natl. Cancer Inst.* 47:935.

Stoudt, H.W., A. Damon, and R. McFarland. 1965. *Weight, height, and selected body dimensions of adults.* Vital Health Statistics, series 11, no. 8. DHEW, Washington, D.C.

Trichopoulos, D., B. MacMahon, and P. Cole. 1972. Menopause and breast cancer risk. *J. Natl. Cancer Inst.* 48:605.

Wallace, R., B. Sherman, J.A. Bean, J.P. Leeper, and A.E. Treloar. 1978. Menstrual cycle patterns and breast cancer risk factors. *Cancer Res.* 38:4021

Waterhouse, J., C. Muir, P. Correa, J. Powell, and W. Davis. 1976. Cancer incidence in five continents, volume III. *IARC Sci. Publ.* 15.

COMMENTS

SEGALOFF: I'm very distressed. You started off by telling us that the only thing we should believe is mortality figures. Now you have presented us with an entire theory based on incidence. If the only thing I should believe is mortality statistics—and I might add that's all I do believe—I don't believe any of the rest of it.

PIKE: The problem with most incidence figures is that time trends in them are often misleading. The figures shown are not time trends. It should be noted that between the First, Second, and Third National Cancer Surveys, there were only small changes, presumably because they used the same method.

PETRAKIS: I'd like to challenge Malcolm Pike's data in another way, because you don't put any confidence limits around the data in terms of incidence in Japanese. Looking at the number of cases that you have in Los Angeles and the numbers you have in the Bay area and in Hawaii, you have about 10-20 cases—you may have 40 in one age group—and you're making a rate per 100,000 out of that. I just wonder if that's really that valid.

In Japan, you claim there's been a 100% increase in breast cancer incidence, but there was practically nothing to start with. I just wonder if it's really reaching those epidemic proportions that the implication carries. When you really look at it, I don't think it's that convincing. What's your confidence interval? How low would it be and how high will it be? And you'll find that it's huge. I just wonder as a statistician if you would accept that.

PIKE: Even though any one particular figure or point on a graph may not be reliable, the general picture is clear. All studies of Japanese migrants show that when the Japanese emigrate they slowly adopt the breast cancer rate of their adopted country. The rate at which they do this is really not all that important. The mere fact of it clearly demonstrates that it's something that you do that changes your breast cancer rates, not something that you are.

Body Size and Breast Cancer Risk

FRITS de WAARD
Department of Epidemiology
Institute of Social Medicine
University of Utrecht
Utrecht, The Netherlands

When we ventured our hypothesis on two etiologies of breast cancer (de Waard et al. 1960, 1964), the idea was based on our observation tht some women were able to produce estrogens from extraovarian sources. These women were obese, hypertensive, and (or) diabetic. Obesity turned out to be the key factor (de Waard and Baanders-van Halewijn 1969), and the biochemical evidence that adipose tissue is able to convert androstenedione into estrone was provided by MacDonald and Siiteri (1974) and Poortman et al. (1973).

Meanwhile, we had designed a prospective study in the Netherlands to find out whether obesity and the associated phenomenon of estrogenic smears in postmenopausal women predicted breast cancer risk. The outcome was somewhat different from expected (de Waard and Baanders-van Halewijn 1974). Whereas high body weight proved to be a risk factor, indeed, we observed an independent effect of body height. Moreover, our cytohormonal assessment of estrogen status apparently did not predict breast cancer risk (de Waard 1975). Therefore, doubt was growing as to whether overweight (namely, weight corrected for height) through an estrogen mechanism was a causal factor in breast cancer development. Our mind became open for other biologic mechanisms.

The risk of high body weight and height was confirmed in a number of case-control studies in Europe, North and South America, and East Asia (see Lin et al. 1971; Mirra et al. 1971; de Waard et al. 1977; Staszewski 1977; Paffenbarger et al. 1980). We estimated that the fraction in breast cancer risk attributable to body weight and height was considerable, namely, 50% of the difference in incidence between the Netherlands and Japan can be accounted for by these variables (de Waard et al. 1977).

RECENT FINDINGS REGARDING ESTROGEN RECEPTORS

In the same year that we published the results of our first prospective study (de Waard and Baanders-van Halewijn 1974), a second one was initiated. This was a periodic screening program for the citizens of Utrecht and its suburbs, born 1911-1925, in which all cases of breast cancer (including interval cancers) were documented by the local registry. Weight and height were measured at each of four screening examinations (clinical exam plus xeromammography) in the city population and at each of two such examinations in the suburban population.

In the period between December 1974 and January 1, 1980, 258 cases of mammary cancer were registered. In two-thirds of them, estrogen receptors were measured by one laboratory. We analyzed the effect of weight and height on breast cancer risk, distinguishing between estrogen-receptor-positive (ER^+) and estrogen-receptor-negative (ER^-) cases. It was found that risk of ER^+ breast cancer rose with increasing weight (W), not with height (H), and therefore also with overweight as defined by Quetelet index (W/H^2). These findings fitted perfectly well with the old hypothesis on the etiologic role of extraovarian estrogens. Apparently, the effect of body height may go through entirely different biologic mechanisms, e.g., relationship with age at menarche.

Another finding, quite unexpected, was that the risk of an ER^- breast cancer sharply decreased with increasing degrees of obesity. The explanation was sought in the mechanism of clonal selection. In lean women, estrogen-dependent cancer cells receive no stimulus for growth postmenopausally so that clones of ER^- cancer cells have a relative growth advantage and eventually will predominate in the tumor. Experimental work (Sluyser et al. 1976) supports this concept.

These findings have led us to believe that the natural history of breast cancer is mainly or exclusively a matter of growth of cancer induced much earlier, presumably before menopause. They can be fitted into the hypothesis of two etiologies for breast cancer if we distinguish between two sources of estrogen (ovarian and extraovarian sources respectively) promoting the process of mammary carcinogenesis.

Two approaches seem possible to test this hypothesis. If induction of cancer is rare after menopause, a disease model results which predicts that breast cancer becoming clinically manifest in early postmenopausal years grows more rapidly than breast cancer becoming manifest at a later age. In our periodic screening program, this disease model can be tested epidemiologically, as explained elsewhere (Collette 1980; de Waard 1981).

The second approach is based on the idea that the effect of obesity on ER^+ cancer diagnosed after the menopause will be the same before diagnosis as after diagnosis. If a program of weight reduction could be shown to alter the growth rate and prognosis of clinical breast cancer, it would also tend to slow down its growth rate in the preclinical phase; in other words, it would postpone or even prevent the clinical appearance of breast cancer. There is both clinical and experimental evidence that weight reduction is effective in this way (Waxler 1954; Donegan et al. 1978).

AGE AT MENOPAUSE

Late age of menopause is associated with increased risk of mammary cancer (Trichopoulos et al. 1972). In our periodic screening program, we have not yet analyzed the effect of this factor. We have, however, by means of the so-called status quo method studied age at menopause according to body weight and height, Quetelet index, and smoking habits. Increased weight and Quetelet index tend to defer menopause (Fig. 1), whereas height does not show an effect. Smoking accelerates the occurrence of menopause, probably because smokers are less heavy (Figs. 2 and 3).

Some years ago we have suggested (de Waard 1973) that estrogen levels at climacteric age are determined partly by an extraovarian contribution to total estrogen production. Obese women, on the basis of that contribution, could have higher estrone levels in circulating blood, even before menopause. As

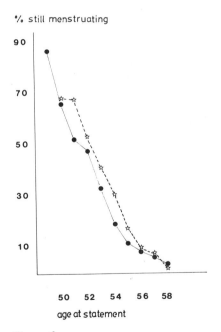

% still menstruating

Figure 1
Percentage of normal women still menstruating (defined as at least one period over the last 12 months) by age at statement and relative weight (Quetelet index): Obese (☆, Quetelet index ≥ 29) versus lean (●, Quetelet index < 23) women, with sample sizes of 1503 and 1549 women respectively. Curve of intermediate group (Quetelet index 23-28) runs between these curves; it has been omitted for reasons of surveyability. See also note under Fig. 2.

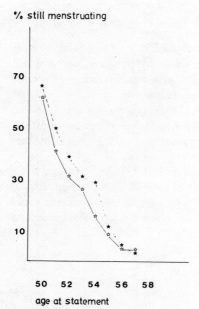

% still menstruating

age at statement

Figure 2

Percentage of normal women still menstruating by age at statement and present smoking habits: Smokers (☆) (*n* = 1887) versus nonsmokers (★) (*n* = 3848). *Notes:* (1) Although the curves look like cumulative frequency distributions, each point is an independent estimate. (2) A statement of being postmenopausal can be made only if there have been no menses for 12 months; thus the curves should be moved backward 1 year to find median age at menopause.

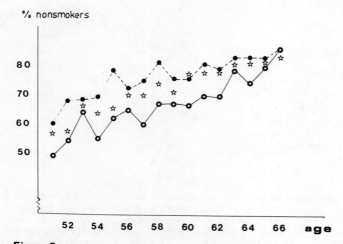

% nonsmokers

age

Figure 3

Percentage of current nonsmokers by age and relative weight (Quetelet index). Total population 11,517 women aged 50-66; subpopulation aged 50-58 used for analysis resulting in Fig. 1 and 2. Quetelet index: (●) ≥ 29; (☆) 23-28; (○) < 23.

aging proceeds, total estrogen will decrease with a decline in ovarian function; when a critical level has been passed, menses (of an anovulatory kind) will stop. Obese women might cross this level at a later age assuming equal ovarian contributions to the estrogen pool and no effective feedback regulation between ovarian and extraovarian estrogen production on the one hand and pituitary function on the other.

SUMMARY

The effect of body size on breast cancer risk should be separated into two components—body weight and height. The effect of weight probably is related to extraovarian estrogen production in adipose tissue; weight determines the growth rate of already induced breast cancer. The effect of late age at menopause is also related to weight and obesity, and possibly mediated by extraovarian surplus of estrogen.

REFERENCES

Collette, H.J.A. 1980. Incidence trends during the course of a periodic screening programme for breast cancer. Paper presented at UICC Symposium, Oslo, August 6-7.

de Waard, F. 1973. Hormonal background of late menopause: An epidemiological approach. In *Symposium on endometrial cancer at St. Thomas Hosp.* (ed. M.G. Brush et al.), p. 141. W. Heinemann, London.

_____ . 1975. Breast cancer incidence and nutritional status, with particular reference to body weight and height. *Cancer Res.* **35**:3351.

_____ . 1981. Etiologic factors in breast cancer, in particular promoting factors. In *Breast cancer* (ed. E.F. Lewison and A.C.W. Montague), p. 22. Williams and Wilkins Company, Baltimore.

de Waard, F. and E.A. Baanders-van Halewijn. 1969. Cross-sectional data on estrogenic smears in a postmenopausal population. *Acta Cytol.* **13**:273.

_____ . 1974. A prospective study in general practice on breast cancer risk in postmenopausal women. *Int. J. Cancer* **14**:153.

de Waard, F., J.W.J. de Laive, and E.A. Baanders-van Halewijn. 1960. On the bimodal age distribution of mammary cancer. *Br. J. Cancer* **14**:437.

de Waard, F., E.A. Baanders-van Halewijn, and J. Huizinga. 1964. The bimodal age distribution of patients with mammary carcinoma. *Cancer* **17**: 141.

de Waard, F., J.P. Cornelis, K. Aoki, and M. Yoshida. 1977. Breast cancer incidence according to weight and height in two cities of the Netherlands and in Aichi prefecture, Japan. *Cancer* **40**:1269.

Donegan, W.L., A.J. Hartz, and A.A. Rimm. 1978. The association of body weight with recurrent cancer of the breast. *Cancer* **41**:1590.

Lin, T.M., K.P. Chen, and B. MacMahon. 1971. Epidemiologie characteristics of cancer of the breast in Taiwan. *Cancer* **27**:1497.

MacDonald, P.C. and P.K. Siiteri. 1974. The relationship between the extraglandular production of estrone and the occurrence of endometrial neoplasia. *Gynecol. Oncol.* **2**:259.

MacDonald, P.C., C.D. Edman, D.L.Hemsell, J.C. Porter, and P.K. Siiteri. 1978. Effect of obesity on conversion of plasma androstenedione to estrone in postmenopausal women with and without endometrial cancer. *Am. J. Obstet. Gynecol.* **130**:448.

Mirra, A.P., P. Cole, and B. MacMahon. 1971. Breast cancer in an area of high parity: Sao Paulo, Brazil. *Cancer Res.* **31**:77.

Paffenbarger, R.S., J.B. Kampert, and Hwa-Gan Chang. 1980. Characteristics that predict risk of breast cancer before and after menopause. *Am. J. Epidemiol.* **112**:258.

Poortman, J., J.H.H. Thijssen, and F. Schwartz. 1973. Androgen production and conversion to estrogens in normal postmenopausal women and in selected breast cancer patients. *J. Clin. Endocrinol. Metab.* **37**:101.

Sluyser, M., S.G. Evers, and A. de Goey. 1976. Sex hormone receptors in mammary tumours of GR mice. *Nature* **263**:386.

Trichopoulos, D., B. MacMahon, and P. Cole. 1972. Menopause and breast cancer risk. *J. Natl. Cancer Inst.* **48**:605.

Waxler, S.H. 1954. The effect of weight reduction on the occurrence of spontaneous mammary tumors in mice. *J. Natl. Cancer Inst.* **14**:1253.

COMMENTS

BULBROOK:　After 20 years in the field I know that if you dine with the devil, or with epidemiologists, you need a very long spoon. You are both still using age-specific incidence curves. In a recent paper by Moolgavkar et al. (1980), they showed an enormous cohort effect in six countries and this should surely alter your views. Your model may work very well for California but may not explain geographical variation at all well. As far as weight is concerned, this may correlate in Holland but it is not generally a risk factor world-wide. It has not been properly studied in conjunction with variables such as parity.

So I would say to both of you that things are not quite as rosy as you would have us believe.

DE WAARD:　I think that in MacMahon's and Cole's international study, weight and height were studied besides parity and age at first pregnancy. I know for certain that the effects of weight and height were adjusted for parity and age at first pregnancy in the Athens paper (Valaoras et al. 1969). Moreover, in our paper on the prospective study (de Waard and Baanders 1974), we found that weight and parity had independent effects on breast cancer risk.

COLE:　Well, all of those effects were adjusted for all of the other variables for which we had information or thought important at that time. Of course, this was more than 10 years ago.

DE WAARD:　The other question raised by Dr. Bulbrook has to do with cohort effects on the shape of the age-specific incidence curve of breast cancer. It is being argued that the hook in the Japanese curve, with the downward trend after age 50, is an artefact of cross-sectional curves and that if one studies age-specific rates for birth cohorts the hook is no longer visible. This is true in countries with low risk where breast cancer incidence is now rising (for example, Japan) just as it did (and does) in the daughters of Japanese migrants to Hawaii and California. However, I am still convinced that the original "Japanese curve" was the base-line incidence of life-long experience before the Westernization of Japan. The original curve (with no increase according to age after menopause) still can be observed in the Chinese of Singapore and Taiwan and the People's Republic of China. The final answer must come from longitudinal observations on low-risk populations in whom there is no rise in breast cancer incidence during the next decades.

PIKE:　Can I answer that? First of all, I thought that I began by explaining to you that the data which the epidemiologists can provide on incidence is bad. It's very important to understand that it's bad because, if you had a new breed of pathologists who decide that, in fact, there's a new disease called breast cancer and they can see it in one or two cells, then of course your incidence goes up. There's nothing you can do about it. So what you should expect a model to do is explain the basic general pattern to explain that. To cross the T's is impossible.

Now, the data that we put up was data that deliberately went back to 1970 or to 1937 because the national studies in this country showed no change for 35 or 40 years. That's not California data; it's U.S. data. And I don't believe that either.

I was trying to show that you could explain most of the effects by very simple time things that we understand—that late menarche is good for you, early babies are good for you, early menopause is good for you—and that we shouldn't try to find major other effects, because those simple effects are enough to explain most of the pattern.

I meant to show you one other thing. I think we now have a clue as to why women who have babies at 35 are more at risk than nulliparous women. We have some new data that shows that having an abortion before you ever have a baby is really bad for you.

DE WAARD: Regarding the effect of weight on breast cancer risk, there are more positive than negative studies, which I'll list for you. Negative: Sweden (Adami et al. 1977); Finland (under age 60, Soini et al. 1977); United States (Wynder et al. 1978). Positive: Brazil (Mirra et al. 1971); Greece (Valaoras et al. 1969); Holland (de Waard et al. 1977); Japan (Hirayama 1978); Taiwan (Lin et al. 1971); Poland (Staszewski 1977); Canada (Miller et al. 1978); United States (Brinton et al. 1979); United States (Ross et al. 1980); United States (Paffenbarger et al. 1980). Marginal effect: Yugoslavia (Ravnihar et al. 1971).

Wynder et al. (1978) maintain that there is no effect to be seen in the data. Actually in their last paper some effects of weight can be discerned among pre- and perimenopausal women. My view is that their control groups from Memorial Hospital have undergone selective bias.

PIKE: The American Cancer Society data for the mortality show a clear weight effect on breast cancer mortality.

MEITES: I'd like to ask Dr. de Waard whether the increased incidence of cancer in women who weigh more is not really due entirely to the fat factor, irrespective of any increase in body weight. I ask this because Charles Aylsworth and I have been working on high-fat diets in rats treated with carcinogen. These animals have not gained in weight as compared with the controls, but a high-fat diet, nonetheless, very definitely increases the incidence of mammary cancer in rats. I'm wondering whether or not the same thing may not be true in women—that it is the fat and not the weight that's responsible for the higher incidence of breast cancer.

DE WAARD: As far as I can see, there are two aspects of Western nutrition that are important: Amount of fat in the diet and obesity. Obesity plays a role only in the postmenopausal woman, stimulating the growth of already-existing cancers. The role of dietary fat may be different, and I think perhaps this may have to do with prolactin. The team at the Naylor Dana Institute has done quite a bit of work on that. However, I haven't studied that aspect of Western nutrition.

References

Adami, H.O., A. Rimsten, B. Stenkvist, and J. Vegelius. 1977. Influence of height, weight and obesity on risk of breast cancer in an unselected Swedish population. *Br. J. Cancer* **36**:787.

Brinton, L.A., R.R. Williams, R.N. Hoover, N.L. Stegens, M. Feinleib, and J.F. Fraumeni, Jr. 1979. Breast cancer risk factors among screening program participants. *J. Natl. Cancer Inst.* **62**:37.

de Waard, F. and E.A. Baanders-van Halewijn. 1974. A prospective study in general practice on breast cancer risk in postmenopausal women. *Int. J. Cancer* **14**:153.

de Waard, F., J.P. Cornelis, K. Aoki, and M. Yoshida. 1977. Breast cancer incidence according to weight and height in two cities in The Netherlands and in Aichi prefecture, Japan. *Cancer* **40**:1269.

Hirayama, T. 1978. Epidemiology of breast cancer with special reference to the role of diet. *Prev. Med.* **7**:173.

Lin, T.M., K.P. Chen, and B. MacMahon. 1971. Epidemiologie characteristics of cancer of the breast in Taiwan. *Cancer* **27**:1497.

Mirra, A.P., P. Cole, and B. MacMahon. 1971. Breast cancer in an area of high parity: Sao Paulo, Brazil. *Cancer Res.* **31**:77.

Miller, A.B., A. Kelly, N.W. Choi, V. Matthews, R.W. Morgan, L. Munan, J.D. Burch, J. Feather, G.R. Horve, and M. Jain. 1978. A study of diet and breast cancer. *Am. J. Epidemiol.* **107**:499.

Moolgavkar, S., N.E. Day, and R.G. Stevens. 1980. Two-stage model for carcinogenesis: Epidemiology of breast cancer in females. *J. Natl. Cancer Inst.* **65**:559.

Paffenbarger, R.S., J.B. Kampert, and Hwa-Gan Chang. 1980. Characteristics that predict risk of breast cancer before and after menopause. *Am. J. Epidemiol.* **112**:258.

Ravnihar, B., B. MacMahon, and J. Lindtner. 1971. Epidemiologic features of breast cancer in Slovenia, 1965-67. *Eur. J. Cancer* **7**:295.

Ross, R.K., A. Paganini-Hill, V.R. Gerkins, T.M. Mack, R. Pfeffer, M. Arthur, and B.E. Henderson. 1980. A case-control study of menopausal estrogen therapy and breast cancer. *J. Am. Med. Assoc.* **243**:1635.

Soini, J. 1977. Risk factors of breast cancer in Finland. *Int. J. Epidemiol.* **6**: 365.

Staszewski, J. 1977. Breast cancer and body build. *Prev. Med.* 6:410.

Valaoras, V.G., B. MacMahon, D. Trichopoulos, and A. Polychronopoulou. 1969. Lactation and reproductive histories of breast cancer patients in greater Athens 1965-1967. *Int. J. Cancer* 4:350.

Wynder, E.L., F.A. MacCormack, and S.D. Stellman. 1978. The epidemiology of breast cancer in 785 U.S. Caucasian women. *Cancer* 41:2341.

SESSION 2:
Endocrinology of Women At Risk to Breast Cancer

Hormone Profiles in Young Women at Risk of Breast Cancer: A Study of Ovarian Function during Theelarche, Menarche, and Menopause and After Childbirth

JAMES B. BROWN
Department of Obstetrics and Gynecology
University of Melbourne
Parkville, Victoria, 3052 Australia

One aim of the present meeting is to consider the roles of three risk factors in breast cancer—early menarche, late first birth, and late menopause. However, our present knowledge of the hormone changes that occur at menarche, the menopause, and after childbirth is completely inadequate for designing experiments to determine these roles, particularly as any differences between populations at high and low risk of breast cancer are likely to be small. The main emphasis of this paper, then, is to present results of our studies on ovarian function in women at these three phases of life.

In a group of 70 menstruating Californian girls aged 15-18 years, it was found that only 33% of the girls aged 15-16 years ovulated during the cycle studied, whereas 50% of the girls aged 17-18 years ovulated (G.E. Gray et al., in prep.). In a study of normal, mainly parous women aged 20-40 years, anovulation was found to be a comparatively rare phenomenon, accounting for approximately 3% of the cycles studied (J.B. Brown, unpubl.). Thus, age and time past the menarche are important factors that must be considered in the study of ovarian function of young women.

In another study conducted by Drs. Trichopoulos and B. MacMahon et al. (in prep.) involving approximately 80 girls aged 15-18 years and belonging to two socioeconomic groups in Athens, it was found that only 12% of the cycles from the girls in the lower socioeconomic group with the lower breast cancer risk were anovulatory, whereas 34% of those in the higher socioeconomic group were anovulatory (Trichopoulos et al. 1980). This difference approached significance and suggested that the duration of anovulatory ovarian activity after menarche might be a breast cancer risk factor. In another study involving 286 young women aged 15-18 years in Finland, Norway, Sweden, Holland, Greece, and Yugoslavia, it was found that the incidences of anovulatory cycles were highest in the Norwegian and Finnish girls and lowest in the Yugoslavian girls, who had the lowest risk of breast cancer. This finding might be due to the effects of the long northern winters on ovarian function and is the first indication that photoperiodicity might be involved in human reproduction as it is in most other animal species (B. MacMahon et al., in prep.).

In the chimpanzee, fertility does not develop for several years after menarche; it is assumed that the first menstrual cycles are anovulatory and that full ovulatory activity does not develop for several years (Short 1976). Therefore, to obtain more information in the human, we have studied ovarian function in groups of women at various stages of their reproductive life.

METHODS

Ovarian function was assessed by measurement of estrogen and pregnanediol excretion in 24-hour collections of urine using the methods of Brown et al. (1968) and of Cox (1963). For the studies on the normal menstrual cycle, specimens were collected daily throughout 61 cycles from 26 parous and 14 nulliparous women aged 20-40 years.

Studies were also performed using single, 24-hour urine specimens obtained from 38 girls and 24 boys aged 2-13 years and analyzing them with methods of high sensitivity (Brown 1976). Six of these girls were studied further by serial weekly assays for various periods of time. Also, 82 perimenopausal women have been studied similarly by weekly assays, as well as 42 women postpartum. In the recent studies, blood has also been collected weekly for the assay of serum follicle-stimulating hormone (FSH) and luteinizing hormone (LH) by radioimmunoassay. Time allows the presentation of only some of the findings here.

THE NORMAL OVULATORY CYCLE

The estrogen and pregnanediol values found in the 61 normal cycles obtained from the 26 parous and 14 nulliparous women aged 20-40 years are shown in Figure 1. The 10th, 50th, and 90th percentiles are shown, and the days are numbered from the day of the midcycle estrogen peak (equals day 0). The well-known patterns of estrogen and progesterone production characteristic of the normal ovulatory cycle are demonstrated. A point of importance in the present context is that raised estrogen values of, say greater than 25 μg/24 hours in the presence of low pregnanediol values, say less than 1 mg/24 hours, occur on average for only 5 days of the normal cycle. This usually applies even when the follicular phase is prolonged. However, sometimes the estrogen values in prolonged cycles may be raised somewhat for a time before the midcycle peak and this may result in midmenstrual bleeding. Such cycles have not been included in the figure.

These results are used for interpreting the patterns obtained in other studies. For example, the finding of a pregnanediol value of 2 mg/24 hours or more, or of two weekly values exceeding 1.5 mg/24 hours, indicates that

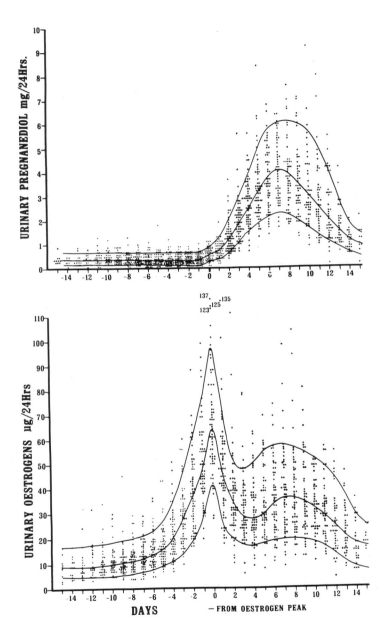

Figure 1

Urinary estrogen and pregnanediol values throughout 61 normal ovulatory cycles in 40 women aged 20-40 years. 10th, 50th, and 90th percentiles are shown. Day of preovulatory estrogen peak = day 0.

ovulation has occurred. Increases in pregnanediol values that do not reach these figures are observed commonly. The interpretation of such values is uncertain; they may be associated with ovulation and a deficient luteal phase or with luteinization of a follicle that has not ovulated.

The lengths of the luteal phases found during the above study, calculated as the interval from day +1 to the day before onset of bleeding, inclusive, are shown in Figure 2. In the normal group aged 20-40 years, the luteal phases were 11-17 days. A luteal phase longer than 17 days, say 19 days for safety, is diagnostic of pregnancy; a luteal phase of less than 11 days, as was found in 2 of the 9 ovulating girls aged 18-19 years is considered to be deficient.

ANOVULATORY CYCLES

Two main patterns of estrogen excretion have been identified in anovulatory cycles. One pattern is shown in Figure 3. Here the estrogen values show a single

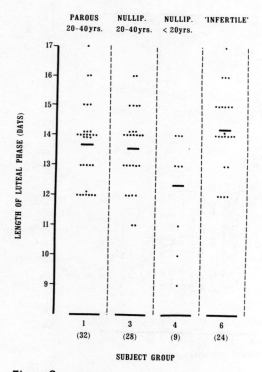

Figure 2

Lengths of luteal phases in 32 ovulatory cycles from parous women aged 20-40 years, in 28 cycles from nulliparous women aged 20-40 years, in 9 cycles from girls aged 18-19 years, and in 24 cycles from women being investigated because of infertility.

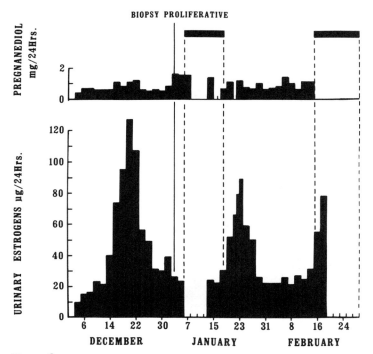

Figure 3
Values throughout two anovulatory cycles of the fluctuating estrogen type. (■) Bleeding.

peak resembling the preovulatory peak of the normal cycle, but this is not followed by a luteal-phase rise in estrogen and pregnanediol excretion; bleeding occurs as an estrogen withdrawal phenomenon. This type of cycle has several characteristics. First, the peak estrogen values may exceed those seen during the normal ovulatory cycle. Second, the pattern of pregnanediol excretion may vary from no rise premenstrually, to a small rise, as in Figure 3, to larger increases which merge through the deficient luteal phase, to the full pattern of the ovulatory menstrual cycle. Many examples of this transition were encountered in the present study. Third, bleeding does not necessarily follow the fall in estrogen values after the peak, but it always follows the fall in pregnanediol values during an ovulatory cycle. In the figure, it is seen that purely estrogenic activity with urinary values exceeding 20 μg/24 hours persisted for 25 days.

The second pattern found in anovulatory cycles is shown in Figure 4. The urinary estrogen values remain elevated at between 15-40 μg/24 hours and bleeding occurs, often at irregular intervals, as an estrogen breakthrough phenomenon. The first pattern is caused by insufficient LH release at midcycle; the second is caused by insufficient FSH release to produce a mature follicle.

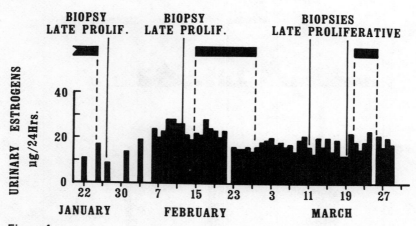

Figure 4

Values throughout anovulatory cycles of the constant estrogen type showing findings at endometrial biopsy. (■) Bleeding.

ABSENT OVARIAN ACTIVITY

Absent ovarian activity is indicated by urinary estrogen values that remain persistently below 10 μg/24 hours.

VALUES FOUND IN CHILDREN

In Figure 5 are shown the sums of estriol, estrone, and estradiol in micrograms per 24 hours found in the 38 girls and 24 boys aged 2-13 years. The values are shown on a logarithmic scale covering the 2000-fold range of values encountered. The lowest total estrogen value recorded was in a 2-year-old boy who was excreting 0.09 μg/24 hours. In the majority of children aged 2-8 years, the total estrogen excretion was within the range 0.1-0.5 μg/24 hours with no differences between the sexes. These compare with values of 0.09-0.43 μg/24 hours ($n = 15$) found in women after bilateral oophorectomy and adrenalectomy, and of 1.8-14.6 μg/24 hours (mean 5.5 μg/24 hours, $n = 39$) found in unablated postmenopausal women. The source of this extraglandular production of estrogens in the ablated women is unknown, but in children, serial assays show that periodic fluctuations occur (subject J.O.) and therefore some of this is probably of ovarian origin.

After the age of 8 years, the general values in both sexes began to rise, and by age 11 years the majority was above 1 μg/24 hours. The values found in the girls rose more rapidly than those in the boys. Of the 3 girls who registered values above 10 μg/24 hours, one was already menstruating (subject B) and the others began menstruating within 2 months of the study (subjects A and C).

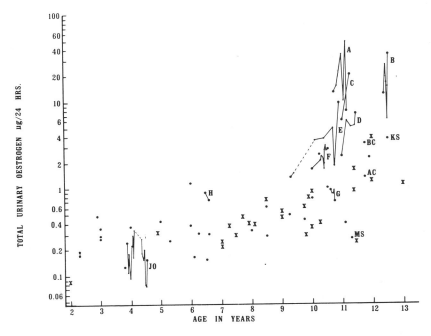

Figure 5
Urinary estrogen values in 38 girls (●) and 24 boys (✕) aged 2-13 years (results on a logarithmic scale). (Data from Brown et al. 1978.)

All girls who recorded that breast development (theelarche) had commenced, including subject H with precocious breast development at age 6.5 years, had estrogen values that were above 0.5 μg/24 hours and were approaching or exceeding 1 μg/24 hours. Thus 1 μg/24 hours is the urinary estrogen value associated with theelarche. Assuming a metabolic clearance rate roughly similar to adults, this represents a production rate of approximately 5 μg/day, and is equivalent to a plasma level of approximately 5 pg/ml which is well below the sensitivity of current radioimmunoassays. This is the only information available on the minimum physiological levels of estrogen production required for breast development. Oophorectomy and adrenalectomy are performed in adult women with metastatic breast cancer to remove all sources of estrogen stimulation of the breast; it can be concluded that such surgery successfully achieves this purpose.

LONGITUDINAL STUDIES OVER MENARCHE

In Figure 6 is shown a longitudinal study in a girl, K.S., who collected urine weekly for intervals between the ages of 12-16 years. The urinary estrogen and

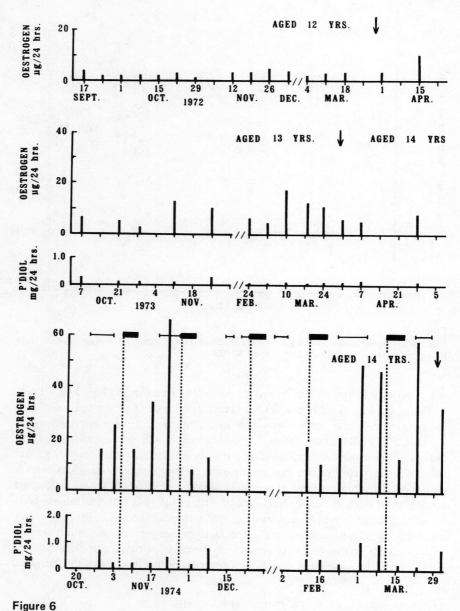

Figure 6

Subject K.S. Urinary estrogen and pregnanediol values measured over 4 years from age 12 to 16 years. Menarche and first ovulation were documented. (↓) Birthdays; (⊢—⊣) production of cervical mucus; (■) bleeding. (Data from Brown et al. 1978.)

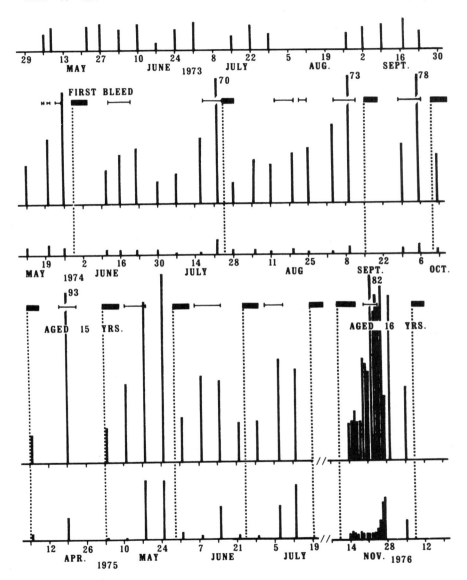

AGED 13 YRS.

FIRST BLEED

pregnanediol values are shown, together with the times of bleeding and the self-observed production of fertile-type cervical mucus. The scales of values used in Figure 6 are expanded during the 4-year period to accommodate the increases in hormone values that occurred over this time. At age 12.5 years, the estrogen values were fluctuating rhythmically between 0.9-5.0 $\mu g/24$ hours. The fluctuations increased in amplitude during the age of 13 years, the highest value recorded being 17 $\mu g/24$ hours in March 1974. In May, the estrogen values peaked to 44 $\mu g/24$ hours, and the subject experienced her first bleed (menarche) 2 days later. The subsequent pattern showed fluctuating estrogen values peaking to 70 $\mu g/24$ hours before bleeds. The periodicity of the bleeds was 8 weeks at first, but this settled to a monthly rhythm.

During the ages of 12 and 13 years, the pregnanediol values remained less than 0.3 mg/24 hours (first year not shown). However, a small rise to 0.4 mg/24 hours was recorded before the first bleed in May 1974, and a value of 0.6 mg/24 hours was recorded before the second bleed in July. These premenstrual rises in pregnanediol excretion increased in amplitude and first exceeded 1 mg/24 hours for 2 consecutive weeks before the ninth bleed in March 1975. In May 1975, the pregnanediol values first exceeded 2 mg/24 hours, our criterion for ovulation, and the luteal phase was of normal duration. Regular ovulatory cycles with normal lengths of luteal phases became established, as demonstrated by the cycle studied at age 16 years.

It can be concluded that cyclical ovarian activity was occurring during the 1-2 years before menarche, that the amplitude of these fluctuations in estrogen production increased until the endometrium had been stimulated sufficiently to bleed (menarche), that the initial menstrual cycles were anovulatory of the fluctuating estrogen type, and that these changed gradually to become fully ovulatory by a year after menarche. It demonstrates the processes by which the ovulatory mechanism matures at the ovarian level. Another point of interest was that the level of estrogen production required for the initiation of menstruation was 10-20 times that required for the initiation of breast development.

The results obtained in M.S., the younger and less-developed sister of K.S. are shown in Figure 7. Collections commenced at the age of 11.5 years when she was still excreting submicrogram amounts of urinary estrogens. These already were fluctuating in the range 0.09-0.30 $\mu g/24$ hours. The values gradually increased and the first reading over 1 $\mu g/24$ hours was recorded in September 1973. After 2 years, the values consistently were above 1 $\mu g/24$ hours and the first value reaching 10 $\mu g/24$ hours was recorded in May 1976, just before her 15th birthday. Menarche occurred in October 1976 and thereafter anovulatory cycles of both constant and fluctuating estrogen patterns were recorded. Bleeding occurred at irregular intervals at first, but became more regular as the fluctuating estrogen type of anovulatory cycle became established. Nevertheless, throughout this time the pregnanediol values remained persistently low. This subject has been studied at intervals since the last recording shown in October, and only now, at the age of 19.5 years, are the pregnanediol values beginning to rise premenstrually and figures exceeding 1 mg/24 hours have been recorded. It would seem that ovulation is now imminent, 4 years after menarche.

Six other girls have been studied by serial assays with similar results. One ovulated 3 months after menarche. In the records of the Royal Women's Hospital, Melbourne, a girl has been documented who conceived and delivered before menarche. Thus, ovulation in relation to menarche is a very variable event in the human. Furthermore, these results show that menarche is the manifestation of underlying dynamic events that have been proceeding with increasing amplitude for years, rather than being due to a sudden change in ovarian function. All these findings need to be considered when searching for hormone risk factors during the adolescent years.

RETURNING FERTILITY AFTER CHILDBIRTH

The return of ovarian activity postpartum has been likened to a second menarche. We have accumulated detailed longitudinal data on 42 women postpartum; the majority of these were breastfeeding their infants. Two examples are shown to illustrate the findings.

Mrs. H.F., whose profile is shown in Figure 8, breastfed her infant until it died at 11 months. The urinary estrogen and pregnanediol values remained uniformly low (less than 5 µg/24 hours and 0.4 mg/24 hours, respectively) over this time. After the infant died and lactation ceased, ovarian activity resumed within 4 weeks. The subject conceived again 3 months later. This pattern shows complete ovarian quiescence during lactation, followed by an immediate return to full ovulatory activity.

The profile illustrated in Figure 9, Mrs. M.S., shows a different sequence of events in a subject who was also lactating. Even at 12 weeks after delivery, cyclic fluctuations in estrogen values were occurring with levels varying between 2-8 µg/24 hours and periodicities of approximately 1 month. The fluctuations increased in amplitude and menstruation commenced in August. The following two cycles were anovulatory, of the fluctuating estrogen pattern, and the premenstrual pregnanediol values were increasing. Ovulation occurred in the October and November cycles with normal lengths of luteal phases. This pattern therefore was similar to those seen in the girls at menarche.

Many variations of these two patterns were encountered. When ovulation commenced within 6 months of delivery, the luteal phases were usually shorter than normal, a finding that is common when the prolactin values are raised.

WANING OVARIAN ACTIVITY AT THE MENOPAUSE

A longitudinal study that commenced in 1972 when the subject was 42 years of age and had recorded the first onset of irregular cycles after a life-time of regularity is shown in Figure 10 (subject 2). All cycles shown up to July 1974 were ovulatory. After this time, a change to anovulatory ovarian function

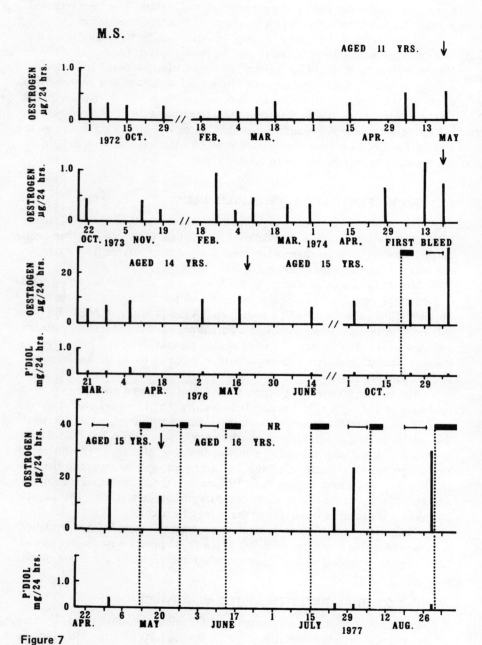

Figure 7

Subject M.S. Urinary estrogen and pregnanediol values measured over 5 years from age 11-16 years. (↓) Birthdays; (⊢—⊣) production of cervical mucus; (■) bleeding. (Data from Brown et al. 1978.)

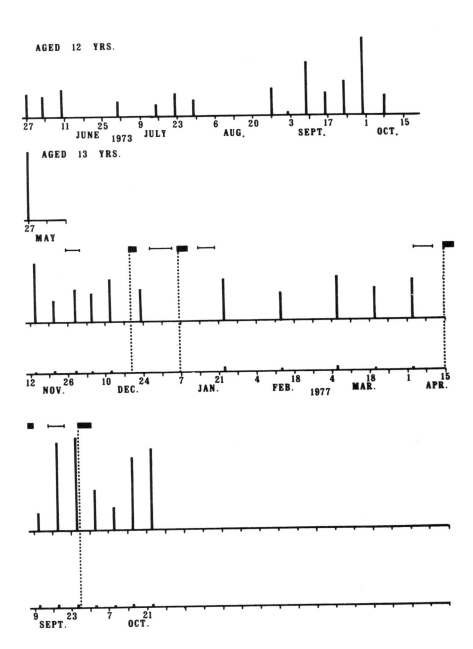

AGED 12 YRS.

27 11 25   9   23   6   20   3   17   1   15
    JUNE 1973 JULY   AUG.   SEPT.   OCT.

AGED 13 YRS.

27
MAY

12 26   10   24   7   21   4   18   4   18   1   15
NOV.   DEC.   JAN.   FEB. 1977 MAR.   APR.

9   23   7   21
SEPT.   OCT.

45

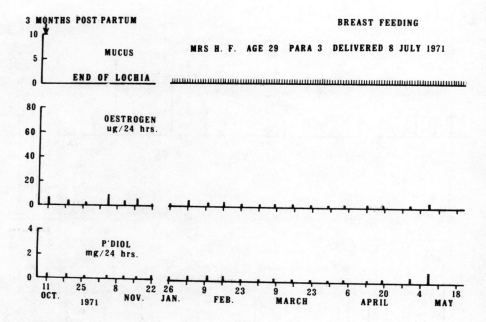

Figure 8

Subject H.F. Values following childbirth with lactation showing return of fertility. Mucus production is shown in this and subsequent figures. (■) Bleeding.

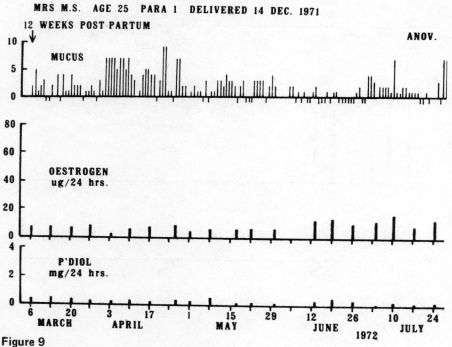

Figure 9

Subject M.S. Values following childbirth with lactation showing return of fertility.

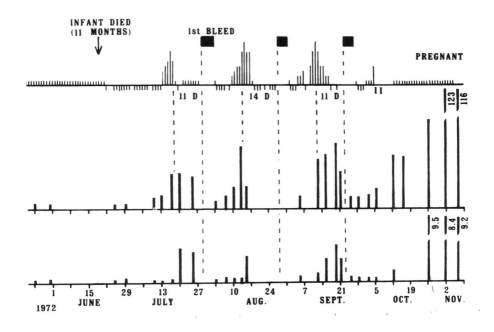

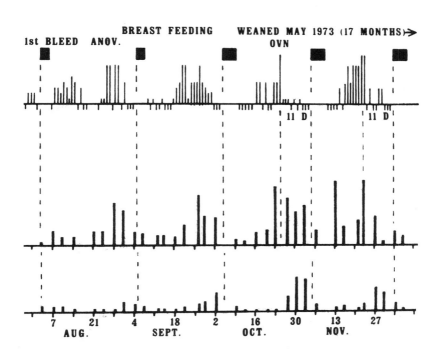

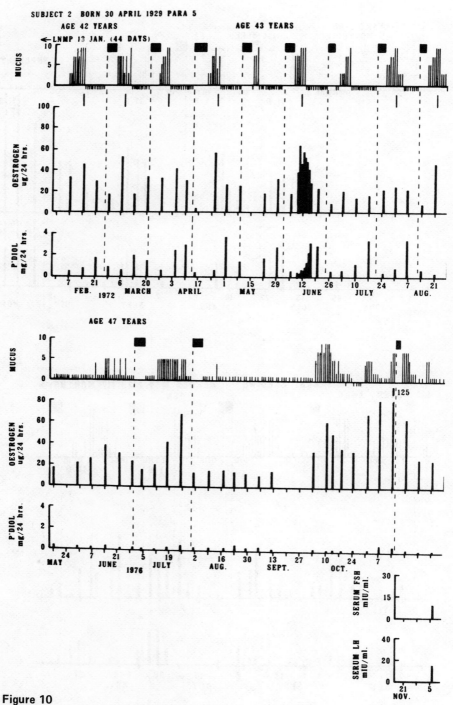

Figure 10
Subject 2. Values measured over 9 years in a woman aged 42-51 years.

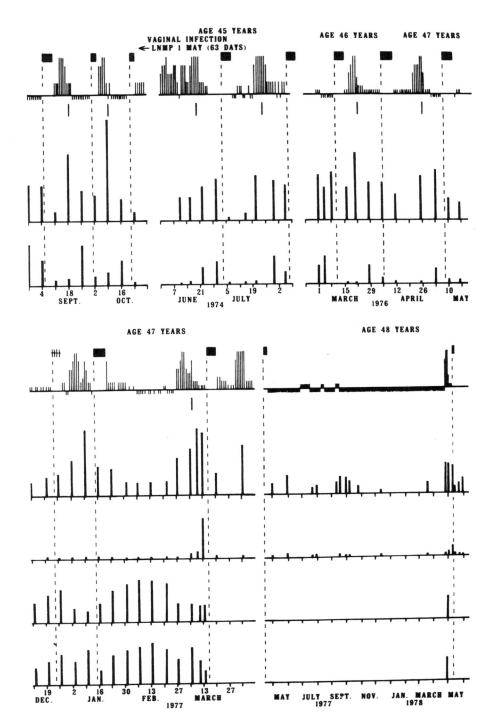

AGE 45 YEARS
VAGINAL INFECTION
← LNMP 1 MAY (63 DAYS)

AGE 46 YEARS   AGE 47 YEARS

4   18   2   16
SEPT.   OCT.

7   21   5   19   2
JUNE   1974   JULY

1   15   29   12   26   10
MARCH   1976   APRIL   MAY

AGE 47 YEARS

AGE 48 YEARS

19   2   16   30   13   27   13   27
DEC.   JAN.   FEB.   MARCH
1977

MAY   JULY   SEPT.   NOV.   JAN.   MARCH   MAY
1977   1978

occurred. The cycle documented in February-March 1976 was ovulatory with urinary pregnanediol values of 2.7 mg/24 hours. During the next two cycles, the luteal-phase pregnanediol values began to decrease, the maximum values recorded being 1.8 mg/24 hours during the March cycle and 1.4 mg/24 hours in April. Thereafter, the pregnanediol values remained low within the range 0.2-0.4 mg/24 hours, and a series of anovulatory cycles was recorded lasting for between 3-15 weeks and with peak estrogen values of between 40-125 μg/24 hours. These events were the exact reverse of those documented at onset of ovulation in the girls. A rise in pregnanediol excretion to 3.9 mg/24 hours was observed in March 1977. This was the first ovulatory episode for nearly a year, but the luteal phase lasted for only 8 days. During the next year, sporadic episodes of cyclic ovarian activity were recorded, but no estrogen value reached 20 μg/24 hours and amenorrhea persisted for more than a year. Thus by definition, the bleed that occurred in April 1977 was the menopause. In May 1978, increased ovarian activity was again observed and this was followed by bleeding, which was investigated by curettage. Serum FSH and LH values were measured weekly between December 1977 and March 1978; these fluctuated between high-normal menstrual cycle levels and postmenopausal levels, the fluctuations being the exact inverse of the estrogen levels. The continuation of this study is shown in Figure 11. Bleeding occurred in September and October, and spotting occurred in August 1978 and in July 1979, each preceded by rises in estrogen excretion of between 35-70 μg/24 hours. The estrogen values have now settled at the rather high value of approximately 20 μg/24 hours and amenorrhea has persisted for more than 1 year. The subject is considerably overweight, and these high values are presumably due to this. The FSH and LH values are now within the normal postmenopausal range. However, it should be noted that even the small rise in estrogen values that occurred before the last spotting on July 1970 was sufficient to depress the FSH values back into the premenopausal range. It has been a common experience in this study to see such definite estrogenic effects on the hypothalamus and uterus being caused by quite small increases in the amounts of estrogens produced, presumably by the ovarian follicles, whereas larger amounts of base-line estrogen produced by extraglandular production are required for these effects.

This and the companion studies show that the menopause, like menarche, is not a single event, but is the result of underlying dynamic changes in ovarian activity that may persist or occur sporadically for some considerable time after the recorded date of the menopause. We have not yet encountered the situation where normal ovarian activity stops suddenly to initiate the menopause. All of these factors must be considered when planning further studies aimed at elucidating the roles of early menarche, anovulation, childbirth, and late menopause as risk factors in the development of both endometrial and breast cancers.

Furthermore, when considering the so-called deficient luteal phase, our studies show that this occupies quite a wide grey zone between frankly anovulatory cycles of the fluctuating estrogen type and frankly ovulatory cycles that satisfy defined biochemical criteria of ovulation, in our case a pregnanediol value exceeding 2 mg/24 hours. This grey zone almost certainly results from variations in responsiveness of the Graafian follicle to variations in LH release, the prolactin levels being one of the factors involved in this process. Furthermore, when assessing the potential fertility of a cycle, we have found that the length of the luteal phase is just as, or more, important than the levels of hormones found, and this can only be calculated by having a midcycle marker for timing ovulation. I urge that such a midcycle marker should be included in any future studies comparing hormone profiles in different populations at high and low risk of breast cancer, otherwise an important parameter, namely length of the luteal phase, will be missing when interpreting the results.

SUMMARY

In summary, the following points merit emphasis.

1. During the normal ovulatory cycle, raised estrogen values in the absence of raised progesterone values occur for an average of 5 days only. Two types of luteal deficiency occur: One in which a normal length of luteal phase (11-16 days) is associated with lower than normal levels of pregnanediol excretion ($<$ 1.5 mg/24 hours), the other in which normal or subnormal levels of pregnanediol excretion are associated with a shortened length of luteal phase ($<$ 10 days). The latter is the greater bar to fertility because it does not allow sufficient time for implantation before the corpus luteum regresses and bleeding occurs. Thus, length of luteal phase is just as important in fertility as the level of progesterone production and this can only be determined by the use of a reliable midcycle marker of ovulation.

2. Two types of anovulatory cycles have been identified, one with constant, raised ovarian estrogen production, the other with fluctuating production. The latter type merges from a frank anovulatory cycle without any increase in progesterone production, through the inadequate luteal phase to the full ovulatory cycle. In this sequence, the dividing line between failure of follicle rupture (anovulation) and the release of an ovum (ovulation) has not been defined but currently is being studied by ultrasound.

3. No human yet has been encountered who does not excrete estrogens in the urine as measured by methods of sufficiently high sensitivity. The source of this estrogen is important when considering its biological activity. These studies show that, weight for weight, estrogen (estradiol) produced, usually cyclically, by the ovarian follicle is considerably more biologically active than estrogen (estrone) derived from extraglandular production, whether judged by endometrial stimulation (bleeding), its effect on suppressing the pituitary production of FSH, or by the production of cervical mucus. Studies using urine show that cyclical estrogen production, presumably from the ovaries, commences in girls at an early age at levels that are

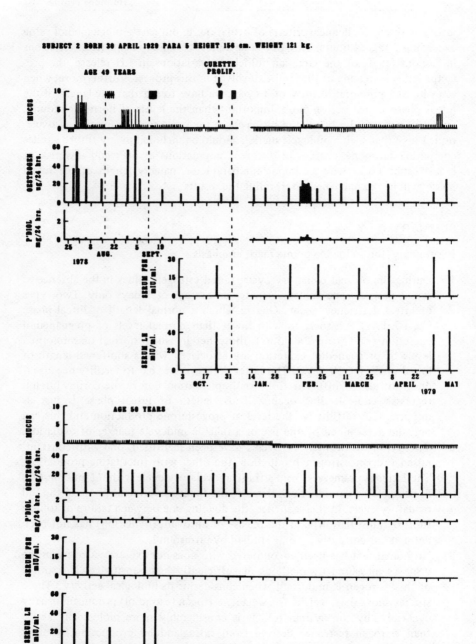

Figure 11
Subject 2. Values measured over 9 years in a woman aged 42-51 years.

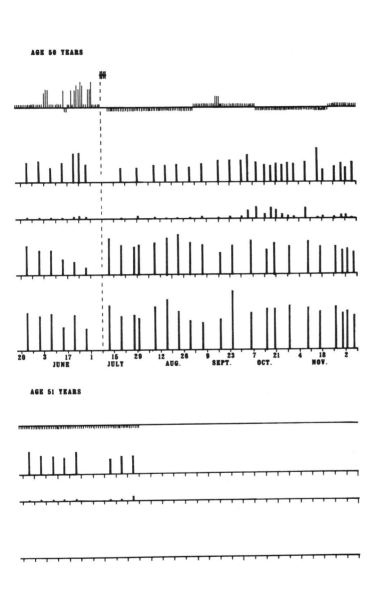

AGE 50 YEARS

20   3   17   1   15   29   12   26   9   23   7   21   4   18   2
      JUNE   JULY   AUG.   SEPT.   OCT.   NOV.

AGE 51 YEARS

3   17   31   14   28   12   26
     AUG.   SEPT.   OCT.

immeasurable by current radioimmunoassays using blood. This cyclical production gradually increases in amplitude, causing theelarche (breast growth) as the production rates pass through 2-5 μg of estradiol per day, and menarche (endometrial stimulation leading to bleeding) when the production rates reach 10-20 times the theelarche figure.

4. Anovulatory cycles are much more common in teenage girls, after childbirth, and during the approach to the menopause. As with menarche, menopause is not a single event. Ovarian activity wanes over a period of time. Even several years after menopause, sporadic elevations in urinary estrogen output above the base line provided by extraglandular production may be seen. These elevations, which may be relatively small, are accompanied by depression of serum FSH values and sometimes by spotting or bleeding. That the ovaries are the source of these increases recently has been demonstrated by the finding of follicles by ultrasound at such times.

REFERENCES

Brown, J.B. 1976. Determination of estriol, estrone, and estradiol-17β in non-pregnancy urine by spectrophotometry or fluorimetry. In *Methods of hormone analysis* (ed. H. Breuer et al.), p. 446. Georg Thieme Verlag, Stuttgart.

Brown, J.B., P. Harrisson, and M.A. Smith. 1978. Oestrogen and pregnanediol excretion through childhood, menarche and first ovulation. *J. Biosoc. Sci. (Suppl.)* 5:43.

Brown, J.B., S.C. MacLeod, C. Macnaughtan, M.A. Smith, and B. Smyth. 1968. A rapid method for estimating oestrogens in urine using a semi-automatic extractor. *J. Endocrinol.* 42:5.

Cox, R.I. 1963. Gas chromatography in the analysis of urinary pregnanediol. *J. Chromatogr.* 12:242.

Short, R.V. 1976. Special aspects—rhythms. In *Subcellular mechanisms in reproductive neuroendocrinology* (ed. F. Naftolin et al.). Elsevier Scientific, Amsterdam.

Trichopoulos, D., B. MacMahon, and J. Brown. 1980. Socioeconomic status, urine estrogens and breast cancer risk. *J. Natl. Cancer Inst.* 64:753.

COMMENTS

SIITERI: I'd like to ask a question. As you know, Dr. Frisch at Harvard has put forth the idea that puberty is related to body size, and in particular percent fat composition. Although this is an intriguing idea, we don't know what the mechanism(s) may be.

How do you view extraglandular estrogen production in the pre-pubertal or, more importantly, premenarchial, girl? Jim [Brown], you showed that estrogen excretion began to rise about the time of adrenarche, when the adrenal gland was putting out androstenedione, which could have been converted to estrone. If you have an obese young lady, she will make more estrogen from that androstenedione than a thin young lady will. I have hypothesized somewhere or other in the literature that this estrogen, in fact, could serve to "prime the pump" at the level of the pituitary to initiate normal cyclical function. How do you feel about that?

BROWN: In our studies, we did not document adrenarche, but most girls have some degree of breast development before they record growth of pubic hair, and then menarche occurs 1-5 years later. We found that estrogen production was already occurring at an early age and that the values gradually increased with age until they were sufficient to induce breast growth and eventually menarche. The blood androgen values reported by others show a similar trend. Apparently, the concept that androgen or estrogen production begins at a certain time (for example, at adrenarche) is an artefact due to the fact that the analytical methods applied have not been sensitive enough to measure the amounts being produced before that time. There is nothing in our data to support the concept of "priming the pump;" it is a continuous process. Certainly, part of the estrogen rise must be due to extraglandular production from the rising adrenal androgens. However, the finding of periodic fluctuations in estrogen production at an early age suggests that some of the estrogen is being produced in the ovaries. It is a useful rule that fluctuating estrogen production usually equates with ovarian activity whereas extraglandular production usually equates with noncyclical output.

PIKE: What is the relationship between the age at which your anovulatory cycles cease and the age at menarche? All the slides that you both showed had either age, bone age, or time from menarche as the horizontal axis; but Dr. Korenman's "estrogen window" hypothesis needs an early age of menarche to be associated with a longer period of anovulation if it is to help explain age at menarche as a breast cancer risk factor. The data that I know of shows quite the opposite; that is, the earlier you have menarche the sooner you settle down.

BROWN: Well, we get the impression that it's age from menarche that matters, rather than age at menarche.

HENDERSON: But the recent paper of Wallace et al. (1978) on their follow-up study in Minneapolis, where they looked at regularity of cycling in relation to age of menarche, showed that the earlier the age of menarche the quicker after menarche you were regular.

References

Wallace, R., B. Sherman, J.A. Bean, J.P. Leeper, and A.E. Treloar. 1978. Menstrual cycle patterns and breast cancer risk factors. *Cancer Res.* 38:4021.

Endocrine Maturation in the Course of Female Puberty

REIJO VIHKO AND DAN APTER
Department of Clinical Chemistry
University of Oulu
SF-90220 Oulu 22, Finland
and Department of Medical Chemistry
University of Helsinki
SF-00170 Helsinki 17, Finland

Female puberty is characterized by a number of endocrine changes that are initiated several years before the first hallmarks of pubertal somatic changes appear (Styne and Grumbach 1978). One step in the pubertal process in girls is the first menstruation (menarche), which, however, does not indicate advanced endocrine maturity. Rather, profound endocrine changes occur following menarche (Apter and Vihko 1977). It is also obvious that acquisition of reproductive ability, as evidenced by ovulation, takes place in most girls approximately 2 years following menarche. The first ovulatory cycles then show evidence of insufficient luteal function, as compared with cycles in women over 20 years of age.

In the following, we will present our data on changes in levels of serum peptide (adrenocorticotropin [ACTH], follicle-stimulating hormone [FSH], luteinizing hormone [LH], and prolactin) and steroid (pregnenolone, progesterone, 17-hydroxyprogesterone, cortisol, dehydroepiandrosterone [DHEA], androstenedione, testosterone, 5α-dihydrotestosterone [5α-DHT], androsterone, and estradiol) hormone concentrations in the course of puberty in girls. Part of the data results from longitudinal studies. The main emphasis will be on the hormonal changes associated with the appearance of menarche and with the maturation of the menstrual cycle.

SUBJECTS AND METHODS

Subjects

The subjects at the beginning of the longitudinal study were 200 healthy schoolgirls, 7-17 years of age (Apter and Vihko 1977). The pubertal stages were graded according to Tanner (1962). X-ray examination of the hand and wrist was performed in every subject and bone age was estimated according to Greulich and Pyle (1959). All blood specimens were drawn at 0800-1000 hours. In postmenarcheal girls, two specimens were drawn, on days 6-9 and 20-23 of the same menstrual cycle. Of the original group, 70% took part in the second examination performed 1.5 years after the first one.

The hormonal patterns of adolescent cycles were investigated in 20 girls, 13-17 years of age, who had their menarche 0.2-4.5 years before the start of the study. The first blood specimen was obtained on days 1-3 of the menstrual cycle. During the first 10 days of the cycle, specimens were drawn every second day and then every day during the 10 following days, and then again every second day until the appearance of the next menstrual bleeding.

Hormone Determinations

Peptide hormones were determined by direct radioimmunoassays (RIA) (Hammond et al. 1977b; Apter et al. 1979) using CEA-IRE-Sorin (CIS) kits. Dehydroepiandrosterone (Hammond et al. 1979) and estradiol (Hammond et al. 1977a) were quantified by RIA of serum extracts. The other steroids were also determined by RIA, but following chromatography of serum extracts on Lipidex-5000™ (Apter et al. 1976).

RESULTS AND DISCUSSION

Prepubertal Changes

The possible role of the adrenals has been a main issue in discussions about the onset of puberty in recent years. Our results corroborate the results of a number of studies (Hopper and Yen 1975; Sizonenko and Paunier 1975; Ducharme et al. 1976; Korth-Schutz et al. 1976) that show an early rise in circulating DHEA concentrations as shown in Figure 1. There was a threefold increase in serum DHEA levels in girls from 7.5 to 10.5 years of age. In addition to DHEA, another steroid with a 3β-hydroxy-5-ene structure, pregnenolone, showed an early increase (Fig. 2). In contrast to this, the changes in serum ACTH (Fig. 3) and cortisol (Fig. 2) concentrations were very minor. These findings are compatible with the suggestion that there might be a separate unidentified pituitary hormone that stimulates adrenal androgen production (Grumbach et al. 1978). The suggested central role of adrenarche in the initiation of pubertal development has recently been questioned seriously on the basis of clinical conditions in which, despite deficient adrenal function, the onset and progression of puberty have been normal (Sklar et al. 1980).

Adrenarche in girls is immediately followed by gonadarche, the activation of the gonads, which is the result of increasing stimulation by gonadotropic hormones. The FSH levels increased from the youngest age group in this study, 7.5 years, onwards (Fig. 3). This is consistent with the findings of Peters et al. (1976) on ovarian morphology; after the age of 6 years in particular, they saw more follicles reach late antral size as age advanced. Serum LH started to increase 2-3 years later than FSH (Fig. 3).

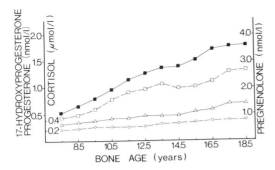

Figure 1
Serum DHEA (○), estradiol (■), testosterone (▲), and 5α-DHT (△) concentrations in pubertal girls. The changes have been expressed in a mixed longitudinal manner, in which the ratios of changes in hormone concentrations and bone age in each individual are calculated first. The mean annual changes then are added to or subtracted from the previous age group, beginning from the mean actual concentrations of the bone age group of 13.5 years, which includes the largest number of subjects. This point is the only one representing the actual mean hormone concentration of the age group; others reflect relative changes (for details, see Apter 1980).

Serum prolactin displayed a slow increase from the youngest age group onwards (Fig. 3). By a bone age of 13.5 years, its concentration had increased approximately 50% compared with the values seen in the youngest age group.

Gonadal Activation

Serum FSH concentrations reached adult early follicular phase levels by 11.5 years of bone age (Fig. 3). The increase in serum LH continued until 13.5 years, when a distinct peak was seen.

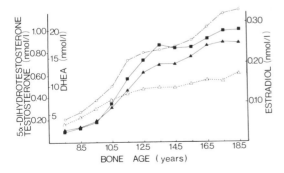

Figure 2
Serum pregnenolone (■), 17-hydroxyprogesterone (□), progesterone (△), and cortisol (○) concentrations in pubertal girls, expressed as in Fig. 1.

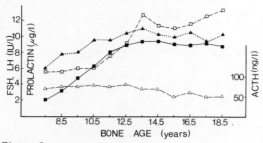

Figure 3
Serum prolactin (▲), LH (□), FSH (■), and ACTH (△) concentrations in pubertal girls, expressed as in Fig. 1.

Reflecting a sign of clear gonadal activation, serum estradiol was significantly increased at 10.5 years of bone age compared with the younger age groups (Fig. 1). The steep increase in its concentration continued until 13.5 years, the bone age group when menarche took place. The testosterone level very closely paralleled that of estradiol, suggesting that the pubertal testosterone rise is mainly ovarian in origin (Fig. 1). This is supported further by the finding that the pubertal rise of serum testosterone is very small in patients with Turner's syndrome (D. Apter et al., in prep.). Serum androstenedione concentration showed a steep increase between 9.5-12.5 years of bone age (Apter 1980). Serum 5α-DHT displayed a somewhat different pattern than testosterone and androstenedione. Although in the adult this steroid is formed mainly by peripheral conversion from testosterone and androstenedione (Ito and Horton 1971), its serum concentration during puberty was by no means a constant percentage of testosterone or androstenedione levels. A gradual, slow rise was observed from the youngest age group onwards, and it resulted in a decrease in the DHT: testosterone ratio in the course of puberty.

The concentration of serum sex-hormone-binding globulin (SHBG) also displays clear-cut changes in association with the changes of circulating estrogens and androgens. In girls, after 9-10 years of age, serum SHBG concentrations decreased to about one-half the prepubertal values (Vermeulen 1977; Bartsch et al. 1980), and, in boys, this decline was more pronounced still (Vermeulen 1977). This suggests that in girls, too, androgen action dominates over estrogen action in the regulation of serum SHBG concentrations during pubertal development.

Anovulation-Ovulation

In our group, the mean age at menarche was 12.9 years of chronological age and 13.4 years of bone age. There is evidence that the great majority of cycles are anovulatory following menarche, and the percentage of ovulatory cycles slowly increases during the following years (Treloar et al. 1967; Döring 1969). Table 1 summarizes the distribution of 209 adolescent cycles into ovulatory and anovulatory ones, based on the serum progesterone concentration on days 20-23 of the cycle. We chose a progesterone concentration exceeding 6.4 nmoles/liter (2 ng/ml), which is more than 10 times the concentration seen at the beginning of the cycle, to signify an ovulatory cycle. Correspondingly, a progesterone concentration of less than 1.6 nmoles/liter (0.5 ng/ml) was considered to signify an anovulatory cycle. It is to be observed, however, that the distribution of maximal progesterone levels is rather continuous in adolescent menstrual cycles (Apter et al. 1978), and, therefore, classification based on serum progesterone concentrations is somewhat arbitrary. Among these 209 cycles (Table 1), there were 19 cycles (9% of all) with a progesterone concentration of 1.6-6.4 nmoles/liter in the latter part of the cycle. They were excluded from the comparisons of ovulatory and anovulatory cycles. As can be seen in Table 1, 82% of the cycles were anovulatory during the first gynecological year, 50% during the third, and 15% 6.0-7.5 years after menarche.

The concentrations of a number of steroids and of gonadotropins display differences when ovulatory and anovulatory cycles are compared (Table 2). Especially interesting are the differences between androgen levels. Testosterone concentrations did not differ between the follicular and luteal phases of ovulatory cycles, whereas, in the anovulatory cycles, testosterone increased significantly towards the end of the cycle. At the two time points when specimens were drawn, the serum testosterone concentration was higher in anovulatory cycles when compared with the ovulatory ones (Table 2). The pattern of serum

Table 1

Distribution of Early Adolescent Cycles into Ovulatory and Anovulatory Types in Relation to Gynecological Age (Years Since Menarche)

Gynecological age (years)	Number of cycles	Ovulatory	Anovulatory	Percent anovulatory
0.0-0.9	35	4	29	82
1.0-1.9	44	13	24	54
2.0-2.9	32	14	16	50
3.0-3.9	29	11	14	48
4.0-4.9	37	23	12	32
5.0-5.9	19	14	4	21
6.0-7.5	13	10	2	15

A serum progesterone concentration of more than 6.4 nmoles/liter (2.0 ng/ml) was considered to signify an ovulatory cycle, and a concentration of less than 1.6 nmoles/liter (0.5 ng/ml), an anovulatory one, in samples taken on days 20-23 of the cycles.

The difference between the number of cycles and the sum of ovulatory and anovulatory ones represents cycles with luteal-phase serum progesterone concentrations of 1.6-6.4 nmoles/liter. These cycles were not included in either group.

Table 2

Serum Steroids (nmole/liter) and Gonadotropins (IU/liter) in Ovulatory (n = 53, except for androstenedione, n = 26) and Anovulatory (n = 70, except for androstenedione, n = 38) Adolescent Cycles in Samples Taken on Days 6-9 and 20-23 of the Cycle

Serum hormone	Day of cycle		ovulatory		anovulatory	
				Nature of cycle		
			ovulatory		anovulatory	
Progesterone	6-9	$p \ll 0.001$	0.54	N.S.	0.51	$p < 0.01$
	20-23		18.18	$p \ll 0.001$	0.63	
Estradiol	6-9	$p \ll 0.001$	0.22	N.S.	0.21	$p < 0.01$
	20-23		0.59	$p < 0.001$	0.33	
Testosterone	6-9	N.S.[a]	0.75	$p < 0.05$	0.85	$p < 0.001$
	20-23		0.76	$p < 0.01$	1.06	
Androstenedione	6-9	N.S.	2.70	N.S.	2.85	$p < 0.01$
	20-23		2.78	$p < 0.05$	3.63	
5α-DHT	6-9	$p < 0.00$	0.60	N.S.	0.62	N.S.
	20-23		0.73	N.S.	0.63	
DHEA	6-9	N.S.	19.20	N.S.	21.30	N.S.
	20-23		20.00	N.S.	21.20	
FSH	6-9	$p \ll 0.001$	8.90	N.S.	8.90	N.S.
	20-23		4.60	$p < 0.001$	8.30	
LH	6-9	$p < 0.05$	13.10	N.S.	12.70	$p < 0.001$
	20-23		11.40	$p < 0.05$	16.20	

[a] Not significant.

androstenedione concentrations was very similar to that of testosterone, whereas serum 5α-DHT concentrations were not significantly different when ovulatory and anovulatory cycles were compared. DHEA concentrations did not show any differences between ovulatory and anovulatory cycles, nor in different phases of both types of cycles (Table 2).

There were also differences in gonadotropin levels between ovulatory and anovulatory cycles. The FSH levels were significantly lower in the latter part of the ovulatory cycles, whereas in anovulatory cycles, FSH levels were very similar at the beginning and close to the end of the cycle. The differences in gonado-tropin levels were accentuated in the case of serum LH. Its concentration was lower in the latter part of the ovulatory cycles, but higher in the latter part of the anovulatory cycles, when compared with concentrations prevailing on days 6-9 of the cycle. In accordance with these results, serum FSH and LH were significantly higher on days 20-23 in the anovulatory cycles than in the ovulatory ones (Table 2). Serum prolactin concentrations did not differ between ovulatory and anovulatory cycles, neither were there any differences in its levels in the samples taken on days 6-9 or 20-23 of the cycle (Apter 1980).

To obtain detailed information of the hormonal characteristics of adolescent menstrual cycles, we investigated 20 girls, 0.2-4.5 years after menarche, with serum specimens taken every day or every other day over one menstrual cycle (Apter et al. 1978). The adolescent cycles investigated could be divided into three different categories based on serum progesterone levels in the latter part of the cycle and on the length of the luteal phase. The three different types were normal ovulatory cycles, short luteal-phase cycles, and anovulatory cycles.

In 10 cycles (Fig. 4), the duration of the luteal phase was 11-13 days and the maximum serum progesterone concentration was 10-48 nmoles/liter (5-15 ng/ml). These cycles therefore were considered to be normal ovulatory ones. The oldest girls investigated belonged to this group, and their mean gynecological age (years since menarche) was 2.9 years. It is to be observed, however, that the mean progesterone level during the luteal phase was lower, the luteal phase shorter, and the follicular phase longer than in a group of adult (21-35 years) women investigated in a similar manner (Punnonen et al. 1975). A negative correlation existed between the FSH levels early in the follicular phase and the total length of the follicular phase. When serum FSH increased slowly at the beginning of the cycle, the ovarian estradiol secretion increase took place later, which resulted in a late LH surge (Apter et al. 1978).

Short luteal-phase cycles seem to be rather common amongst adolescents. Four of twenty adolescent cycles investigated had a short luteal phase of 4-8 days duration. In such cycles, the progesterone concentration clearly was lower than in the luteal phase of normal cycles.

Six of the 20 adolescent cycles investigated using frequent blood specimen collection were anovulatory. In this group, which was the youngest, serum progesterone concentrations did not exceed 3.2 nmoles/liter (1.0 ng/ml). According to the hormone measurements, the reasons for anovulation were

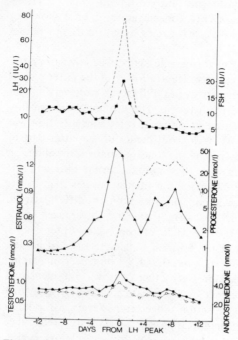

Figure 4

Daily mean concentrations on serum LH (□), FSH (■), estradiol (▲), progesterone (∇), testosterone (●), and androstenedione (○) in 10 adolescent menstrual cycles considered to be ovulatory. The cycles were synchronized by taking the day of the LH peak as day 0. The scale for progesterone concentration is logarithmic.

variable. In one girl (Fig. 5), the lack of ovulation was due most likely to immaturity of the positive gonadal-pituitary feedback mechanism, i.e., lack of an LH surge after a "periovulatory" estradiol peak. In another, midcycle LH and FSH surges were seen following the increased estradiol, but no increase in serum progesterone was observed. In the majority of anovulatory cycles, the hormonal background behind anovulation seems to be different. In four cycles studied by us, no follicular maturation, reflected by increasing serum estradiol, was seen (Fig. 6). Instead, in these cycles, testosterone and androstenedione levels tended to be elevated together with LH. This finding is in accordance with the results described above for the large number of cycles in which specimens were taken on days 6-9 and 20-23 of the cycle, and which revealed increased testosterone and androstenedione levels in the latter part of anovulatory cycles.

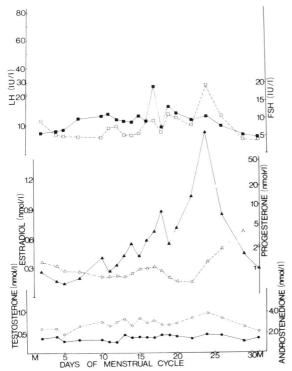

Figure 5
Serum LH (□), FSH (■), estradiol (▲), progesterone (△), testosterone (●), and androstenedione (○) during one anovulatory menstrual cycle in a 13.3-year-old girl. (M) The first
day of menstruation.

CONCLUDING REMARKS

Gonadotropins are secreted from birth onwards and are always essential for
ovarian follicular development (Ross 1974). Even during childhood, follicles
begin to grow but they do not reach full maturity. Instead, they undergo atresia
continuously in an asynchronous manner (Peters et al. 1976). After about 7
years of age, under the stimulation of increasing serum FSH concentrations,
accelerating follicular maturation takes place. Androgens are produced by the
first maturing follicles. In animals, it has been shown that experimentally
increased intraovarian androgen concentrations produced atresia (Louvet et al.
1975). In addition, atretic follicles produce increased amounts of androgen
(McNatty et al. 1979). This had led us to suggest that a certain critical ovarian
follicular androgen concentration is achieved during early pubertal development,
leading to the arrest of follicular development and subsequent follicular atresia
(Vihko and Apter 1980). Repetitions of this process lead to a cyclic endocrine
pattern in girls, with cyclic ovarian follicular growth as the driving force. No

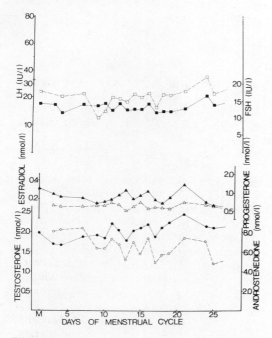

Figure 6

Serum LH (□), FSH (■), estradiol (▲), progesterone (△), testosterone (●), and androstene-dione (○) during the initial third of one anovulatory cycle in a 14.2-year-old girl. (M) The first day of menstruation. Note the high levels of testosterone and androstenedione.

hypothalamic cyclic centers seem to be involved (Knobil 1980). Sometime in midpuberty, there is sufficient estrogen priming of the endometrium, followed by estrogen withdrawal, to lead to the first menstrual bleeding, menarche. The first menstrual cycles are anovulatory and are characterized by increased serum levels of testosterone, androstenedione, and LH. This resembles the pattern seen in the polycystic ovary (PCO) syndrome, where, however, the changes are more exaggerated. This pattern seems to be a normal step in the maturation of the menstrual cycle. It remains to be seen, however, whether aberrancies in the conversion of anovulatory cycles into ovulatory ones may result later in patho-logical developments.

The next step in the maturation of the normal menstrual cycle is charac-terized by increased production of estradiol. Eventually a follicle under FSH stimulation escapes the critical microenvironment leading to atresia, and it produces sufficient estradiol finally to elicit the preovulatory gonadotropin surge. When ovulation later takes place, the first luteal phases are usually incom-plete, being of short duration, and the serum progesterone level is subnormal. In the large majority of girls, normal ovulatory ovarian function is reached within 5 years of menarche, at about 17-18 years of bone age. However, even at this age, the luteal phase is shorter and progesterone secretion is somewhat lower than in an adult (21-35 years of age) population.

REFERENCES

Apter, D. 1980. Serum steroids and pituitary hormones in female puberty. A partly longitudinal study. *Clin. Endocrinol.* 12:107.

Apter, D. and R. Vihko. 1977. Serum pregnenolone, progesterone, 17-hydroxy-progesterone, testosterone and 5α-dihydrotestosterone during female puberty. *J. Clin. Endocrinol. Metab.* 45:1039.

Apter, D., L. Viinikka, and R. Vihko. 1978. Hormonal pattern of adolescent menstrual cycles. *J. Clin. Endocrinol. Metab.* 47:944.

Apter, D., O. Jänne, P. Karvonen, and R. Vihko. 1976. Simultaneous determination of five sex hormones in human serum by radioimmunoassay after chromatography on Lipidex-5000. *Clin. Chem.* 22:32.

Apter, D., A. Pakarinen, G.L. Hammond and R. Vihko. 1979. Adrenocortical function in puberty: Serum ACTH, cortisol and dehydroepiandrosterone in girls and boys. *Acta Paediatrica Scandinavica* 68:599.

Bartsch, W., H.-J. Horst, and K.-M. Derwahl. 1980. Interrelationships between sex hormone-binding globulin and 17β-estradiol, testosterone, 5α-dihydro-testosterone, thyroxine and triiodothyronine in prepubertal and pubertal girls. *J. Clin. Endocrinol. Metab.* 50:1053.

Ducharme, J.R., M.G. Forest, E. de Peretti, M. Sempé, R. Collu, and J. Bertrand. 1976. Plasma adrenal and gonadal sex steroids in human pubertal development. *J. Clin. Endocrinol. Metab.* 42:468.

Döring, G.K. 1969. The incidence of anovulatory cycles in women. *J. Reprod. Fertil.* 6:77.

Greulich, W. and S. Pyle. 1959. *Radiographic atlas of skeletal development of the hand and wrist.* Stanford University Press, Stanford.

Grumbach, M.M., G.E. Richards, F.A. Conte, and S.L. Kaplan. 1978. Clinical disorders of adrenal function and puberty: An assessment of the role of the adrenal cortex in normal and abnormal puberty in man and evidence for an ACTH-like pituitary adrenal androgen stimulating hormone. In *The endocrine function of the human adrenal cortex* (ed. V.H.T. James et al.), p. 583. Academic Press, New York.

Hammond, G.L., L. Viinikka, and R. Vihko. 1977a. Automation of radio-immunoassays for some sex steroids with use of both iodinated and tritiated ligands. *Clin. Chem.* 23:1250.

Hammond, G.L., M. Koivisto, K. Kouvalainen, and R. Vihko. 1979. Serum steroids and pituitary hormones in infants with particular reference to testicular activity. *J. Clin. Endocrinol. Metab.* 49:40.

Hammond, G.L., M. Kontturi, P. Määttälä, M. Puukka, and R. Vihko. 1977b. Serum FSH, LH and prolactin in normal males and patients with prostatic diseases. *Clin. Endocrinol.* 7:129.

Hopper, B.R. and S.S.C. Yen. 1975. Circulating concentrations of dehydro-epiandrosterone and dehydroepiandrosterone sulfate during puberty. *J. Clin. Endocrinol. Metab.* 40:458.

Ito, T. and R. Horton. 1971. Dihydrotestosterone in human peripheral plasma. *J. Clin. Endocrinol. Metab.* 31:362.

Knobil, E. 1980. The neuroendocrine control of the menstrual cycle. *Recent Progr. Horm. Res.* 36:53.

Korth-Schutz, S., L.S. Levine, and M.I. New. 1976. Serum androgens in normal prepubertal and pubertal children and in children with precocious adrenarche. *J. Clin. Endocrinol. Metab.* 42:117.

Louvet, J.-P., S.M. Harman, J.R. Schreiber, and G.T. Ross. 1975. Evidence for a role of androgens in follicular maturation. *Endocrinology* 97:366.

McNatty, K.P., A. Makris, C. DeGrazia, R. Osathanondh, and K.J. Ryan. 1979. The production of progesterone, androgens and oestrogens by human granulosa cells in vitro and in vivo. *J. Steroid Biochem.* 11:775.

Peters, H., R. Himelstein-Braw, and M. Faber. 1976. The normal development of the ovary in childhood. *Acta Endocrinologica* 82:617.

Punnonen, R., S. Nummi, O. Ylikorkala, U. Alapiessa, P. Karvonen, and L. Viinikka. 1975. A composite picture of the normal menstrual cycle. *Acta Obstet. Gynecol. Scand.* 51:63.

Ross, G.T. 1974. Gonadotrophins and preantral follicular maturation in women. *Fertil. Steril.* 25:522.

Sizonenko, P.C. and L. Paunier. 1975. Hormonal changes in puberty. III. Correlation of plasma dehydroepiandrosterone, testosterone, FSH and LH with stages of puberty and bone age in normal boys and girls and patients with Addison's disease or hypogonadism or with premature or late adrenarche. *J. Clin. Endocrinol. Metab.* 41:894.

Sklar, C.A., S.L. Kaplan, and M.M. Grumbach. 1980. Evidence for dissociation between adrenarche and gonadarche: Studies in patients with idiopathic precocious puberty, gonadal dysgenesis, isolated gonadotropin deficiency, and constitutionally delayed growth and adolescence. *J. Clin. Endocrinol. Metab.* 51:548.

Styne, D.M. and M.M. Grumbach. 1978. Puberty in the male and female: Its physiology and disorders. In *Reproductive endocrinology* (ed. S.S.C. Yen and R. B. Jaffe), p. 189. W.B. Saunders Company, Philadelphia/London/Toronto.

Tanner, J.M. 1962. *Growth at adolescence*, 2nd edition. Blackwell Scientific Publications, Oxford.

Treloar, A.E., R.E. Boynton, B.G. Behn, and B.W. Brown. 1967. Variation of the human menstrual cycle through reproductive life. *Int. J. Fertil.* 12:77.

Vermeulen, A. 1977. Transport and distribution of androgens at different ages. In *Androgens and antiandrogens* (ed. L. Martini and M. Motta), p. 53. Raven Press, New York.

Vihko, R. and D. Apter. 1980. The role of androgens in adolescent cycles. *J. Steroid Biochem.* 12:369.

COMMENTS

SIITERI: I'm glad there are no neuroendocrinologists here, because to suggest that the cycle begins in the ovary, as Reijo [Vihko] has done, certainly wouldn't sit well with them. But I like it. As you know, puberty has been related to body size, and in particular to fat composition; however, we don't understand the mechanism.

VIHKO: As far as the weight at menarche is concerned, it was from 37 kg to 64 kg in our group. Therefore, it is very difficult to believe in a critical weight at which menarche should take place.

In studies on pubertal development is is not easy to point out causal relationships. When the age advances, the weight increases and serum steroid and peptide hormone concentrations also increase. It is therefore very difficult to identify something other than only an age-related phenomenon. However, an interesting observation was made in the youngest groups of prepubertal girls with a bone age of below 9.5 years. In these groups, luteinizing hormone (LH) correlated with body weight, as well as with the calculated fat amount and body fat percentage, although in these prepubertal age groups, LH did not correlate with age. Hence, these relationships were not primarily age-related parallel phenomena.

SIITERI: That's very interesting.

HENDERSON: I also noticed in your data that the prolactin rise preceded the estrogen rise. This is contrary to standard doctrine and would suggest that prolactin secretion, at least at that time, is controlled separately.

VIHKO: The increase in serum prolactin before menarche was gradual and relatively small, but there is no doubt that the difference between the age groups of 7.5 years and 8.5 years was statistically significant. This is amongst the first of the endocrine changes observed and clearly precedes the first significant increases in serum estradiol.

Reproductive Endocrinology and Breast Cancer in Women

STANLEY G. KORENMAN
Department of Medicine
UCLA-San Fernando Valley Program
VA Medical Center
Sepulveda, California 91343

There is considerable evidence that the reproductive endocrine system contributes to the etiology and pathogenesis of breast cancer. In addition to the differential rate between the sexes, this includes well-established epidemiological evidence that early menarche, late menopause, and late first birth increase the risk of breast cancer dramatically (MacMahon et al. 1973; Gray et al. 1979).

The influence of Westernization in increasing breast cancer incidence has been attributed to nutritional influences on menarche and menopause, obesity, later marriage, pregnancy and first-term birth, greater carcinogen exposure particularly due to fat or meat ingestion, and to other factors as described elsewhere in this volume.

Endocrine and other environmental factors are interdependent variables. Nutrition contributes to control over the age of menarche, which appears to be dependent on attainment of a certain body mass or adiposity (Frisch and McArthur 1974). Heavy cigarette smoking is associated with an earlier age of menopause (Pike, this volume). Education, job opportunities, contraceptive availability, and social customs influence the age at marriage, the age at first birth and parity, and therefore, the lifelong hormonal exposure of individuals. Menstrual cycles and hormone secretions are affected by intensive exercise (Dale et al. 1979; Shangold et al. 1979; Brisson et al. 1980; Warren 1980), drug use, particularly heroin (Gaulden et al. 1964), and other factors. Various stresses, such as entering a nunnery or college, have also been reported to be associated with a high incidence of temporary amenorrhea.

All of these factors and others could individually or collectively influence the hormonal milieu in such a way as to alter the likelihood of breast cancer.

A review of the endocrine epidemiology of breast cancer (Korenman 1980) demonstrated a lack of consistent findings and considerable likelihood of serious population biases. The hypothesis was developed (Table 1) that the endocrine environment simply influenced susceptibility to carcinogens and that breast cancer risk, therefore, would be linked more closely to the duration of mammary exposure to a supporting endocrine environment than to the level of a particular

Table 1
Estrogen-window Hypothesis

1. Human breast cancer is induced by carcinogens in a susceptible mammary gland.
2. Unopposed estrogenic stimulation is the most favorable state for induction.
3. There is a long latency between induction of tumor and clinical expression.
4. The duration of the estrogen window determines risk.
5. Inducibility declines with establishment of normal ovulatory menses and becomes very low during pregnancy.

hormone. By analogy to the 7,12-dimethylbenz[a]anthracene (DMBA) rat model (Welsch and Meites 1978), the most conducive environment for tumor induction would be estrogenic stimulation in the absence of the differentiating and inhibitory effects of progesterone or the hormonal consequences of the latter half of pregnancy. During certain periods of normal reproductive life, there would be open windows for carcinogenesis. Abnormal conditions and environmental influences would alter the duration of these estrogen windows. This concept evolved from a previous analysis of breast cancer risk data (Sherman and Korenman 1974c) in which luteal inadequacy per se was considered to be the preeminent risk factor.

The estrogen-window hypothesis was supported by data obtained from studies of irradiation-induced mammary carcinoma (Boice and Monson 1977; Tokunaga et al. 1979) and by review of the lifetime changes in reproductive cycles (Treloar et al. 1967; Sherman and Korenman 1975; Sherman et al. 1976; Korenman et al. 1978). The present analysis will focus on normal and abnormal reproductive function, with particular attention to our knowledge of how the mammary gland is regulated by the principal reproductive hormones.

HORMONAL INTERACTIONS IN THE REGULATION OF MAMMARY FUNCTION

It is remarkable how little we know about the intimate nature of the regulation of mammary function.

The mammalian reproductive cycle in females, unlike equilibrium-tending endocrine systems, is directed toward the climactic events of ovulation and either implantation or corpus luteum regression. These events require complex hormonal interactions at the level of the hypothalamus, pituitary, and ovary, as well as overriding cerebral cortical controls. Secondary hormonal targets, such as the breast, reflect these interactions in a complexly integrated manner that reflects not only the level and duration of stimuli but the responsiveness of the tissue and the interactions between the different cell types. Under normal circumstances, the mammary gland is influenced predominantly by the interactions between estrogens, progesterone, and prolactin that are listed in Table 2.

Table 2

Interactions between Estrogens, Progesterone, and Prolactin

1. Estrogens
    Stimulate ductal proliferation in mammary gland
    Stimulate prolactin secretion at both hypothalamic and pituitary levels
    Increase prolactin receptors in breast
    Inhibit dopamine production in hypothalamus
    Suppress gonadotropins
    Stimulate LH production at midcycle
    Induce progesterone receptors
2. Progesterone
    Stimulates lobuloalveolar proliferation in mammary gland
    Enhances dopamine production
    Inhibits prolactin secretion
    Inhibits lactation during pregnancy
    Inhibits estrogen receptor in uterus, pituitary gland, and hypothalamus
    Facilitates estradiol inactivation
3. Prolactin
    Stimulates lactation and mammary cell division
    Inhibits hypothalamic dopamine production
    Stimulates its own receptors
    Stimulates estrogen receptors in breast
    Inhibits gonadotropin secretion
    Inhibits granulosa and luteal cell estrogen and progesterone secretion
    Inhibits prolactin secretion

Endogenous and exogenous estrogens stimulate mammary ductal proliferation in everyone if there is not a high concentration of an androgen. Mammary gland carcinoma is conditioned by estrogens (Horowitz and McGuire 1978; Kelly et al. 1980) to respond to progesterone and prolactin through stimulation of receptors for both hormones, though suppression may occur with high doses of estrogens (Kledzik et al. 1976). Stimulation of prolactin secretion also takes place, with data demonstrating an effect principally on the pituitary to inhibit dopamine response (Labrie et al. 1980; West and Dannies 1980), thus reducing inhibition of prolactin secretion. Because prolactin stimulates its own receptors (reviewed in Kelly et al. 1980), it may well be that the estrogen-mediated increase of mammary prolactin receptors occurs secondarily. The complex regulation by estrogens of gonadotropin production is central to the control of ovarian function and therefore to the secretion of progesterone. Local ovarian effects of estrogens and androgens also play a significant role in follicular maturation. These levels of regulation will not be discussed further.

We know little about the mechanism by which estrogens control mammary cellular proliferation and the biological consequences of their alteration of transcription. Whereas estrogens produce a great many secondary responses throughout the body, there appears to be little evidence that estrogens are mutagenic in their own right, so that their predominant carcinogenic effects appear to be to promote cellular susceptibility to neoplastic transformation.

Progesterone

Progesterone has both positive and negative effects on mammary development. In the prepared tissue, it stimulates lobuloalveolar proliferation. However, it is the main inhibitor of lactation during pregnancy (Davis et al. 1972) and inhibits estrogen action at least by suppressing its receptors in the uterus (Hsieh et al. 1975; Bhakoo and Katzenellenbogen 1977), hypothalamus (Labrie et al. 1980), and pituitary (Haug 1979). Inhibition of the biological actions of estrogens by this mechanism have been demonstrated (Brenner et al. 1974; Mester et al. 1974; Warner et al. 1980). The question of whether progestational agents stimulate or inhibit either basal or estrogen-stimulated prolactin secretion in vivo is not settled. Progesterone also opposes estrogen action by facilitating inactivation of estradiol. In human endometrium, progesterone stimulates the production of 17β-hydroxysteroid dehydrogenase (Tseng and Gurpide 1975; Pollow et al. 1975). A variable level of this enzyme in human breast and breast cancer tissue was demonstrated, peaking in both tissues in the early secretory phase of the menstrual cycle (Pollow et al. 1977). It should be emphasized that the function of progesterone in the breast is not understood and that it cannot simply be limited to control of estrogen receptors or estrogen-metabolizing enzymes, because the two hormones synergize in the uterus and mammary gland in producing the differentiated cell population necessary for their respective reproductive functions. Progesterone is not a mutagen. Although there is no established primary disorder of progesterone excess, there is a substantial number of patients who have anovulatory, short, or inadequate luteal cycles and therefore represent cases of long-term progesterone deficiency (see below). Whether or not this relates to breast cancer incidence is a principal question of this symposium.

Prolactin

Prolactin is a potent stimulator of lobuloalveolar proliferation and of lactation. It stimulates the production of estrogen receptors as well as its own. However, prolactin has other important influences, suppressing and stimulating, at least in some species, both granulosa and luteal cell hormone production (McNatty et al. 1974; Day et al. 1980; Veldhuis et al. 1980), as well as suppressing gonadotropin secretion (Robyn et al. 1977). Prolactin effects are well described in humans in the syndromes of infertility associated with a short luteal phase and of amenorrhea-galactorrhea where the prolactin-induced suppression of hormone secretion by both the ovaries and the pituitary gonadotropes can be reversed by dopaminergic agonists, particularly bromoergocryptine (Franks et al. 1975; Bohnet and Schneider 1977; Corbey et al. 1977; Van Look et al. 1977), which inhibit prolactin secretion. The overall effect of primary prolactin excess on the breast, therefore, is associated with estrogen and progesterone deficiency.

Conditions of Estrogen Excess

With these complex interrelationships among the principal reproductive hormones that control the mammary gland and our lack of knowledge as to how proliferative stimuli are controlled in a cell, it is possible to hypothesize that unopposed estrogenic stimulation is most likely to produce susceptibility to a transforming event. It is estrogens that produce primary proliferation of the duct epithelium, the cell most susceptible to neoplastic transformation, and at the same time stimulate progesterone responsiveness, prolactin secretion, and prolactin responsiveness. The other hormones, particularly progesterone, have strong inhibitory effects on estrogen action.

Having hypothesized that unopposed estrogens or estrogen excess is the most likely endocrine cause of breast cancer risk, it was appropriate to ask when during normal reproductive life or under what pathological conditions would such a condition prevail. These are listed in Table 3.

Prior to menarche, there is a significant rise of estradiol and estrone production, which operates on a susceptible gland to initiate breast development. Probably as a result of estrogenic stimulation, prolactin secretion also rises. Little progesterone is secreted. The period of time between breast budding and menarche is at least a year, but may be several years. This is reviewed magnificently by Styne and Grumbach (1978).

Table 3
Conditions of Estrogen Excess or Unopposed Estrogens

A. Premenarchial puberty
B. Nonovulatory postmenarchial cycles
C. Some varieties of hypothalamic and postpill amenorrhea
D. Short luteal-phase cycles
E. Long follicular-phase cycles
F. Euestrogenic amenorrhea of obesity
G. Polycystic ovary syndrome
H. Early amenorrhea-galactorrhea syndrome
I. Premenopausal anovulation and luteal inadequacy
J. Estrogen administration
K. Estrogen-secreting tumors
L. Precocious puberty in females
M. Klinefelter's syndrome
N. Other male hypergonadotropic hypogonadism
O. Testicular feminization (type 1)
P. Gynecomastia of any cause

The onset of menarche has been reported to be associated with anovulation for up to several years, as noted elsewhere in this volume. At present, the perimenarchial period is also a time of maximum physical training for young women, as runners, ballet dancers, swimmers, etc. Menarche may be delayed in such individuals, although estrogenic stimulation is under way, most probably as a result of delayed attainment of an appropriate percent body fat (Frisch and McArthur 1974; Warren 1980). Even after menarche, many cycles in trained athletes are associated with diminished progesterone secretion (Dale et al. 1979).

Although "unopposed" estrogens prevail in postmenarchial hypoestrogenic amenorrhea, the degree of mammary stimulation is unknown but probably low (Yen 1978). Other cases of dysfunctional uterine bleeding in the adolescent period may be associated with substantial estrogen production without evidence of ovulation (Fraser et al. 1973).

Short luteal-phase cycles (Sherman and Korenman 1974a) are a common cause of endocrine infertility in young women who are otherwise normal and whose sexual partner is fertile. The cycles may be short or of normal length, but the luteal phase is 10 days or less and may be only a few days. Their characteristic features are normal estrogen secretion in the follicular phase in the face of normal luteinizing hormone (LH) and reduced follicle-stimulating hormone (FSH) levels. Follicular maturation may be delayed. After an estrogen burst and a normal LH peak, corpus luteum formation is grossly defective with very low levels of progesterone and estrogens, a brief rise of basal body temperature (BBT) followed by menses. These cycles may be repetitive or sporadic. They are often, but not always, associated with excessive prolactin secretion (Askel 1980). Because the dopaminergic agonist bromoergocryptine suppresses prolactin secretion and usually normalizes the cycle promptly, it is considered that the disorder represents a primary prolactin hypersecretion (del Pozo et al. 1979), however, it must be kept in mind that gonadotropin secretion may be stimulated by dopaminergic agonists. Such subjects are hard to identify in epidemiological surveys because cycle length is so often normal or near normal. They do constitute a group with unopposed estrogen and excessive prolactin stimulation and are candidates for late first pregnancy and relative infertility. The incidence of such cycles falls with reproductive life, so that total fertility may not be reduced.

Long follicular-phase cycles characterize some of the prolonged cycles of young women (Sherman and Korenman 1975). They terminate in a full ovulation but demonstrate prolonged unopposed estrogenic stimulation. Prolactin levels have not been reported in these cycles. Subjects with cycles such as these are excluded routinely from case-control studies of breast cancer risk, possibly creating biased sampling.

The amenorrhea of obesity has not been fully characterized, but it may be related to the reproductive endocrine state in patients with the polycystic ovary (PCO) syndrome. It is associated with infertility and prolonged unopposed estrogen stimulation. There has been no epidemiologic study characterizing such women nor have full endocrine characterizations of such subjects been reported. The amenorrhea may be terminated by an ovulation and a luteally inadequate secretory phase (Sherman and Korenman 1974b). It is likely that these women have elevated estrone levels that are derived from increased aromatization of androstenedione and (or) from increased androstenedione production. Low sex-hormone-binding-globulin (SHBG) levels typical of obesity (Glass et al. 1977; O'Dea et al. 1979) would make both their estradiol and testosterone more available. This would result in suppressed FSH secretion and elevated LH secretion.

Remarkably, inadequate luteal-phase cycles have been noted to be prominent defects in women with benign breast disease (Sitruk-Ware et al. 1977). PCO disease is now thought similarly to be a hyperestrogenic, hyperandrogenic syndrome associated with androstenedione overproduction and conversion to excessive concentration of both estrone and testosterone (Baird 1976; Korenman and Sherman 1976; Yen et al. 1976). The consequence is amenorrhea, mild androgen excess, and progesterone deficiency. Their menses probably are associated with luteally inadequate cycles. These patients have a high risk of cystic endometrial hyperplasia and of endometrial carcinoma at a younger age than usual. Unfortunately, there are no data regarding breast cancer in this group of women. However, androgen excess exerts a powerful inhibitory effect on the breast as well as other tissues and surely modifies the response to estrogen excess.

The amenorrhea-galactorrhea syndrome is the result of prolonged, substantial prolactin oversecretion due to pituitary adenoma. Profound gonadotropic and ovarian suppression eventuate. In the early stages, follicular-phase levels of estrogens are accompanied by prolactin hypersecretion and lactation (Jacobs and Daughaday 1973; del Pozo et al. 1974; Van Look et al. 1977).

Prior to the menopause, there is a variable period of time during which menstrual cycles are irregular in most women (Treloar et al. 1967). These cycles are long or short in duration. The short cycles are ovulatory and have normal luteal phases and short follicular phases (Sherman and Korenman 1975). The long cycles, which become more prevalent as menopause approaches, have been shown to be more or less euestrogenic but luteally inadequate or anovulatory (Sherman et al. 1976). At this time a period of unopposed estrogenic stimulation of up to 8 years may occur. When cycle intervals were compared to age of menopause, it was found that late menopause was associated with a longer period of long and presumably luteally inadequate cycles (Wallace et al. 1978). Late menopause, of course, has been correlated with risk of breast cancer.

We will not consider other conditions of unopposed estrogens except to indicate that estrogen administration invariably increases prolactin secretion.

DISCUSSION

It is remarkable just how ignorant we are of the biological consequences of the hormonal stimuli regulating mammary function. When tissue complexity, genetic heterogeneity, and metabolic regulation of tissue responsiveness are considered, the problems seem awesome indeed. The role of hormones in cell transformation and maintenance of the transformed state is mysterious. We lack a feasible tool for moment-by-moment assessment of the endocrine status of the breast similar to vaginal cytology. It was possible, therefore, to deal only theoretically with how the complex endocrine interrelations characterizing normal and abnormal reproductive cycles might affect the breast.

Studies of human reproductive endocrinology are useful in helping epidemiologists who wish to investigate the endocrine factors in breast cancer risk to be aware of the numerous pitfalls that lie in their way.

1. Normal cycle length or even menstrual discomfort is not proof of cycle normalcy.
2. Nutrition, adiposity, drugs, hormones, physical activity, and emotional state play important and changing roles in reproductive cycles.
3. It is inappropriate to compare reproductive hormones in populations of different ages because cycle length and, therefore, follicular phase length declines with age.
5. There is great cycle variability at both extremes of reproductive life, and this may be very important in risk assessment. It is inappropriate to bar subjects with irregular or abnormal cycles from investigations since they may be the carriers of excess risk.
6. Prior cycle does not predict current cycle.
7. Recalled reproductive cycle and hormonal history are suspect.

The estrogen window hypothesis is readily testable given the appropriate population and sufficient funding. The focus should be on duration of luteal inadequacy in euestrogenic women, preferably those without androgen excess or exposure to known carcinogens prospectively in a high-risk group, if possible. A positive result could strengthen the argument for progestogen administration in the perimenopausal period and lead to more aggressive diagnostic assessment of oligomenorrhea in young women.

REFERENCES

Askel, S. 1980. Sporadic and recurrent luteal phase defects in cyclic women: Comparison with normal cycles. *Fertil. Steril.* 33:372.

Baird, D.T. 1976. Pituitary-ovarian relationships in disorders of menstruation. In *The endocrine function of the human ovary* (ed. V.H.T. James and G. Giusti), p. 349. Academic Press, London.

Bhakoo, H.S. and B.S. Katzenellenbogen. 1977. Progesterone inhibition of estrogen-stimulated uterine biosynthetic events and estrogen receptor levels. *Mol. Cell Endocr.* 8:121.

Bohnet, H.G. and H.P.G. Schneider. 1977. Prolactin as a cause of anovulation. In *Prolactin and human reproduction* (ed. P.G. Crosignani and C. Robyn), p. 153. Academic Press, New York.

Boice, J.D. Jr. and R.R. Monson. 1977. Breast cancer in women after repeated fluoroscopic examinations of the chest. *J. Natl. Cancer Inst.* 39:823.

Brenner, R.M., J.A. Resko, and N.B. West. 1974. Cyclic changes in oviductal morphology and residual cytoplasmic estradiol binding capacity induced by sequential estrogen-progesterone treatment of spayed rhesus monkeys. *Endocrinology* 95:1094.

Brisson, G.R., M.A. Yolle, D. De Carufel, M. Desharnais, and M. Tanaka. 1980. Exercise-induced dissociation of the blood prolactin response in young women according to their sports habits. *Horm. Metab. Res.* 12:177.

Corbey, R.S., R.M. Lequin, and R. Pollard. 1977. Hyperprolactinemia and secondary amenorrhea. In *Prolactin and human reproduction* (ed. P.G. Crosignani and C. Robyn), p. 203. Academic Press, New York.

Dale, E., D.H. Gerlach, and A.L. White. 1979. Menstrual dysfunction in distance runners. *Obstet. Gynecol.* 51:47.

Davis, J.W., J. Wikman-Coffelt, and C.L. Eddington. 1972. The effect of progesterone on biosynthetic pathways in mammary tissue. *Endocrinology* 91:1011.

Day, S.L., H.J. Kirchick, and L. Birnbaumer. 1980. Effect of prolactin on luteal function in the cyclic rat: Positive correlation between luteinizing hormone-stimulated adenylyl cyclase activity and progesterone secretion; role in corpus luteum rescue of the morning surge of prolactin on day 3 of pseudopregnancy. *Endocrinology* 106:1265.

del Pozo, E., H. Wyss, G. Tolis, H. Friesen, R. Wenner, L. Vetter, and A. Vettwiter. 1974. Clinical and hormonal response to bromocryptin (CB-154) in the galactorrhea syndromes. *J. Clin. Endocrinol. Metab.* 39:18.

del Pozo, E., H. Wyss, G. Tolis, J. Alcaniz, A. Campara, and F. Naftolin. 1979. Prolactin and deficient luteal function. *Obstet. Gynecol.* 53:282.

Franks, S., M.A.F. Murray, A.M. Jequier, S.J. Steele, J.D.N. Nabarro, and H.S. Jacobs. 1975. Incidence and significance of hyperprolactinaemia in women with amenorrhea. *Clin. Endocrinol.* 4:597.

Fraser, I.S., E.A. Michie, L. Wide, and D.T.Baird. 1973. Pituitary gonadotropins and ovarian function in adolescent dysfunctional uterine bleeding. *J. Clin. Endocrinol. Metab.* 37:407.

Frisch, R.E. and J.W. McArthur. 1974. Menstrual cycles: Fatness as a determinant of minimum weight for height necessary for their maintenance or onset. *Science* 185:949.

Gaulden, E.C., D.C. Littlefield, O.E. Putoff, and L.L. Seivert. 1964. Menstrual abnormalities associated with heroin addiction. *Am. J. Obstet. Gynecol.* 90:155.

Glass, A.R., R.S. Swerdloff, G.A. Bray, W.T. Dahms, and R.L. Atkinson. 1977. Low serum testosterone and sex hormone binding globulin in massively obese men. *J. Clin. Endocrinol. Metab.* 45:1211.

Gray, G.E., M.C. Pike, and B.E. Henderson. 1979. Breast cancer incidence and mortality rates in different countries in relation to known risk factors and dietary practices. *Br. J. Cancer* 39:1.

Haug, E. 1979. Progesterone suppression of estrogen-stimulated prolactin secretion and estrogen receptor levels in rat pituitary cells. *Endocrinology* 104:429.

Horwitz, K.D. and W.L. McGuire. 1978. Estrogen control of progesterone receptor in human breast cancer. *J. Biol. Chem.* 253:2223.

Hsieh, H.A.W., E.J. Peck, and J.H. Clark. 1975. Progesterone antagonism of the estrogen receptor and the estrogen induced uterine growth. *Nature* 254: 337.

Jacobs, L.S. and W.H. Daughaday. 1973. Pathophysiology and control of prolactin secretion in patients with pituitary and hypothalamic disease. In *Human prolactin* (ed. J.L. Pasteels and C. Robyn), p. 189. Elsevier, New York.

Kelly, P.A., J. Djiane, and A. DeLean. 1980. Interaction of prolactin with its receptor: Dissociation and down-regulation. In *Central and peripheral regulation of prolactin function* (ed. R.M. MacLeod and U. Scapagnini), p. 173. Raven Press, New York.

Kledzik, G.S., C.V. Bradley, S. Marshall, G.A. Campbell, and J. Meites. 1976. Effects of high doses of estrogen on prolactin-binding activity and growth of carcinogen-induced mammary cancers in rats. *Cancer Res.* 36:3265.

Korenman, S.G. 1980. The endocrinology of breast cancer. *Cancer* 46:874.

Korenman, S.G. and B.M. Sherman. 1976. Hormonal regulation of the menstrual cycle: Abnormal cycles. In *Endocrinology of the ovary* (ed. R. Sholler), p. 347. SEPE Press, Paris.

Korenman, S.G., B.M. Sherman, and J.C. Korenman. 1978. Reproductive hormone function: The perimenopausal period and beyond. *Clin. Endocrinol. Metab.* 7:625.

Labrie, F., L. Ferland, T. DiPaulo, and R. Veilleux. 1980. Modulation of prolactin secretion by sex steroids and thyroid hormones. In *Central and peripheral regulation of prolactin function* (ed. R.M. MacLeod and U. Scapagnini), p. 97. Raven Press, New York.

MacMahon, B., P. Cole, and J. Brown. 1973. Etiology of human breast cancer: A review. *J. Natl. Cancer Inst.* 50:21.

McNatty, K.P., R. Sawers, and A.S. McNeilly. 1974. A possible role for prolactin in the central of steroid secretion by the human Graafian follicle. *Nature* 250:653.

Mester, I., D. Matel, A. Psyphoyof, and E.E. Baulieu. 1974. Hormonal control of oestrogen receptor in uterus and receptivity for ovo implantation in the rat. *Nature* 250:776.

O'Dea, J.P., R.G. Wieland, M.C. Hallberg, L.A. Llerena, E.M. Zorn, and S.M. Genuth. 1979. Effect of dietary weight loss on sex steroid binding, sex steroids and gonodotropins in obese postmenopausal women. *J. Lab. Clin. Med.* 93:1004.

Pollow, K., E. Boquoi, J. Baumann, M. Schmidt-Gollwitzer, and B. Pollow. 1977. Comparison of the in vitro conversion of estradiol-17β to estrone of normal and neoplastic human breast tissue. *Mol. Cell. Endocr.* 6:333.

Pollow, K., H. Lubbert, E. Boquoi, G. Kreuzer, R. Jeske, and B. Pollow. 1975. Studies on 17β-hydroxysteroid dehydrogenase in human endometrium and endometrial carcinoma. *Acta Endocrinol.* 79:134.

Robyn, C., P. Delvoye, C. Van Exter, M. Vekemans, A. Caufriez, P. De Noyer, J. Delogne-Desnoeck, and M.L. Hermite. 1977. Physiological and pharmacological factors influencing prolactin secretion and their relation to human reproduction. In *Prolactin and human reproduction* (ed. P.G. Crosignani and C. Robyn), p. 71, 96. Academic Press, New York.

Shangold, M., R. Freeman, B. Thysen, and M. Gatz. 1979. The relationship between long distance running, plasma progesterone and luteal phase length. *Fertil. Steril.* 31:130.

Sherman, B.M. and S.G. Korenman. 1974a. Measurement of plasma LH, FSH, estradiol and progesterone in disorders of the human menstrual cycle: The short luteal phase. *J. Clin. Endocrinol. Metab.* 38:89.

_____. 1974b. Measurement of serum LH, FSH, estradiol and progesterone in disorders of the human menstrual cycle: The inadequate luteal phase. *J. Clin. Endocrinol.* 39:145.

_____. 1974c. Inadequate corpus luteum function: A pathophysiological interpretation of human breast cancer epidemiology. *Cancer* 33:1306.

_____. 1975. Hormonal characteristics of the human menstrual cycle throughout reproductive life. *J. Clin. Invest.* 55:699.

Sherman, B.M., S.H. West, and S.G. Korenman. 1976. The menopausal transition: Analysis of LH, FSH, estradiol and progesterone concentrations during menstrual cycles of older women. *J. Clin. Endocrinol.* 42:629.

Sherman, B., R. Wallace, J. Bean, L. Schlabaugh, and A. Treloar. 1981. Relationship of body weight to menarchal and menopausal age: Implications for breast cancer risk. *J. Clin. Endocrinol. Metab.* (in press).

Sitruk-Ware, L.R., N. Sterkers, I. Mowszowicz, and P. Mauvais-Jarvis. 1977. Inadequate corpus luteum function in women with benign breast diseases. *J. Clin. Endocrinol. Metab.* 44:771.

Styne, D.M. and M.M. Grumbach. 1978. Puberty in the male and female. Physiology and disorders. In *Reproductive endocrinology* (ed. S.S.C. Yen and R.B. Jaffe), p. 189. Saunders Publishers, Philadelphia.

Tokunaga, M., J.E. Norman Jr., M. Asano, S. Tokuoka, H. Ezaki, I. Nishimori, and Y. Tauji. 1979. Malignant breast tumors among atomic bomb survivors, Hiroshima and Nagasaki 1950-74. *J. Natl. Cancer Inst.* 62:1347.

Treloar, A., R.D. Boynton, B.G. Benn, and B.W. Brown. 1967. Variation of the human menstrual cycle through reproductive life. *Int. J. Fertil.* 12:77.

Tseng, L. and E. Gurpide. 1975. Induction of human endometrial estradiol dehydrogenate by progestins. *Endocrinology* 97:825.

Van Look, P.F.A., A.S. McNeilly, W.M. Hunter, and D.T. Baird. 1977. The role of prolactin in secondary amenorrhea. In *Prolactin and human reproduction* (ed. P.G. Crosignani and C. Robyn), p. 217. Academic Press, New York.

Veldhuis, J.D., P. Klase and J.M. Hammond. 1980. Divergent effects of prolactin upon steroidogenesis by porcine granulosa cells in vitro: Influence of cytodifferentiation. *Endocrinology* 107:42.

Wallace, R.B., B.M. Shrman, J.A. Bean, J.P. Leeper, and A.E. Treloar. 1978. Menstrual cycle patterns and breast cancer risk factor. *Cancer Res.* 38:4021.

West, B. and P.S. Dannies. 1980. Effect of estradiol on prolactin production and dihydroergocryptine-induced inhibition of prolactin production in primary cultures of rat pituitary cells. *Endocrinology* 106:11108.

Warner, M.R., L. Yau, and J.M. Rosen. 1980. Long term effects of perinatal injection of estrogen and progesterone on the morphological and biochemical development of the mammary gland. *Endocrinology* 106:823.

Warren, M.P. 1980. The effects of exercise on pubertal progression and reproductive function in girls. *J. Clin. Endocr.* **51**:1150.

Welsch, C. and J. Meites. 1978. Prolactin and mammary carcinogenesis. In *Endocrine control in neoplasia* (ed. R.K. Sharma and W.E. Criss), p. 71. Raven Press, New York

Yen, S.S.C. 1978. Chronic anovulation due to CNS hypothalamic-pituitary dysfunction. In *Reproductive endocrinology* (ed. S.S.C. Yen and R.B. Jaffe), p. 341. W.B. Saunders Company, Philadelphia.

Yen, S.S.C., C. Chaney, and H.L. Judd. 1976. Functional aberrations of the hypothalamic-pituitary system in polycystic ovary sundrome: A consideration of the pathogenesis. In *The endocrine function of the human ovary* (ed. V.H.T. James et al.), p. 373. Academic Press, London.

COMMENTS

LIPPMAN: Stan [Korenman], could you try to relate this notion of unopposed estrogen action in a way that fits population data, that is, as opposed simply to fitting the notions of enocrine causation of unopposed estrogens?

KORENMAN: There is evidence, some of which you heard today, that obesity is associated with a later menopause and a long period of irregular cycles. I have not heard or seen any data on the hormonal changes in thin people around menopause. Do they have a long period of anovulation? Hirayama didn't think that Japanese women have this long period; he thought they had a sudden cessation of menses (T. Hirayama, pers. comm.).

Concerning the duration of the perimenarchial period, the most solid information (Sherman et al. 1981) indicated an earlier menarche, per se, in heavier women. The problem is that these researchers never dealt with the premenstrual period; which may have lasted longer in the heavy girls. I think that this hypothesis is consistent with the population data.

ZUMOFF: I'm puzzled about something that you said. I read the most recent summary by Tokunaga's group about radiation susceptibility. I reread it again last night. My reading is that the premenopausal women did not have increased susceptibility to breast cancer from radiation. In fact, if anything, it was slightly decreased.

KORENMAN: There are two age periods to consider here and the age of menopause was not defined.

ZUMOFF: I just read it last night.

KORENMAN: The data are:

Age	Risk ratio
< 10	0.95
10-15	5.00
15-19	2.30
20-29	1.85
30-39	1.23
40-49	0.83
50+	1.39

This number for the 50+ group was not statistically significant, but it's not low. It's never going to be statistically significant. The 40-49 year olds would be premenopausal women and their relative risk was not statistically significantly less than one.

PIKE: The interpretation of the relative risk of the 0.83 in this 40-49 year age group is confounded by the fact that most exposed women in this age group never menstruated again after the date of the atomic bomb, i.e., they had an induced menopause presumably associated with the known reduced risk of breast cancer (Sawada 1959).

It should also be pointed out that the figures in Dr. Korenman's table are relative risks. Absolute risks from the radiation show very little age effect (except of course the 40-49 year age group). This lack of an age effect on absolute risk is *not* what is reported in the summary of the latest published paper from the Radiation Effects Research Foundation (see Fig. 2 in Tokunaga et al. 1979); this is because in this figure person years at risk under age 30 are excluded. The data prior to this later "correction" are very different and a plot of them is given in Figure 1 of the same paper, and dealt with at greater length in an earlier radiation effects Research Foundation Technical Report (Tokunaga et al. 1978). When calculated prior to the "correction," the relative risks still show some age effects in the face of constant absolute risks, because the base line (nonexposed) rates are age dependent, being lower in the age groups who were younger at the time of the bomb.

SEGALOFF: But isn't it true, that these people have spent their years being exposed to the different diet and everything else that the rest of the Japanese are exposed to, and that they have ended up with the kids that looked down on these parents that you referred to?

KORENMAN: Wait a second. These were people who lived in the same town at the same time. Most of them moved into the town after the bombing.

SEGALOFF: But they don't get their cancers until later.

KORENMAN: These ages are the ages of exposure at the time of the bomb, not the age of cancer.

ZUMOFF: And the effect on them of the subsequent change in diet and everything should be different for the ones at every age group with which they start.

KORENMAN: That's correct. But they're comparing them with the cohorts of the same age, so that should be blanked out if you want to see the radiation effect. That's what was shown putatively—the selective carcinogenic effect of the radiation.

References

Tokunaga, M., J.E. Norman, M. Asano, S. Tokuoka, H. Ezaki, I. Nishimori, and Y. Tsugi. 1978. *Malignant breast tumors among atomic bomb survivors, Hiroshima, Nagasaki; 1950-1974.* Technical Report RERF TR 17-77. Radiation Effects Research Foundation, Hiroshima.

_____. 1979. Malignant breast tumors among atomic bomb survivors, Hiroshima, Nagasaki; 1950-1974. *J. Natl. Cancer Inst.* 62:1347.

Sawada, H. 1959. *Sexual function in female atomic bomb survivors, 1947-1957.* Hiroshima Technical Report 34-59. Atomic Bomb Casualty Commission, Hiroshima.

Sherman, B., R. Wallace, J. Bean, L. Schlabaugh, and A. Treloar. 1981. Relationship of body weight to menarchal and menopausal age: Implications for breast cancer risk. *J. Clin. Endocrinol. Metab.* (in press).

Increased Availability of Serum Estrogens in Breast Cancer: A New Hypothesis

PENTTI K. SIITERI, GEOFFREY L. HAMMOND*, AND
JEFFREY A. NISKER†
Reproductive Endocrinology Center
Department of Obstetrics, Gynecology and Reproductive Sciences
University of California
San Francisco, California 94143

Progress toward understanding the role of endogenous estrogens in human breast cancer has been painfully slow. Whereas overwhelming evidence implicates estrogens as having a profound influence on breast tumor development in experimental animals, human studies have not yet identified abnormalities in serum or urinary estrogens that distinguish the women who have or will develop breast cancer. This failure simply may reflect our ignorance of some yet to be discovered facet of estrogen physiology or, as is more likely, may be due to our inability to discern subtle differences that may be important when amplified by temporal or other factors (see Pike et al., this volume). Comparatively speaking, the human breast appears to be extremely sensitive to estrogens. Pubertal breast growth and development occurs in the human, but not in other primates, and is stimulated by very low levels of estrogens (see Vihko and Apter, this volume). Short and Drife (1977) have suggested that this difference in sensitivity of the breast to estrogens may account, in part, for the virtual absence of breast cancer in the lower primates. Other obvious differences in diet and exposure to carcinogens may be equally important. Of particular interest in the present context is the apparently unique ability of the human to produce biologically significant amounts of extraovarian estrogen.

As pointed out by Korenman (this volume), exposure of the breast to unopposed estrogen during the premenarchial or perimenopausal years appears to increase risk for breast cancer. During these periods, as well as in adult anovulatory women, estrogen is produced primarily by conversion of adrenal androstenedione to estrone (E_1) in peripheral tissues with the ovaries contributing only small amounts (Siiteri and MacDonald 1973). Therefore, serum levels of estrogens differ both qualitatively and quantitatively from those found in

---

*Current address: Steroid Research Laboratory, Department of Medical Chemistry, Siltavuorenpenger 10 A, SF-00170 Helsinki 17 Finland.

†Current address: University of Western Ontario, Victoria Hospital-South Street Colborne 3, London, Ontario N6B 1B9 Canada.

normal cycling females. The levels of E_1 and estradiol (E_2) generally are lower but they do not rise and fall cyclically. Furthermore, there is a reversal in the E_1/E_2 ratio. Whether the latter is important, aside from the chronic nature of the estrogen stimulus, remains unclear (Siiteri et al. 1974). The term "unopposed estrogen," as used by gynecologists, implies the presence of estrogen but no progesterone due to the absence of ovulation and corpus luteum formation. Although extensive studies have demonstrated that progesterone is antiestrogenic in the uterus by virtue of its ability to suppress estrogen receptor (ER) levels (Clark and Peck 1979), similar evidence for the breast is meager. Nevertheless, it seems probable that the ratio of progesterone to estrogen is important in regulation of breast growth, as is the ratio of estrogen to androgen in the development of gynecomastia in males (Siiteri and MacDonald 1973; Aiman et al. 1980).

The manner in which estrogens promote breast cancer is unknown. Endogenous estrogens may act by any one of at least three mechanisms. They may be either carcinogens or promotors in the classical sense or they may stimulate the growth of previously transformed cells. There is little evidence to suggest that endogenous estrogens are carcinogens and it is generally assumed that they are promotors. Although a distinction between a promotor mechanism and hormonal stimulation of tumor growth is difficult to make, both possibilities should be kept in mind when considering the relationship of endocrine events to epidemiologic data. For example, the notion of a long latent period (15-20 yr) of human breast cancer arose, at least in part, from epidemiologic observations indicating that ovarian estrogen-related factors that influence risk for breast cancer early in life (age at menarche and first pregnancy) may not be expressed until many years later when estrogen was thought to be unimportant. Because we now know that anovulatory and postmenopausal women have the capacity to produce extraovarian estrogen, an estrogen-associated carcinogenic event may occur at any time in certain individuals. Although many factors influence the extent of extraglandular estrogen production, the increased efficiency observed in obese subjects (Edman and MacDonald 1974; MacDonald et al. 1978) has been of particular interest because obesity also has been associated with increased risk for endometrial and breast cancer. However, studies of extraglandular estrogen production have not demonstrated quantitative differences in breast (Poortman et al. 1973; Kirschner et al. 1978) or endometrial (Judd et al. 1976; MacDonald et al. 1978) cancer patients when compared to controls who were carefully matched for weight. These results do not negate the importance of excess weight and elevated peripheral estrogen production in promoting cancer of estrogen target tissues, because obese women quite obviously vary in their exposure to carcinogens. We recently have studied another mechanism whereby obesity appears to increase the impact of estrogens on target tissues.

SERUM BINDING OF E_2

Human serum contains a protein known as sex-hormone-binding globulin (SHBG), sex-steroid-binding protein (SBP), or testosterone-estradiol-binding globulin (TEBG) that binds gonadal steroids (Mercier-Bodard et al. 1976; Rosner 1976; Petra 1979). SHBG is unique in that it binds both androgens and estrogens with high affinity as compared with albumin. Studies with the purified protein have shown that it has the highest affinity for dihydrotestosterone (DHT) ($K_D \cong 10^{-9}$ M) whereas testosterone ($K_D \cong 3 \times 10^{-9}$ M) and E_2 ($K_D \cong 1 \times 10^{-8}$ M) are bound less avidly. Other potent circulating androgens such as 3β, 17β-5α-androstandiol also are bound with about the same affinity as testosterone. Many physiologic studies have led to the concept that only the free or unbound fraction of steroid hormones in serum is available to target cells (Anderson 1974). For example, estimates of "apparent free" testosterone levels correlate better with the clinical degree of androgen excess than do the total serum levels (Anderson 1974). Similar conclusions have been reached for cortisol and thyroid hormones that bind with high affinity to cortisol-binding globulin (CBG) and thyroxine-binding globulin (TBG) in serum.

Because of the relatively weak binding of E_2 to SHBG, the potential influence of fluctuations in serum SHBG levels on the availability of serum E_2 has received little attention as compared with testosterone. Anderson (1974) suggested that the binding interaction was important because he found that the percentage of free E_2 is increased at low levels of SHBG. More recently, other workers have suggested that the binding of E_2 to SHBG is not of any consequence under physiologic conditions (Vigersky et al. 1979). The failure of the latter authors to detect the interaction of E_2 with SHBG at $37°C$ by a variety of techniques may be explained by the fact that the serum had been diluted $1:5$, whereas Anderson's studies were carried out with undiluted serum. The difficulty in observing E_2 binding to SHBG in diluted serum as compared with testosterone binding is due not only to the lower affinity of E_2 for SHBG but also to its higher affinity for serum albumin.

We have developed a new, simple method for the measurement of the percentage of free E_2 as well as other steroids in serum under conditions that closely reflect the in vivo situation (Hammond et al. 1980). This technique, centrifugal ultrafiltration-dialysis, is carried out with undiluted serum under equilibrium conditions at $37°C$. We have confirmed Anderson's observations that the percentage of free E_2 is increased when SHBG levels are depressed. As shown in Figure 1, both the percentage of free testosterone and E_2 are inversely related to the binding capacity of SHBG when sera from men, women, and pregnant women are compared. As shown in Figure 2, sera obtained from postmenopausal women with or without endometrial cancer exhibit a highly significant inverse correlation between SHBG capacity and percent free E_2 (Nisker et al. 1980b). Reduced serum SHBG-binding capacity is inversely

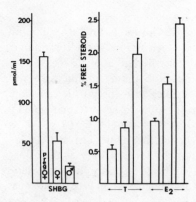

Figure 1

SHBG binding capacity (pmole/ml) and percent free testosterone (T) and E_2 in serum from pregnant women (preg ♀), women (♀), and men (♂). Values shown are the mean ± S.D. of 8 subjects in each group.

correlated with excess body weight (Fig. 3) in premenopausal and postmenopausal women. Indeed, virtually all women who weigh more than 50 pounds above their ideal body weight have an SHBG binding capacity that is only 20–30% of that found in normal weight women. Although no significant differences in either SHBG binding capacity or percentage of free E_2 were found in women with endometrial carcinoma when compared with appropriate weight-matched controls (Nisker et al. 1980b; Davidson et al. 1981), it is evident that

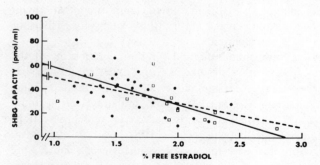

Figure 2

The relationship between the percentage of free E_2 and SHBG capacity in the serum of 13 postmenopausal patients with endometrial carcinoma (□, broken regression line) and 29 postmenopausal reference subjects (●, solid regression line). A significant correlation was observed both for the postmenopausal patients with endometrial carcinoma ($r = -0.63$, $p < 0.001$) and the reference population ($r = -0.60$, $p < 0.001$). There was no significant difference between the regression lines generated by these two groups. (Reprinted, with permission, from Nisker et al. 1980b.)

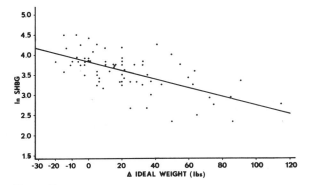

Figure 3
Relationship between the natural logarithm of serum SHBG binding capacity and deviation from ideal body weight in normal women ($r = -0.642$; $p < 0.001$). Ideal body weight was estimated from the relationship Δ ideal weight = 105 lbs + 5 (height$_{ins}$ – 60).

obesity plays a dual role in increasing estrogen exposure of target tissues. In addition to increasing estrogen production, the depressed SHBG levels increase the percentage of serum E_2 that is free and presumably available.

Few previous studies have examined SHBG levels or percent free E_2 in breast cancer patients. Bulbrook (Wang and Bulbrook 1969) compared the binding of E_2 and many other steroids in serum from normal and breast cancer patients, but found no differences. Similar results were obtained by Kirschner (Kirschner et al. 1978). However, both studies utilized conventional dialysis of diluted serum, and, therefore, important differences may have been obscured. In a preliminary study of breast cancer patients, we have found a similar relationship between obesity, reduced SHBG, and increased free E_2. In addition, however, some normal-weight breast cancer patients with normal SHBG levels were found to have elevated percentage of free E_2 (Fig. 4). As a result, the mean difference in percentage of free E_2 between patients (2.15) and controls (1.52) was significantly different ($p < 0.001$). These results indicated that the percentage of free E_2 in serum may be elevated by factors other than reduced SHBG concentrations. Amongst these possibilities are an altered SHBG binding site such that the affinity for steroids is reduced, competition for the normal binding site by androgens or other substances which increase the percentage of free E_2, or a reduction in serum albumin concentration. To study these possibilities, we have examined the kinetics of DHT binding in serum from normal women and those with breast cancer. However, no differences in K_D were observed between patients and controls. At present, we cannot explain the elevation of percentage free E_2 in the presence of normal SHBG levels, nor do we know the frequency with which this abnormality occurs.

While the term "free" or nonprotein bound is commonly employed to describe the biologically active fraction of a hormone in serum, this concept is

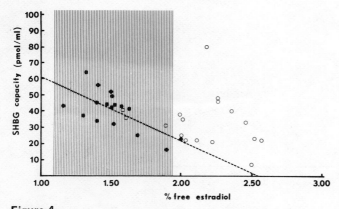

Figure 4

Individual values of SHBG capacity (pmole/ml) and percentage of free E_2 in serum or plasma samples taken from patients with breast cancer (○) and a reference group of normal women (●), matched individually for age, weight, height, deviation from ideal weight, and menstrual status. (−−−−−) Regression line between SHBG capacity and percentage of free E_2 for the normal reference group; (▓) mean ± 2 S.D. of the percentage of free E_2 in blood samples from the reference population only.

not supported by definitive evidence. Early studies of glucocorticoid and andro-gen binding in serum under different conditions (pregnancy, hyperthyroidism, hyperandrogenism) used conventional techniques of dialysis or ultrafiltration. Although the importance of changes in binding protein levels was demon-strated, such methods separate free steroid from that bound to both albumin and SHBG and usually are carried out under nonphysiologic conditions. The question of whether the much larger albumin-bound fraction of serum steroid is available to target tissues has received little attention until recently. This is due in part to the difficulty of estimating the distribution of the hormone between SHBG (or corticosteroid-binding globulin [CBG]), albumin, and the free fraction as it occurs in vivo. Vermeulen (1977) calculated the serum dis-tribution of testosterone from data obtained by equilibrium dialysis, K_Ds, and serum concentrations of SHBG and albumin. In serum from male, female, and pregnant female sources, 60%, 80%, and 94%, respectively, of testosterone was bound to SHBG due to the corresponding increase in SHBG levels. More recently, Dunn et al. (1981) have extended this approach using a computer model to include binding parameters for 21 steroids and measurements of SHBG-bound and albumin-bound fractions made under nearly physiologic conditions. Their estimates of the percentage of free E_2 and testosterone agree remarkably well with our direct measurements in male and female serum (Fig. 1).

In unpublished studies (G.L. Hammond and P.K. Siiteri), we have been able to calculate the distribution of E_2 and other steroids between the free, albumin-bound, and SHBG-bound fractions from measurements of the percent-age free steroid performed on native serum before and after heat treatment

(60°C X 45 min) to destroy SHBG binding. These results indicate that the percentage of serum E_2 that is bound to albumin is 25-35 times greater than the percentage of free E_2 over the physiologic range of SHBG concentrations. In view of the virtually instantaneous dissociation of steroids that are bound to albumin (Westphal 1971), we have defined the sum of the percentage of free and albumin bound as the percent available steroid. As shown in Fig. 5, alterations of SHBG concentrations have a profound effect on the percent available E_2. The percent available ranges from about 20% in pregnancy or hyperthyroidism to 80-90% in hypothyroid or obese subjects. The normal range is approximately 40-60%. Also shown are results from two unusual breast cancer patients in whom 100% of serum E_2 was available despite relatively normal SHBG levels.

DISCUSSION

By using a new method for measuring the percentage of free steroids in serum that closely approximates physiologic conditions, we have shown unequivocally that E_2 binding to SHBG is of potential physiologic importance. Serum SHBG appears to play a central role in regulating not only androgen but also estrogen

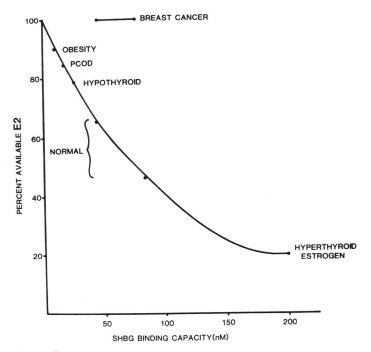

Figure 5
Relationship of the sum of percent free and percent albumin bound (percent available) serum E_2 and SHBG levels in various conditions.

availability to target cells. That this is not a trivial effect is illustrated by the data in Figure 5, where the percent available E_2 varies nearly twofold over the range of SHBG concentrations encountered in normal and obese women. Therefore, it is possible that available E_2 is elevated in breast cancer patients or subjects at risk, even though total serum E_2 levels are normal. This possibility is suggested by our preliminary results (Fig. 3) and also by epidemiological and endocrinological findings, which may be rationalized on the basis of their effects on serum SHBG and increased E_2 availability.

Obesity increases target tissue exposure to estrogen in at least three ways. First, increased adrenal secretory activity makes more androstenedione available for conversion to E_1 in periperhal tissues. Second, the efficiency of androstenedione-to-E_1 conversion is elevated in obese subjects. Third, and probably most important, serum SHBG is markedly depressed in virtually all subjects who weigh more than 50 pounds above their ideal body weight. Therefore, up to 100% greater than normal amounts of serum E_2 are available potentially to target tissues in obese women. This may be particularly important in premenarchial, adult but anovulatory and postmenopausal women because the chronically elevated estrogen is unopposed by progesterone. Increased E_2 availability may also be of importance in ovulatory obese women if a critical ratio of E_2 and progesterone is exceeded.

Reduced SHBG levels in obese subjects first was described by DeMoor (DeMoor and Joossens 1970) more than 10 years ago, but the mechanism underlying this abnormality is unknown. The reduction in serum SHBG binding capacity seems paradoxical because it is known that estrogens stimulate SHBG synthesis, presumably in the liver (Anderson 1974). However, large amounts of estrogen as found in pregnancy or given pharmacologically are required to elicit this effect, whereas no changes are found during the normal menstrual cycle (Wu et al. 1976). Reduced serum SHBG binding capacity and elevated "free" androgens are commonly observed in hyperandrogenic conditions (Anderson 1974) such as polycystic ovarian (PCO) disease. Excessive adrenal androgens may also depress SHBG levels in obese women. Obesity is known to be associated with increased adrenal secretion of cortisol (Migeon et al. 1973), but few studies of adrenal androgen secretion have been made in obese subjects. However, it has been demonstrated that puberty occurs earlier in obese girls and that they have elevated serum levels of adrenal androgens (Genazzani et al. 1978).

We recently have demonstrated that the percentage of free E_2 and the percent available E_2 (Fig. 5) is also elevated in PCO disease (Nisker et al. 1980a). The mean levels of free E_2 (1.5 pg/ml) and available E_2 (60 pg/ml) in 12 PCO disease patients were three- and fourfold higher, respectively, than those found in normal women during the early follicular phase of the menstrual cycle. The initiating event(s) in the etiology of PCO disease has been variously ascribed to abnormalities in hypothalamic, pituitary, ovarian, or adrenal function (Yen 1978). Chronically elevated extraglandular estrogen production from excessive androstenedione secretion by the ovary has been demonstrated (Siiteri and MacDonald 1973) and likely explains chronically elevated secretion of luteinizing hormone (LH) by the pituitary. We proposed that the initiation of LH hypersecretion in young women may be due to increased estrogen availability because of low SHBG levels caused by ovarian and (or) adrenal hypersecretion of androgens and (or) obesity (Nisker et al. 1980a). Thus, the pituitary, as well as other estrogen target tissues such as the breast, may be exposed to excessive estrogen in conditions where androgens appear to predominate.

In this regard, it is of interest that a high proportion of anovulatory women with symptoms of excessive androgens was found in premenopausal breast cancer patient studies by Grattarola (Grattarola 1973) and similar observations have been made in endometrial cancer (Wynder et al. 1966).

Serum SHBG levels also are influenced by thyroid hormones. They are elevated markedly in hyperthyroidism (Anderson 1974), but relatively little data is available for hypothyroid patients (Tulchinsky and Chopra 1973). However, highly significant positive correlations between serum SHBG binding capacity and both serum thyroxine (T_4) ($r = 0.61$) and triiodothyronine (T_3) ($r = 0.72$) have been found in 103 normal, euthyroid, and hyperthyroid subjects (R. Cowan and W. Campbell, pers. comm.). Interestingly, a similar relationship was not found for either T_4 or T_3 and serum CBG-binding capacity. At present, we can only speculate as to whether the depressed SHBG levels found in obesity result from a defect in thyroid hormone action in the liver, such as reduced T_4 to T_3 conversion or excessive androgen production or both. It is important to note, however, that virtually all data on SHBG in serum have been obtained by measurements of its binding capacity and not the protein itself. It is possible that the depressed levels of SHBG binding found in obesity may be artefactual due to interference with binding assays by steroid or other lipids.

A possible relationship between thyroid disorders and breast cancer has been the subject of speculation and controversy for many years. It began when Beatson (1896) combined oophorectomy and administration of thyroid extract as treatment for young women with breast cancer. Many clinical studies of thyroid therapy for breast cancer have been carried out since then with uniformly negative results. On the other hand, epidemiologic and retrospective studies of patients almost uniformly have suggested that hypothyroidism predisposes women to breast cancer (Repert 1952; Loeser 1954; Liechty et al. 1963). Furthermore, a history of hypothyroidism has been associated with a much more rapid recurrence rate and lower survival of breast cancer patients (Moosa 1973). More recently, plasma thyroid-stimulating hormone (TSH) was found to be significantly higher in patients with early or advanced breast cancer than in women hospitalized for unrelated illnesses (Mittra and Hayward 1974; Aldinger et al. 1978). The biochemical basis of the relationship between hypothyroidism and breast cancer is obscure, although it has been speculated that subnormal thyroid hormone levels somehow enhance the sensitivity of mammary epithelial cells to prolactin (Mittra et al. 1976).

We suggest that the link between hypothyroidism and breast cancer may be due to subnormal serum SHBG levels, which increases estrogenic stimulation of the breast. A considerable body of data supports this suggestion. The relative proportion of the urinary androgen metabolites androsterone (3α-hydroxy-5α-androstan-17-one) and etiocholanolone (3α-hydroxy-5β-androstan-17-one) is markedly influenced by thyroid status. The $5\alpha/5\beta$ ratio is high (>2.0) in hyperthyroid and low (<0.25) in hypothyroid states (Hellman et al. 1959; Beale et al. 1973). The effect of thyroid hormone appears to be exerted on the hepatic 5α-reductase enzyme, because the administration of T_3 to patients with anorexia nervosa normalizes their markedly depressed $5\alpha/5\beta$ ratio (Bradlow et al. 1976). In extensive studies of urinary androgen excretion by breast cancer patients, Bulbrook and his colleagues noted many years ago that the $5\alpha/5\beta$ ratio in Japanese women is significantly higher than in British women (Bulbrook et al. 1967). Recently, this observation has been confirmed with modern analytical methods for both normal premenopausal and postmenopausal women (Thomas et al. 1977). In addition, they found that the $5\alpha/5\beta$ ratio was lower than normal in Japanese breast cancer patients and further, that serum TSH levels were negatively correlated with the $5\alpha/5\beta$ ratio in Japanese patients and controls. These data are consistent with the notion that hypothyroidism predisposes to breast cancer. Furthermore, they suggest that the strikingly different breast cancer incidence rates between Japanese and British, or American, women may arise from differences in SHBG levels and estrogen availability. Unfortunately, we know of no measurements of SHBG in breast cancer patients that bear on this question.

Thyroid hormones also exert a powerful influence on the metabolism of estrogens. Fishman and his colleagues have shown that 16α-hydroxylation of E_2 to yield estriol (E_3) is favored over 2-hydroxylation in hypothyroidism, whereas the reverse is true in hyperthyroidism (Fishman et al. 1965). These workers have also shown that increased 16α-hydroxylation of E_2 occurs in both male (Zumoff et al. 1966) and female (Hellman et al. 1971) patients with breast cancer. Therefore, Fishman has proposed that hypothyroidism may enhance the estrogenic milieu and predispose women to breast cancer and other diseases because of increased formation of E_3 which appears to have greater estrogenic activity than 2-hydroxy-E_1 or E_2 (Fishman and Martucci 1978). However, an equally plausible explanation relates to the greater availability of serum E_2 in hypothroidism, because not only is E_2 much more active than E_3, it is present in much higher concentrations in both premenopausal and postmenopausal women.

Both hypo- and hyperthyroidism are associated with menstrual abnormalities (Burrow 1978). Hyperstimulation of the endometrium resulting in menorrhagia is commonly found in hypothyroid women and is often reduced or eliminated by treatment with thyroid hormones. Conversely, oligomenorrhea or amenorrhea may be associated with hyperthyroidism. In addition, mean LH levels in both follicular and luteal phases are elevated two-threefold suggesting deficient negative feedback by estrogens (Akande and Hockaday 1972). The fourfold difference in the availability of serum E_2 between hyper- and hypothyroid states as shown in Figure 5 may explain these abnormalities. Low serum SHBG in hypothyroid women may cause hyperstimulation of the uterus whereas the impact of serum E_2 is reduced in hyperthyroid women with high SHBG levels. Whether or not a particular individual is affected also depends upon her production rate and total serum level of E_2. A normal serum level may be hyperestrogenic in one individual but hypoestrogenic in another.

Both positive and negative feedback systems operate to regulate ovarian secretion to maintain the total, and presumably the available, serum E_2 at appropriate levels throughout the normal menstrual cycle. It would appear that the very high or low SHBG levels associated with the extremes of thyroid status interfere with these control mechanisms sufficiently to disrupt reproductive function. Lesser deviations from normal SHBG levels can be expected to have more subtle effects on estrogen target tissues and require long periods of time before they are expressed as some abnormality. This is particularly true in postmenopausal and anovulatory women in whom extraovarian estrogen production is not subject to feedback regulation. We have recently compared two carefully matched groups ($n = 25$) of postmenopausal women with and without hip fractions (Davidson et al. 1981 unpubl. results). The mean difference in body weight between groups was only 10.6 pounds, yet they had significantly different serum SHBG, percent free testosterone and percent free E_2 levels. Thus it appears that even subtle differences in body weight may produce major effects on sex steroid target tissues that are mediated by a reduction in serum SHBG.

SUMMARY

Although we still do not know how estrogens promote cancer, i.e. whether they act directly as carcinogens, or promotors and (or) indirectly by stimulating prolactin secretion, there seems little doubt that chronic stimulation of mammary epithelial cells by some critical level of estrogen is an essential feature. This is most evident from the large sex difference (females/males $\cong 100/1$) in breast cancer incidence which appears to decrease if males are exposed to more than normal amounts of estrogen. However, it is not clear whether the role of estrogens is related to qualitative or quantitative differences in production, metabolism, or transport. By and large, previous studies have not convincingly demonstrated elevated production or serum levels of estrogens in breast cancer patients or women at increased risk. The studies of Fishman and his associates (Fishman et al. 1965) suggest that there are differences in estrogen metabolism that may be related to thyroid status and they have hypothesized that this metabolic difference produces a hyperestrogenic state due to increased formation of E_3.

In this paper, we presented an alternative hypothesis that accommodates much of what is known about the endocrinology of breast cancer. We propose that the availability of E_2 in human serum to the breast is increased when SHBG levels are depressed. Thus, a hyperestrogenic stimulus to the breast may exist in women who are obese, hypothyroid, or hyperandrogenic despite serum E_2 levels that are considered normal. In addition, it appears that a similar situation exists in some women with apparently normal SHBG levels because of abnormal binding of E_2. Chronic stimulation of the breast epithelium in these situations over a sufficient period of time may lead to benign breast disease and set the stage for cancer in those women who are exposed to an effective dose of virus, irradiation, or carcinogen.

Although much more data is required to substantiate this hypothesis, it is attractive because, on the one hand, it can explain many of the endocrine abnormalities previously associated with breast cancer in terms of an estrogen effect and, on the other hand, it can account for the failure to find gross differences in serum estrogen levels. Furthermore, it suggests many potentially fruitful lines of investigation. While genetically determined differences in serum levels of CBG have been described (DeMoor and Louwagie 1980), similar studies have apparently not been carried out with SHBG. A low serum SHBG trait or production of a defective form of SHBG might explain the familial aspects of breast cancer. The latter possibility is suggested by our preliminary studies (Fig. 5). Future epidemiological studies will hopefully address factors that influence SHBG levels. In addition to those already discussed, others include, for example, the influence of various contraceptive preparations. Estrogen administration elevates SHBG levels, however only E_2-related compounds bind to SHBG whereas synthetic compounds such as DES do not. Furthermore, some synthetic progestins such as norethynodrel bind avidly and cause displacement of androgens and estrogens (Victor et al. 1976) whereas others, such as medroxyprogesterone acetate do not bind but may suppress SHBG synthesis (Forest and Bertrand 1972). These confounding effects make analyses of population data based simply on "pill" consumption quite meaningless because various components may promote or inhibit the action of endogenous estrogens. It is quite clear that future investigations of breast cancer etiology require the close cooperation of endocrinologists and epidemiologists.

REFERENCES

Aiman, J., P.F. Brenner, and P.C. MacDonald. 1980. Androgen and estrogen production in elderly men with gynecomastia and testicular atrophy after mumps orchitis. *J. Clin. Endocrinol. Metab.* **50**:380.

Akande, E.O. and T.D.R. Hockaday. 1972. Plasma oestrogen and luteinizing hormone concentrations in thyrotoxic menstrual disturbance. *Proc. R. Soc. Med.* **65**:789.

Aldinger, K.A., P.N. Schultz, G.R. Blumenschein, and N.A. Samaan. 1978. Thyroid-stimulating hormone and prolactin levels in breast cancer. *Arch. Intern. Med.* **138**:1638.

Anderson, D.C. 1974. Sex-hormone-binding globulin. *Clin. Endocrinol.* 3:69.

Beale, R.N., D. Croft, and D. Powell. 1973. Some effects of thyroid disease on neutral steroid metabolism. *J. Endocrinol.* 57:317.

Beatson, G.T. 1896. On the treatment of inoperable cases of carcinoma of the mamma—suggestions for a new method of treatment with illustrative cases. *Lancet* 2:104, 162.

Bradlow, H.L., R.M. Boyar, J. O'Connor, B. Zumoff, and L. Hellman. 1976. Hypothyroid-like alterations in testosterone metabolism in anorexia nervosa. *J. Clin. Endocrinol. Metab.* 43:571.

Bulbrook, R.D., B.S. Thomas, J. Utsunomiya, and E. Hammagushi. 1967. The urinary excretion of 11-deoxy-17-oxosteroids and 17-hydroxycorticosteroids by normal Japanese and British women. *J. Endocrinol.* 38:401.

Burrow, G.N. 1978. The thyroid gland and reproduction in *Reproductive endocrinology* (ed. S.C.C. Yen and R.B. Jaffe), p. 373. W.B. Saunders Company, Philadelphia.

Clark, J.H. and E.J. Peck, Jr. 1979. *Female sex steroids, receptors and function.* Springer-Verlag, New York.

Davidson, B.J., J.C. Gambone, L.D. Lagasse, T.W. Castaldo, G.L. Hammond, P.K. Siiteri, and H.L. Judd. 1981. Free estradiol in postmenopausal women with and without endometrial cancer. *J. Clin. Endocrinol. Metab.* (in press).

DeMoor, P. and J.V. Joossens. 1970. An inverse relation between body weight and the activity of the steroid binding β-globulin in human plasma. *Steroidologia* 1:129.

DeMoor, P. and A. Louwagie. 1980. Association of aberrant transcortin levels with HLA antigens of the B and C loci: High transcortin levels are frequently found in patients with lymphatic leukemia, hairy cell leukemia, or non-Hodgkin lymphoma. *J. Clin. Endocrinol. Metab.* 51:868.

Dunn, J.F., B.C. Nisula, and D. Rodbard. 1981. Transport of steroid hormones: Binding of 21 endogenous steroids to both testosterone binding globulin and corticosteroid binding globulin in human plasma. *J. Clin. Endocrinol. Metab.* (in press).

Edman, C.D. and P.C. MacDonald. 1974. Slow entry into blood of estrone produced in extraglandular sites in obesity and endometrial neoplasma. *Gynecol. Invest.* 5:27 (abst.).

—————. 1978. Effect of obesity on conversion of plasma androstenedione to estrone in ovulatory and anovulatory young women. *Am. J. Obstet. Gynecol.* 130:456.

Fishman, J. and C. Martucci. 1978. Differential biological activity of estradiol metabolites. *Pediatrics* 62 (suppl.):1128.

Fishman, J., L. Hellman, B. Zumoff, and T.F. Gallagher. 1965. Effect of thyroid on hydroxylation of estrogen in man. *J. Clin. Endocrinol. Metab.* 25:365.

Forest, M.G. and J. Bertrand. 1972. Studies of the protein binding of dihydrotestorone (17β-hydroxy-5α-androstan-3-one) in human plasma (in different physiological conditions and effect of medroxyprogesterone). *Steroids* 19:197.

Genazzani, A.R., C. Pintor, and R. Corda. 1978. Plasma levels of gonadotropins, prolactin, thyroxine and gonadal steroids in obese prepubertal girls. *J. Clin. Endocrinol. Metab.* 47:974.

Grattarola, R. 1973. Androgens in breast cancer. I. Atypical endometrial hyperplasia and breast cancer in married premenopausal women. *Am. J. Obstet. Gynecol.* 116:423.

Hammond, G.L., J.A. Nisker, L.A. Jones, and P.K. Siiteri. 1980. Estimation of the percent free steroid in undiluted serum by centrifugal ultrafiltration-dialysis. *J. Biol. Chem.* 255:5023.

Hellman, L., B. Zumoff, J. Fishman, and T.F. Gallagher. 1971. Peripheral metabolism of ^{3}H-estradiol and the excretion of endogenous estrone and estriol glucosiduronate in women with breast cancer. *J. Clin. Endocrinol. Metab.* 33:138.

Hellman, L., H.L. Bradlow, B. Zumoff, D.K. Fukushima, and T.E. Gallagher. 1959. Thyroid-androgen interrelations and the hypocholesteremic effect of androsterone. *J. Clin. Endocrinol.* 19:936.

Judd, H.L., W.E. Lucas, and S.S.C. Yen. 1976. Serum 17β-estradiol and estrone levels in postmenopausal women with and without endometrial cancer. *J. Clin. Endocrinol. Metab.* 43:272.

Kirschner, M.A., F.B. Cohen, and C. Ryan. 1978. Androgen-estrogen production rates in postmenopausal women with breast cancer. *Cancer Res.* 38:4029.

Liechty, R.D., R.E. Hodges, and J. Burket. 1963. Cancer and thyroid function. *J. Am. Med. Assoc.* 183:30.

Loeser, A.A. 1954. A new therapy for the prevention of post-operative recurrence in genital and breast cancer. *Br. Med. J.* 2:1380.

MacDonald, P.C., C.D. Edman, D.L. Hemsell, J.C. Porter, and P.K. Siiteri. 1978. Effect of obesity on conversion of plasma androstenedione to estrone in postmenopausal women with and without endometrial cancer. *Am. J. Obstet. Gynecol.* 130:448.

Mercier-Bodard, C., J.-M. Renoir, and E.-E. Baulieu. 1976. Sex steroid binding plasma protein (SBP) in the pregnant woman. In *Protides of the biological fluids* (27th Colloquim, Bruges, 1975), p. 233. Pergamon Press, Oxford.

Migeon, C.J., D.C. Green, and J.P. Eckert. 1973. Study of adrenocortical function in obesity. *Metabolism* 12:718.

Mittra, I. and J.L. Hayward. 1974. Hypothalamic-pituitary-thyroid axis in breast cancer. *Lancet* i:885.

Mittra, I., J.L. Hayward, and A S. McNeilly. 1976. Hypothalamic-pituitary-prolactin axis in breast cancer. *Lancet* i:889.

Moosa, A.R., D.A. Price-Evans, and A.C. Brewer. 1973. Thyroid status and breast cancer. Reappraisal of an old relationship. *Ann. R. Coll. Surg. Engl.* 53:178.

Nisker, J.A., G.L. Hammond, and P.K. Siiteri. 1980a. "Elevated percent free (%F) estradiol (E2) in women with polycystic ovarian disease (PCOD)." Paper presented at 27th Annual Meeting of the Society for Gynecologic Investigation, Denver, Colorado, March 19-22.

Nisker, J.A., G.L. Hammond, B.J. Davidson, A.M. Frumar, N.K. Takaki, H.L. Judd, and P.K. Siiteri. 1980b. Serum sex hormone-binding globulin capacity and the percentage of free estradiol in postmenopausal women with and without endometrial carcinoma. *Am. J. Obstet. Gynecol.* **138**:637.

Petra, P.H. 1979. The serum sex steroid-binding protein. Purification, characterization, and immunological properties of the human and rabbit proteins. *J. Steroid Biochem.* **11**:245.

Poortman, J., J.H.H. Thijssen, and F. Schwartz. 1973. Androgen production and conversion to estrogens in normal postmenopausal women and in selected breast cancer patients. *J. Clin. Endocrinol. Metab.* **37**:101.

Repert, R.W. 1952. Breast carcinoma study: Relation to thyroid disease and diabetes. *J. Mich. Med. Soc.* **51**:1315.

Rosner, W. 1976. The binding of steroid hormones in human serum. In *Trace components of plasma: Isolation and clinical significance* (ed. G.A. Jamieson and T.J. Greenwalt), vol. 5. Alan R. Liss, Inc., New York.

Short, R.V. and J.O. Drife. 1977. The aetiology of mammary cancer in man and animals. *Symp. Zool. Soc. Lond.* **41**:211.

Siiteri, P.K. and P.C. MacDonald. 1973. The role of extraglandular estrogen in human endocrinology. In *Handbook of physiology* (ed. S.R. Geiger et al.), p. 615. The American Physiological Society, New York.

Siiteri, P.K., B.E. Schwarz, and P.C. MacDonald. 1974. Estrogen receptors and the estrone hypothesis in relation to endometrial and breast carcinoma. *Gynecol. Oncol.* **2**:228.

Thomas, B.S., R.D. Bulbrook, J.L. Hayward, S. Kumaoka, O. Takatani, O. Abes, and J. Utsunomiya. 1977. Urinary steroid profiles in normal women and in patients with breast cancer in Britain and Japan: Relation to thyroid function. *Eur. J. Cancer* **13**:1287.

Tulchinsky, D. and I.J. Chopra. 1973. Competitive ligand-binding assay for measurement of sex hormome-binding globulin (SHBG). *J. Clin. Endocrinol. Metab.* **37**:873.

Vermeulen, A. 1977. Transport and distribution of androgens at different ages. In *Androgens and antiandrogens* (ed. L. Martini and M. Mottra), p. 53. Raven Press, New York.

Victor, A., E. Weiner, and E.D. Johansson. 1976. Sex hormone binding globulin: The carrier protein for d-Norgestrel. *J. Clin. Endocrinol. Metab.* **43**:244.

Vigersky, R.A., S. Kono, M. Sauer, M.B. Lipsett, and D.L. Loriaux. 1979. Relative binding of testosterone and estradiol to testosterone-estradiol-binding globulin. *J. Clin. Endocrinol. Metab.* **49**:899.

Wang, D.Y. and R.D. Bulbrook. 1969. The binding of steroids to plasma proteins in normal women and women with breast cancer. *Eur. J. Cancer* **5**:247.

Westphal, U. 1971. *Steroid protein interactions.* Springer-Verlag, New York.

Wu, C.-H., T. Motohashi, H.A. Abdel-Rahman, G.L. Flickinger, and G. Mikail. 1976. Free and protein-bound plasma estradiol-17β during the menstrual cycle. *J. Endocrinol. Metab.* **43**:436.

Wynder, E.L., G.C. Escher, and N. Mantel. 1966. An epidemiological investigation of cancer of the endometrium. *Cancer* **19**:489.

Yen, S.C.C. and R.B. Jaffe (ed.). 1978. *Reproductive endocrinology,* chapter 14. W.B. Saunders Company, Philadelphia.

Zumoff, B., J. Fishman, J. Cassouto, L. Hellman, and T.F. Gallagher. 1966. Estradiol transformation in men with breast cancer. *J. Clin. Endocrinol. Metab.* **26**:960.

COMMENTS

KORENMAN: Can I make a comment very pertinent to this? It's interesting that obese people are hyperestrogenic and yet they have low SHBG capacity. We've done a study recently (although not using your latest technique) of weight loss in men to try to determine what happens to both their estrogen and their SHBG capacities as they lose weight. We found that within 2 weeks of initiating a diet, the SHBG capacity very rapidly goes back up to normal. Their estrogens, which are elevated, particularly E_1, take months of weight loss to get back down to their basal levels. There is a dissociation between the effects on the serum estrogen and the effect on SHBG capacity.

When we talk about nutritional factors, I think that it's very relevant to recognize that there are two elements—hypernutrition and obesity. They are really two different factors. As soon as you put a person on a diet, those factors related to hypernutrition change. When the person loses a lot of weight, the factors related to obesity stay the same. That dissociation has not been used in epidemiological or physiological studies, but it really makes a difference. If anyone wants to talk about it more, we can go into the parameters that change it acutely and the parameters that change it chronically.

SIITERI: In women, this situation is even more complicated, because in some of them SHBG is back up to normal in a couple of weeks, as you say, but in others it is not. In one example of prolonged weight loss, a woman who lost about 150 pounds of weight over a period of 2 years was just barely getting into the normal range of serum SHBG.

TOPP: The people with breast cancer have 100% of their E_2 available. What is your interpretation of that?

SIITERI: That is the key question right now. We have measured the binding capacity using DHT as the probe. So, we can get an assay with DHT. We also can measure the off rate without any problems using DHT. We can't measure either of these with E_2. So it would appear at the moment that there is an abnormality in the binding site; the site will bind androgen, but it will not bind estrogen. Now, that's a tough thing to say because there's no precedent for that in terms of our chemical knowledge of the binding site.

BULBROOK: It is curious how much interest there is now in SHBG. Dr. Murayama and his colleagues in Tokyo claim that measuring SHBG by agar gel electrophoresis is a good index of response to therapy in advanced breast cancer. John Moore in the Imperial Cancer Research Fund has found a good correlation between plasma levels of SHBG and disease-free interval after mastectomy—the higher the binding, the longer the interval.

HENDERSON: Are these postmenopausal women?

SIITERI: By and large, yes. We're expanding these studies now, but at the present time I can't give you the frequency of how often we have this abnormality. I can tell you that all women with breast cancer don't have this abnormality. Some of them behave normally.

WELSCH: I would like to address my question to Stan Korenman. I've been intrigued with your estrogen window hypothesis ever since you developed it a number of years ago. There are some data in the literature, however, that disturb me because they do not appear to fit your interesting proposal. For example, there are a number of radioautographic labeling index ([^{3}H]thymidine) studies on the human breast that show that the mitotic activity of the ductal epithelium is greater in the luteal phase of the menstrual cycle than in the follicular phase of the cycle. These data do not appear to support your hypothesis. It is conceivable, however unlikely, that the mitogenic stimulus of the follicular phase would not assert itself until the luteal phase of the cycle. Would you care to comment on these data?

KORENMAN: There are at least two or three studies showing labeling indexes higher. Are these data for humans?

WELSCH: Yes. One would expect that the mitotic activity of the human breast epithelium would be higher in the follicular phase of the cycle than in the luteal phase of the cycle if your hypothesis is correct.

KORENMAN: I really haven't seen the data. I've looked for it. You must have a source that I did not identify. What about in pregnancy? Are there any parallel data in the stages of pregnancy?

WELSCH: I do not believe these reports examined the mitotic activity of breast epithelium in pregnant women. I do not know of any studies that have.

KORENMAN: I tried to find human breast data on this, but there was none.

WELSCH: Master et al. (1977) and Meyer (1977) reported this a couple of years ago. There was another report (Milligan et al. 1975) that showed increased breast volume in the luteal phase of the cycle.

KORENMAN: That's interesting. I just don't know.

HENDERSON: It seems to me that there's a crucial piece of information missing. Can you distinguish between the effect of estrogen, that is, just accumulated estrogen, on the one hand, and estrogen with and without other hormones around? The idea that progesterone might be an important antiestrogen in the breast is based primarily on studies on endometrial tissue. There is not very much known about breast tissue in this regard.

MEITES: Stan [Korenman], your idea certainly is not confined to the effects of estrogen on breast tissue alone. As we know, estrogen also influences the pituitary. There are antipituitary effects of progesterone exerted on the pituitary, for example, on secretion of prolactin, as Stan brought out. This may have an indirect influence, or possibly even a direct influence, on mammary cancer.

KORENMAN: I agree with you. You can go even further than that. The liver is a major target for estrogen, and among the components of that target are microsomal hydroxylases, which are responsible for activating procarcinogens to carcinogens. Perhaps the estrogens and progesterones, both independently and together, have very complex effects on those enzymes which may activate compounds like B[a]P and 7,12-dimethylbenz[a]-anthracene (DMBA).

ROSEN: Stan, those are different enzyme systems, so that's a quantum leap. The P-448 that activates carcinogens is not the same as the microsomal hydroxylases involved in steroid metabolism.

KORENMAN: You don't think it has an effect?

ROSEN: I don't think you can make that extrapolation. It's a nice concept but I don't think the data support your statement that the same enzyme systems are involved in both steroid metabolism and carcinogen activation.

KORENMAN: These are not necessarily steroid-metabolizing cytochromes, but there's a tremendous increase in some of the cytochrome.

LIPPMAN: Obviously, everybody is really intrigued by your observations, Dr. Siiteri, but there is a problem that I see. It's too confused. A lot of controls come to my mind, and obviously they come to yours. There are, for example, these blind panels, a variety of malignants from which one can get sera. There are the cohort studies that I think Dr. Zumoff has been involved in with children at high risk, that is, young adults from families at high risk vs their controls.

SIITERI: Yes. We just haven't had the time to do all that is necessary.

LIPPMAN: You have for six of these patients. I wonder if you tried to identify an abnormal SHBG. There's no precedent for that, of course, unless you thought of it from a genetic point of view.

SIITERI: I tried to point out that we are, in fact, ahead of the chemical knowledge about this binding protein. So we have to do what we can with indirect kinds of studies. We are looking at differences in specificity, and just about everything you could think of doing with a receptor, as well as differences in association rates and dissociation rates of binding. Everything we have done so far really says the binding site reads androgen but not estrogen. I just don't know how to deal with that. Now, we really need radioimmunoassay for SHBG to see how it correlates with the binding assays. It's interesting to note that one could say that it is inconsistent to have a low binding capacity in obesity because there is more E_2 available. Well, you know, you could turn that argument around and say, "They have low SHBG levels because the fat cells are picking up the SHBG." It has been suggested that the protein is a carrier, not only for the circulation, but also to transport steroids into cells. Furthermore, there is data suggesting that adipose cells are responsive to estrogens.

SIRBASKU: But isn't it possible to use affinity chromatography rather quickly on something like that?

LIPPMAN: With a purification scheme.

SIITERI: There are several purification methods published. I believe five groups claim they have a pure protein, but there are major differences in molecular weight, amino acid composition, and in the carbohydrate composition. I didn't get into this business to start isolating the protein. I hope somebody else does it and tells me what it's like.

SIRBASKU: But even the slight differences in proteins, like transferrin and a lot of other serum proteins, are known to all have exactly those same characteristics.

SIITERI: That's correct. You put it on the right kind of a gel and you can get five or six peaks.

ROSEN: Regarding the concept of available steroid and mechanism of estrogen action, has anybody done clear-cut animal studies to look at the receptor-bound steroid as a function of free steroid and translocation into the nucleus as a function of what you're calling "available" steroids? Has anyone asked the question of whether or not this relationship is meaningful? You're talking about the correlations. But you can do that study and get a hard fact out of it.

SIITERI: Yes. I neglected to mention the very important work of Pardridge at UCLA (Pardridge et al. 1980), who is very much interested in this question, not only with regard to steroids but a whole variety of substances that are in blood. He has worked out a nice double isotope method to measure the uptake of steroids, including E_2, from human serum in a single passage through a rat brain. The conclusion he has reached thus far is that free plus albumin-bound steroids penetrate the brain. Whether or not this is true for the uterus and breast is not known.

We have measured binding of 10 different steroids in male and female serum. The percent bound to SHBG or CBG has a remarkable inverse correlation with the metabolic clearance rate of the steroid. This indicates that if the steroid is bound to either SHBG or CBG, it isn't cleared in the liver because the line intersects with 2800 liters a day, which happens to be splanchnic blood flow.

Thus, the lower the binding to SHBG or CBG, the higher the metabolic clearance rate (MCR). Progesterone is interesting because it binds to CBG with about the same affinity as cortisol, but it has a much higher MCR. This apparently is due to the higher affinity of progesterone for albumin.

KORENMAN: There's an interesting point that Pardridge made, and that is that different tissues clear at different rates. For example, the liver clears much better than the brain.

PETRAKIS: There is some in the breast fluid itself that's secreted and remains in the breast ducts all the time. You are looking at the urine and the blood, and yet the stuff is sitting in the breasts, where it should be working.

SIITERI: Give me more samples.

References

Master, J.P.W., J.O. Drife, and J.J. Scarisbrick. 1977. Cyclic variation of DNA synthesis in human breast epithelium. *J. Natl. Cancer Inst.* 58:1263.

Meyer, J.S. 1977. Cell proliferation in normal human breast ducts, fibroadenomas, and other ductal hyperplasia measured by nuclear-labeled tritiated thymidine: Its effects on menstrual flow, age, and oral contraceptive hormones. *Hum. Pathol.* 8:67.

Milligan, D., J.O. Drife, and R.V. Short. 1975. Changes in breast volume during normal menstrual cycles and after oral contraceptives. *Br. Med. J.* 4:494.

Pardridge, W.M., L.J. Mietus, A.M. Frumar, B.J. Davidson, and H.L. Judd. 1980. The effect of human serum on transport of testosterone and estradiol into rat brain. *Am. J. Physiol.* 239:E103.

SESSION 3:
Review of Studies Attempting to Establish Endogenous Hormones as Important in Human Breast Cancer

Estrogens and Progesterone in Human Breast Cancer

PHILIP COLE
Epidemiology Program of the Comprehensive Cancer Center
University of Alabama in Birmingham
Birmingham, Alabama 35294

During the last few years, I have been gaining the impression that efforts to elucidate the role of endogenous hormones in the etiology of breast cancer have not been yielding progress. A review of the literature to prepare this presentation, I regret to say, has only reinforced that view. Why have we made so little progress in the last few years? The possible reasons that I see are:

1. The endocrinologic components of some of our studies lack sophistication. This, of course, is true only of those studies conducted by epidemiologists, or so we are led to believe.
2. The epidemiologic component of some of our studies has lacked sophistication. This, of course, is true only of those studies conducted by endocrinologists, or so we are led to believe.
3. We endocrinologists and epidemiologists have been more eager to criticize one another than to collaborate.
4. We have failed to perceive etiologic distinctions and still use the expression "breast cancer" to encompass a heterogenous group of etiologic entities.
5. Although I consider it unlikely, perhaps we are all asking the wrong questions.

So let me try to pose what I consider the questions to be, at least with respect to the estrogens and progesterone. I will phrase these questions in the context of the idea that endogenous estrogens are at least part of the cause of at least some cases of human breast cancer.

1. Is it simply the total amount of estrogens that is important?
2. Is it the balance among the estrogens that is important? If so, which ones are more harmful?
3. Do other hormones, especially prolactin and progesterone, modify the carcinogenic effects of the estrogens?
4. Do the estrogens, with or without a modifying effect of other hormones, play only some incomplete role, with breast carcinogenesis requiring some external or environmental factor as Korenman (1980) has recently suggested?

5. Are there segments of the menstrual cycle or are there phases in a woman's life (e.g., when her breasts develop or the entire period prior to pregnancy) when the carcinogenic effects of the estrogens are maximal?

Let us consider the first two questions together: Is carcinogenesis a question of the total amount (the total activity) of the estrogens or is it a question of the balance among them? I believe we are more or less evenly divided on this question. However, even those persons who favor the "total" idea over the "balance" idea no longer are indifferent to the question of the possibly different carcinogenic activity of the different estrogens. For now, we all have to give them individual attention even though we are not all equally enthusiastic about doing so. But even among the fraction enthusiasts there is disagreement: Is estriol (E_3) or the estriol ratio important? Or is it mainly a question of the levels of estrone (E_1)? For many years several of us have favored Lemon's idea that the E_3 ratio was of crucial importance with a high ratio being protective (Lemon et al. 1966). And, to its credit, the so-called E_3 ratio, or estrogen-fraction hypothesis, caused many to give thought to the underlying issues. In fact, a moderate amount of evidence was amassed in its favor, and not solely by the Harvard group. In a few words, it was shown that the E_3 ratio was favorable, i.e. elevated, in several low-risk populations and that the ratio declined in populations in transition from low to high risks of breast cancer (MacMahon et al. 1974; Dickinson et al. 1974; Cole et al. 1976; Gross et al. 1977). True, we failed to find a low ratio in young women with breast cancer, although that case-control study of ours had a number of limitations (Cole et al. 1978).

I no longer favor the E_3-ratio hypothesis, but neither do I reject it. The problem with the hypothesis is that it is too specific, not that it is demonstrably wrong. So, for the time being at least, I favor a more general hypothesis that in some way the balance among the estrogen fractions is important, whether or not the total amount of estrogen also is. Naturally, it is with considerable regret that I move from a more specific to a less specific hypothesis, because that direction is contrary to the way in which scientific thought ought to develop.

However, although I believe that our level of knowledge is adequate to justify only a vague and general hypothesis, I find it necessary to have a sharper one if I am going to focus my efforts. So I support as a working hypothesis the idea that E_1 is a cause of human breast cancer. This hypothesis, of course, is fully consistent with the E_3-ratio hypothesis. It is also supported by most of the studies that supported the E_3-ratio hypothesis and even by our case-control study. Furthermore, it is also given strong support by studies of exogenous hormones. I have long ago accepted the idea that E_1, both exogenous and endogenous, is a cause of endometrial cancer. And, we know that endometrial cancer has many risk factors in common with breast cancer. Yet these two diseases have some striking differences, for example there is evidently no age-at-first-birth effect for endometrial cancer. I reconcile these observations by suggesting that the etiologic overlap between these two diseases is only partial. That is, the cases of endometrial cancer and of breast cancer which occur up to about age 55 or 60 have largely the same etiology. After age 50, E_1 continues to be a part of the cause of both cancers; but, in addition, the effects of some other causal web begin to become manifest with respect to breast cancer only, or mainly, in Western countries. Because it has a limited geographic distribution, this other factor probably does not relate to any strong biological determinant of susceptibility; more likely it is a question of a culture-bound exposure.

The third question is "Do other hormones, especially prolactin and progesterone, modify the carcinogenic activities of the estrogens?" With respect to prolactin, I have no opinion to offer for there is only a very small amount of evidence from women that prolactin is involved in the etiology of breast cancer and this evidence does not relate to the specific question of the modification of the effects of estrogens. With respect to progesterone, I favor the view supported by many of you that this hormone reduces the carcinogenic activity of the estrogens. But, when I ask myself why we favor this view, I find that we are on weak ground and that we rest mainly on the findings with respect to exogenous hormones. By that I mean:

1. There is some evidence to the effect that exogenous estrogens given to oophorectomized women raise their breast cancer rates even above those of women with ovaries (who, of course, have some progesterone) (Hoover et al. 1976).
2. There is the possibility that the relatively harmful effects of Oracon, a sequential oral contraceptive, on endometrial cancer may be due to its low dose of a weak progestogen (Cole 1980; Weiss and Sayvetz 1980).

But I also favor the idea because the impression that anovulation plays a role in causing breast cancer is attractive. For example, the data presented by Grattarola 15 years ago have never been refuted. In a case-control study of young women with breast cancer, and using endometrial biopsy, he found that anovulators had about six times the breast cancer risk of ovulators (Grattarola 1964). However, we should not lose sight of the substantial amount of experimental evidence that progesterone is a cocarcinogen, enhancing the effect of several other types of agents.

The fourth question relates to interaction. Do the estrogens play only an initiating role, only a promoting role, or only a growth-enhancing role? In any event, do they fail to play at least one of the three roles necessary to the production of manifest breast cancer and, if so, is the causal web completed by an environmental agent? Korenmen recently has proposed that an environmental agent must be involved because international differences in hormonal profiles are, in his opinion, too small to account for international differences in breast cancer rates (Korenman 1980). Surely, this is not true with respect to breast cancer rates up to age 50 or 60. And although there may be an exogenous factor involved in cases that occur after age 60, I do not see that there must be. For example, it may simply be that we have not been measuring the right hormones.

The fifth and final question was are there certain periods in life when the breast is particularly susceptible or particularly resistant to carcinogenic stimuli and (or) are there ages when the stimuli themselves wax and wane? One affirmative answer to this question is the anovulation hypothesis. That is, Sherman and Korenman proposed that at each end of reproductive life the carcinogenic stimulus, unopposed E_1, is increased as well as during the first half of each normal menstrual cycle and both halves of anovular cycles (Sherman and Korenman 1974). Another affirmative answer invokes the idea that the developing, adolescent breast is especially susceptible. And a possibly related proposal is that a period of relatively high risk is terminated or reduced by a pregnancy. What are the bases of these ideas?

The basis for the idea that the two ends of reproductive life are high-risk periods rests on the observation that early menarche and late menopause are associated with increased risk. But, for neither early menarche nor late menopause is there evidence that there is an accompanying protracted period of anovulation. Perhaps this idea also takes some support from the bimodality of the breast cancer age-incidence curve, which could suggest, indeed, that there are two age periods of maximum exposure and (or) susceptibility. The ideas that the young breast is especially susceptible or heavily exposed and that this terminates with parity are supported by the age-at-first-birth effect (MacMahon et al. 1970) and by the findings from the studies of women exposed to radiation (Boice and Monson 1977), although this type of evidence should be generalized only with caution to hormonal carcinogenesis.

I will conclude with a single comment about the role of endogenous progesterone. Here, even more than with respect to the estrogens, I am amazed at how little and unconvincing are the human data. In fact, you can still make the case that if progesterone is involved in human breast cancer, it is because it exerts a harmful, not a protective effect. For example, progesterone is an effective cocarcinogen in animals, even enhancing the adverse effect of estrogens. In addition, late menarche and early menopause mean a net reduction in progesterone stimulation and a net reduction in breast cancer. Yet, most of us cling to the idea that if progesterone plays a part in breast cancer, it is as an anticarcinogen.

REFERENCES

Boice, J.D., Jr. and R.R. Monson. 1977. Breast cancer in women after repeated fluoroscopic examinations of the chest. *J. Natl. Cancer Inst.* **59**:823.

Cole, P. 1980. Oral contraceptives and endometrial cancer. *N. Engl. J. Med.* **302**:575.

Cole, P., J.B. Brown, and B. MacMahon. 1976. Oestrogen profiles of parous and nulliparous women. *Lancet* ii:596.

Cole, P., D. Cramer, S. Yen, R. Paffenbarger, B. MacMahon, and J. Brown. 1978. Estrogen profiles of premenopausal women with breast cancer. *Cancer Res.* 38:745.

Dickinson, L.E., B. MacMahon, P. Cole, and J.B. Brown. 1974. Estrogen profiles of Oriental and Caucasian women in Hawaii. *N. Engl. J. Med.* 291: 1211.

Grattarola, R. 1964. The premenstrual endometrial pattern of women with breast cancer. *Cancer* 17:1119.

Gross, J., B. Modan, B. Bertini, O. Spira, F. de Waard, J.H.H. Thijssen, and P. Vestergaard. 1977. Relationship between steroid excretion patterns and breast cancer incidence in Israeli women of various origins. *J. Natl. Cancer Inst.* 59:7.

Hoover, R., L.A. Gray, Sr., P. Cole, and B. MacMahon. 1976. Menopausal estrogens and breast cancer. *N. Engl. J. Med.* 295:401.

Korenman, S.G. 1980. Oestrogen window hypothesis of the aetiology of breast cancer. *Lancet* i:700.

Lemon, H.M., H.H. Wotiz, L. Parsons, and P.J. Mozden. 1966. Reduced estriol excretion in patients with breast cancer prior to endocrine therapy. *J. Am. Med. Assoc.* 196:112.

MacMahon, B., P. Cole, T.M. Lin, C.R. Lowe, A.P. Mirra, B. Ravnihar, E.J. Salber, V.G. Valaoras, and S. Yuasa. 1970. Age at first birth and breast cancer risk. *Bull. WHO* 43:209.

MacMahon, B., P. Cole, J.B. Brown, K. Aoki, T.M. Lin, R.W. Morgan, and N.C. Woo. 1974. Urine oestrogen profiles of Asian and North American women. *Int. J. Cancer* 14:161.

Sherman, B.M. and S.G. Korenman. 1974. Inadequate corpus luteum function: A pathophysiological interpretation of human breast cancer epidemiology. *Cancer* 33:1306.

Weiss, N.S. and T.A. Sayvetz. 1980. Incidence of endometrial cancer in relation to the use of oral contraceptives. *N. Engl. J. Med.* 302:551.

Prolactin—An Important Hormone in Breast Neoplasia?

BRIAN E. HENDERSON AND MALCOLM C. PIKE
Department of Family and Preventive Medicine
University of Southern California School of Medicine
Los Angeles, California 90033

In recent years, there has been intense interest in the role of prolactin in breast neoplasia. Multiple pituitary isografts, which increase prolactin secretion, and hypothalamic lesions and drugs, which stimulate prolactin, all increase the incidence of spontaneous and 7,12-dimethylbenz[a]anthracene (DMBA)-induced mammary tumors in rats and mice whereas drug-induced suppression of prolactin release decreases the growth of established tumors. The net result of such animal studies, which will be reviewed in detail elsewhere in this volume (see also Welsch, this volume), has been to establish the critical role of prolactin, as well as estrogen, in creating optimum conditions for the development and growth of breast tumors in rodents.

BREAST CANCER PATIENTS AND THEIR FAMILIES

Attempts to establish such a critical role for prolactin in human mammary neoplasia have not been consistently successful. A number of studies of prolactin levels in breast cancer patients and controls have been reported. Many of these studies have had small numbers of patients and controls and it is not always clear that the investigators have controlled carefully for the marked variation in prolactin levels that occurs during a 24-hr period. Nevertheless, of the 6 patient-control comparisons of premenopausal women we have found in the literature, 5 showed higher levels in patients than in controls (Table 1). The results of a similar study in postmenopausal women by Hill et al. (1976) also showed a clear elevation of prolactin levels in U.S. white and Japanese breast cancer patients but not in South African black breast cancer patients, when compared to controls. Other studies of postmenopausal women have not found such a difference (Boyns et al. 1973; Kwa et al. 1974; McFayden et al. 1976; Ohgo et al. 1976).

The apparent inconsistency between the results of studies of prolactin levels in pre- and postmenopausal women may be explained partially by the fall in these levels that seems to occur with advancing age. Vekemans and Robyn

Table 1

Prolactin Levels in Premenopausal Breast Cancer Patients and Controls

Population	Patients	Controls	Reference
Indians	21[a]	21-42[b]	Sheth et al. (1975)
South African blacks	17	9.5	Hill et al. (1976)
U.S. whites	29	12.5	Hill et al. (1976)
Japanese	24	12	Hill et al. (1976)
U.K. whites	11.4	9.7	Cole et al. (1977)
U.S. whites	15.1	10.1	Malarkey et al. (1977)

[a]Published units for prolactin should be taken only as applying to the particular study and thus are not given.

[b]Both figures are given as control mean values; the lower value would appear to be "correct" in the context of other results given in the paper.

(1975) and del Pozo and Brownell (1979) report that women over age 50 have prolactin levels that are only 50-60% of that of women in their 20s.

Kwa et al. (1974) were the first to demonstrate elevated prolactin levels in family members of women with breast cancer. In our studies of daughters of young breast cancer cases and daughters of controls, we have found a consistent elevation of plasma prolactin levels (Henderson et al. 1975). The most striking difference between the two groups of teenagers was obtained by considering the plasma levels of estrone plus estradiol ($E_1 + E_2$) and of prolactin together. Figure 1 shows the results for the specimens collected on day 6 of the menstrual cycle: Values for 12 of 34 patients' daughters were above the line shown in the figure, compared with only 1 of 30 daughters of controls. Repeat sampling of the follicular phase of the same teenage girls 6 months later produced similar results (Pike et al. 1977).

We subsequently studied the teenage daughters of women with bilateral breast cancer diagnosed by age 50 (Pike et al. 1979). First-degree relatives of such women have been reported to have at least a ninefold increased risk of breast cancer (Anderson 1972, 1974). As a group, these teenage daughters were similar to the girls in our previously published study in age, height, and weight at interview (Henderson et al. 1975). A comparison of the plasma and urine hormone levels in these three groups of teenagers is shown in Table 2. Plasma estrogen and prolactin levels of the daughters of patients were elevated above those of daughters of controls, although only the elevation of the day-11 (follicular phase) estrogen level was statistically significant, and, when the plasma estrogen and prolactin values on day 11 or day 22 were combined, discriminated between both groups. Compared with 20% and 36% of elevated values in daughters of controls, daughters of ordinary patients had 44% and 50% and those of women with bilateral cancer had 43% and 60% of the increased values. Plasma progesterone levels were elevated similarly in both groups of daughters of patients.

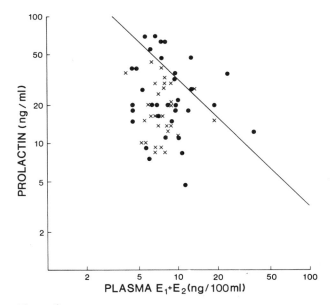

Figure 1
Plasma total estrogen ($E_1 + E_2$) and prolactin levels on day 6 initial sampling in daughters of breast cancer cases (●) and controls (×). (Data from Henderson et al. 1975.)

Urine estrogen values and estriol (E_3) ratios showed less consistent variation among the 3 groups: The follicular urinary E_1 (uE_1) and urinary E_2 (uE_2) were higher in the daughters of patients, but the comparable luteal values were highest in the controls.

PROLACTIN LEVELS AND BREAST CANCER RISK FACTORS

Prolactin levels in women increase at the onset of ovarian activity and are highest during adolescence (Vekemans and Robyn 1975; del Pozo and Brownell 1979). However, no relationship has been found between prolactin levels and age at menarche (Kwa et al. 1976; Gray et al. 1981b; Yu et al. 1981). In the same studies, no consistent relationship was found between body weight and serum prolactin (Kwa et al. 1976; Gray et al. 1981b; Yu et al. 1981). However, in a later study Kwa et al. (1978) reported higher evening prolactin levels in obese postmenopausal women.

In the course of our study of relatives of women with bilateral breast cancer, referred to above, we noted lower levels of plasma prolactin in nulliparous compared with parous women (Pike et al. 1979). As age at first full-term delivery is a major breast cancer risk factor, further study of this possible hormone change was undertaken. We collected two follicular-phase (day 11) blood specimens from a group of Catholic nuns and their nulliparous and parous

Table 2

Mean Plasma and Urinary Hormone Levels in Teenage Daughters of Patients with Breast Cancer and Controls

Cycle day	Hormones	Daughters of controls	Daughters of patients	Daughters of patients with bilateral breast cancer
11	$E_1 + E_2$ (ng/dl)	10.0	12.3	14.0
	$uE_1 + uE_2$ (μg/12 hr)	4.4	5.1	4.7
	$uE_3/uE_1 + uE_2$	0.6	0.6	0.6
	prolactin[a]	21.2	21.5	23.2
	number of subjects	25	25	21
22	$E_1 + E_2$	16.8	16.2	22.0
	$uE_1 + uE_2$	9.4	7.7	9.2
	$uE_3/uE_1 + uE_2$	0.7	0.8	0.6
	prolactin[a]	20.1	22.2	22.9
	progesterone (ng/dl)	2.9	4.3	3.7
	number of subjects	25	24	20

Urine hormone values are preceded by the letter "u." The remaining values were measured in the plasma.

[a] Units for prolactin are not given, as the assay subsequently was changed. The absolute values are, therefore, not directly comparable to those in Tables 3-6 which were tested 2 or more years later using a current method (Gray et al. 1981a,b; Yu et al. 1981).

sisters (Yu et al. 1981). The first specimen was collected between 9:00 AM and 9:30 AM and at least half an hour after the subject arose; the second specimen was drawn 2 hr after the first. An overnight (12-hr) urine specimen was collected ending at 8:00 AM on the morning when the blood sample was taken.

Table 3 presents the mean values of age at interview, oral contraceptive use, and plasma and urine hormone levels for nuns and their parous and nulliparous sisters. The parous sisters were divided into two groups based on their history of estrogen use. The rationale was to separate out the effect, if any, of past exogenous estrogen use on the levels of prolactin and estrogen. The four groups of women were similar in mean height, weight, and age at menarche. For the two groups of parous sisters, the mean age at first full-term pregnancy (FFTP) and the mean number of pregnancies were about the same. Four nuns reported having taken oral contraceptives (OCs) for menstrual irregularities with a mean duration of 7 months. Ninety-six percent of parous sisters who reported a year or more of past estrogen use had used OCs with a mean duration of 4 years.

Table 3
Geometric Mean Levels of Plasma and Urinary Hormones of Nuns and Their Sisters

	Nuns	Parous sisters estrogen use		Nulliparous sisters	Nulliparous	Parous	One-sided p value[a]
		< 1 year	≥ 1 year				
Number of women	70	35	27	18	88	62	
Age at interview (yr)	34.1	32.5	34.1	27.8	32.8	33.2	
Percent OC use ever	6	71	96	39	13	82	
Total number months	6.8	5.8	50.3	5.0	5.3	28.5	
Plasma hormones							
Prolactin (1) (ng/ml)[b]	23.5	17.0	16.6	19.7	22.7	16.8	.0004
Prolactin (2) (ng/ml)[b]	15.4	13.1	11.5	15.4	15.4	12.4	.006
E_1 (1) and (2) (ng/dl)	8.2	7.7	8.2	7.7	8.1	7.9	.32
E_2 (1) and (2) (ng/dl)	11.8	10.6	12.9	12.8	12.0	11.7	.32
Urine hormones							
E_1 (µg/12 hr)	4.3	4.0	4.1	4.3	4.3	4.0	.25
E_2 (µg/12 hr)	2.2	2.0	2.2	2.1	2.2	2.1	.30
E_3 (µg/12 hr)	4.8	4.4	5.0	4.8	4.8	4.6	.46
$E_3/E_1 + E_2$	.73	.73	.79	.74	.73	.75	.42

[a]Comparison of nulliparous and parous, Mann-Whitney rank test.
[b](1) = First sample; (2) = second sample.

We found little difference in hormone levels between the two parous sister groups, or between the nuns and their nulliparous sisters. Between the parous and the nulliparous women, however, we found highly significant differences in mean prolactin levels from both plasma samples. The mean prolactin levels in the nulliparous women was 35% higher ($P = 0.0004$) for the first sample and 24% higher ($P = 0.006$) for the second sample. The elevation of prolactin level in the nulliparous women was maintained across all age groups (Fig. 2).

Similar results were obtained when we adjusted for possible effects of weight and age at menarche on prolactin level. There was no statistically significant relationship between prolactin level and age at FFTP (Fig. 3); however, only 7 of the 62 parous women had their FFTP after the age of 25. There was no effect on prolactin level of second or subsequent full-term pregnancies.

There was no significant difference in the level of circulating E_1 and E_2 among the parous women. There was a positive correlation between the level of plasma and urinary estrogens and age (data not shown). The increase was most pronounced for plasma E_2.

These data clearly demonstrate that a woman's plasma prolactin level may be lowered permanently after her FFTP. The prolactin level is not lowered further by subsequent births, nor is it associated with age at first delivery, at least up to age 30. This effect of FFTP could explain the decrease in prolactin levels in women with age up to about age 35 noted by Vekemans and Robyn (1975) and by del Pozo and Brownell (1979).

This study thus suggests that the protective effect of early FFTP may be mediated, at least in part, by permanently lowering the circulating level of prolactin. The lack of decrease in prolactin level with subsequent full-term deliveries is consistent with the fact that such deliveries do not substantially further lower breast cancer risk (MacMahon et al. 1973).

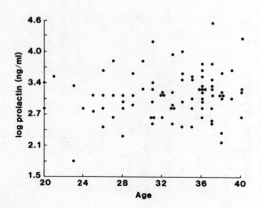

Figure 2
Plasma prolactin level and age at bleeding in nulliparous women

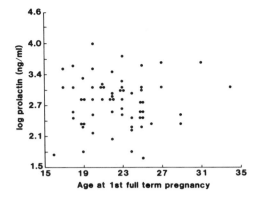

Figure 3
Plasma prolactin level and age at first delivery in parous women

DIET

A high-fat diet increases the incidence of both spontaneous and induced mammary tumors in rodents. Several hypotheses have been suggested to explain these effects, including one that proposes that dietary fat intake has a positive effect on prolactin secretion. It has been demonstrated that rats fed a high-fat diet have elevated proestrus-estrus prolactin levels, and drugs that block prolactin secretion abolish the difference in tumor yield that normally occurs between rats on low- and high-fat diets when a carcinogen such as DMBA is given.

Results of experiments in humans on the effects of diet on prolactin secretion have been conflicting. Hill and Wynder (1976) found that peak nocturnal prolactin levels fell by half in 4 female nurses who followed a lacto-ovo-vegetarian diet for only 2 weeks, their fat intake declining from 40% to 33% of calories.

We, however, failed to produce any change in daytime prolactin levels in 8 women who reduced their dietary fat intake from 41% to 22% of calories for 2 months. The results from our study are given in Table 4. While on the low-fat diet, the subjects almost halved their fat intake and lost an average of nearly 2 kg. Despite this drastic change in dietary fat consumption, there was no significant change in plasma prolactin levels.

Why our results are so different from those of Hill and Wynder (1976) is not clear. Our subjects were on a more extreme diet for a longer period, so that a priori one would have thought that we would have obtained bigger changes than they did. One possibility is that we drew our samples "too late" in the day. These short-term diet changes may only affect peak prolactin levels during sleep, and 9:00 AM levels may still reflect such peak sleep levels, whereas noon-time levels may not. We do not find this an attractive explanation, partly because Hill

Table 4

Mean Nutrient Intake, Weight, and Hormone Levels in 8 Female Subjects on a Low-fat Diet

		Months on diet	
	Prediet	1	2
Energy (Kcal)	1690	1140	1220
Fat (% of calories)	40.9	22.7	21.6
Protein (% of calories)	16.1	20.1	20.4
Carbohydrate (% of calories)	43.0	57.3	58.0
Weight (kg)	67.5	65.9	65.6
Prolactin (ng/ml)	9.1[a]	7.4	8.8

[a]Geometric mean.

and Wynder (1976) also found a 40% reduction in prolactin at 10:00 PM, presumably before the subjects went to sleep.

An alternative explanation is suggested by a more recent paper of Hill et al. (1980). They reported a study in which they fed a Western diet to pre- and postmenopausal rural, black, South African women for 9 and 6 weeks respectively. By doing so, they increased the subjects' fat intakes from 15% to 40% of calories. The effect of this was to increase morning (9:00-9:30 AM) serum prolactin levels in the postmenopausal subjects by 20% and luteal-phase, morning, serum prolactin levels in the premenopausal subjects by more than 25%. The follicular-phase prolactin levels were, however, unchanged by this diet. We have no explanation of why there would be such a cycle phase effect, but, if it is not due to chance, then it could explain the difference between our results and those of Hill and Wynder (1976). Our study only measured prolactin on day 11 of the menstrual cycle (follicular phase), whereas they took measurements 2 weeks apart on unstated cycle days.

We also have examined possible dietary effects on plasma prolactin levels among nonmeat-eating, lacto-ovo-vegetarian Seventh-day Adventist (SDA) teenage girls. Mortality data show that Adventist women have a risk of dying of breast cancer some 30% lower than that of the general California population (Phillips and Kuzma 1977). This lower risk has been attributed to their diet.

Contrary to our expectations, the results of this study showed that the diets of the nonmeat-eating SDAs, when expressed as protein, fat, and carbohydrate, were very similar to those of their meat-eating schoolmates (Gray et al. 1981b). No differences in height, weight, age at menarche, or hormone levels were found (Table 5). More surprising still is the fact that they are very similar to other southern California (OSC) white girls of the same age (Table 6). The Adventists had a slightly earlier age at menarche (SDA vs OSC: 12.5 yr vs 12.9 yr) and were very close in height (164.9 cm vs 165.1 cm) and weight (58.0 kg vs

Table 5

Mean Anthropometric Measurements, Age at Menarche, and Hormone Levels of SDA Teenage Girls

	Vegetarians[a]	Nonvegatarians[a]	Total
Number studied	23	26	49
Height (cm)	165.2	164.7	164.9
Weight (kg)	57.2	58.7	58.0
Quetelet's index[b]	20.9	21.6	21.3
Menarche (years)	12.6	12.5	12.5
	Plasma		
Day 11			
E_1 (ng/dl)	6.3	6.8	6.6
E_2 (ng/dl)	6.0	6.3	6.2
Prolactin (ng/ml)	23.1	22.4	22.7
Day 22			
E_1 (ng/dl)	9.2	9.4	9.3
E_2 (ng/dl)	13.2	11.7	12.4
Prolactin (ng/ml)	25.4	21.9	23.4
Progesterone (ng/ml)	3.2	3.9	3.6
	Urine		
Day 11			
E_1 (μg/12 hr)	2.08	2.15	2.12
E_2 (μg/12 hr)	1.24	1.22	1.23
E_3 (μg/12 hr)	2.68	2.83	2.76
$E_3/(E_1 + E_2)$	0.79	0.84	0.81
Day 22			
E_1 (μg/12 hr)	3.98	4.39	4.19
E_2 (μg/12 hr)	2.45	2.49	2.47
E_3 (μg/12 hr)	6.29	6.22	6.25
$E_3/(E_1 + E_2)$	0.97	0.90	0.93

[a]None of the differences between the vegetarians and the nonvegetarians are statistically significant.

[b](Weight/height^2) $\times$ 10,000.

59.7 kg). The frequency of meat consumption of the OSC girls was about double that of the "nonvegetarian" SDAs, but fat provided only 3% more of their calories.

The day-11 plasma hormone levels were quite similar in the SDAs and OSC girls with mean plasma E_1 plus E_2 values of 12.8 ng/dl and 13.1 ng/dl respectively, and plasma prolactin values of 22.7 ng/ml and 23.3 ng/ml. Urine E_1 plus E_2 values were, however, 18% lower in the SDA girls and their E_3 ratio was 31% higher—0.81 for SDAs vs 0.62 for OSC girls.

Table 6

Mean Anthropometric Measurements, Age at Menarche, Dietary Intake, and Hormone Levels of Teenage Girls in Four Countries

	United States	Chile	Japan	Papua New Guinea	p [a]
Number studied	50	51	50	53	
Height (cm)	165.1	157.1	156.9	154.3	0.0001
Weight (kg)	59.7	50.2	51.4	57.4	0.0001
Quetelet's index	21.9	20.3	20.9	24.4	0.0001
Menarche (years)	12.9	13.1	12.6	14.6	0.0001
Plasma (day 11)					
$\quad$ E_1 (ng/dl)	6.7	5.9	6.1	6.7	0.21
$\quad$ E_2 (ng/dl)	6.4	6.2	6.2	6.9	0.77
$\quad$ Prolactin (ng/ml)	23.3	25.9	25.1	21.1	0.09
Urine (day 11)					
$\quad$ E_1 (μg/12 hr)	2.7	2.6	2.2	2.4	0.27
$\quad$ E_2 (μg/12 hr)	1.3	1.3	1.1	1.0	0.13
$\quad$ E_3 (μg/12 hr)	2.5	3.7	2.3	5.1	0.0001
$\quad$ $E_3/(E_1 + E_2)$	0.62	0.96	0.69	1.45	0.0001
Diet					
$\quad$ Protein (% of calories)	15.6	17.6	(14.6)[b]	12.6	0.0001
$\quad$ Fat (% of calories)	40.2	31.6	(21.4)[b]	15.9	0.0001
$\quad$ Carbohydrate (% of calories)	44.2	50.8	(64.0)[b]	71.5	0.0001

[a] Based on F distribution (3 and 200 degrees of freedom).
[b] Not recorded by us: Data from Kagawa (1978).

In a further study, we obtained dietary and hormone measurements from teenage girls in Japan, Papua New Guinea, and Chile to compare with OSC girls referred to above (Gray et al. 1981a). A 3-day diet record was used in all four countries.

The mean anthropometric measurements, ages at menarche, dietary intake by major nutrient group, and hormone levels are shown in Table 6. There are obvious differences in body build between the subjects from the four countries. The Americans were the tallest; they were 8 cm taller than the girls from Chile and Japan, and 11 cm taller than the girls from Papua New Guinea. The American girls were also the heaviest, but Quetelet's index showed that the Papua New Guinea subjects were the most obese and those in Chile and Japan were the thinnest. The mean age at menarche was almost the same (approximately 13 yr) for the girls from the United States, Chile, and Japan, but the Papua New Guinea subjects had their menarche 18-24 months later than the other subjects.

The total caloric intake was similar in the four countries. However, the proportion of calories consumed from fat was greatest among the American subjects and least among those from Papua New Guinea. Although we do not have complete data on the Japanese girls, it is obvious from other surveys that their fat intake (percent of calories) will be somewhere in the range 20-25%; this is greater than the fat intake of the Papua New Guinea subjects but still at most only 60% that of the U.S. subjects.

The only statistically significant differences in mean hormone levels were in urinary E_3 (uE_3) and the uE_3 ratio. The mean uE_3 and E_3 ratio of Papua New Guinea subjects were considerably higher than those from the girls from the other three countries; the Japanese and U.S. results were close, with the results from Chile being intermediate (and statistically significantly different from both Papua New Guinea and the U.S.-Japan results).

Correlation coefficients were calculated to assess the relationships between the anthropometric measurements, age, age at menarche, the percentage of calories from fat, carbohydrate, and protein, and the hormone levels within each country. No consistent relationships between the hormone levels and any of these other factors were found. Similarly, within a country, the anthropometric measurements and age at menarche were not found to be related to the dietary variables.

Thus, although the average diets of the subjects from the four countries studied were very different, with the proportion of calories from fat varying from 16% to 40%, we found no significant differences in their mean prolactin levels. This is in striking contrast to the recent results of Hill et al. (1980), where they showed that rural blacks in South Africa on a low-fat diet (15% of calories) had prolactin values half those of women in New York. The results do, however, agree with the findings of Hayward et al. (1978) who found no significant differences in prolactin levels in Japanese, British, and Japanese-Hawaiian women.

The Papua New Guinea subjects rose much earlier than the other subjects and this may have led to the falsely elevated prolactin values. However, comparison of the mean prolactin values between the United States, Chile, and Japan still permits us to draw a very important conclusion; viz., that at least with diets leading to the same age at menarche, the percentage of calories from fat has no effect on prolactin levels.

CONCLUSION

The net result of the studies reviewed above is to lend some support to the hypothesis that prolactin is an important hormone in breast neoplasia in humans as it is in rodents. Patients and their high-risk family members tend to show elevated levels of prolactin, although these differences may be difficult to demonstrate in older age groups. A full-term pregnancy lowers the prolactin level. No correlation between weight and prolactin level or between any particular dietary nutrient has been demonstrated consistently in humans.

There is some evidence that would seem to be contradictory to a major role for prolactin in breast neoplasia. Thus, it has been pointed out by MacMahon et al. (1973) that prolactin levels are very high during pregnancy and lactation and yet these two conditions do not increase the risk of breast cancer (unless the first pregnancy is after age 35). It is possible that the mix of steroid and polypeptide hormones at these periods is such that these high levels of prolactin lead to glandular differentiation rather than growth promotion. Women using drugs, such as reserpine, that elevate prolactin levels were thought initially to have an increased risk of breast cancer, but recent studies suggest this is not true (Mack et al. 1975). It may be that the role of prolactin is to enhance the mitogenic effect of estrogen rather than to be a primary mitogen itself.

REFERENCES

Anderson, D.E. 1972. A genetic study of human breast cancer. *J. Natl. Cancer Inst.* 48:1029.

————. 1974. Genetic study of breast cancer: Identification of a high risk group. *Cancer* 34:1090.

Boyns, A.R., E.N. Cole, K. Griffiths, M.M. Roberts, R. Buchan, R.G. Wilson, and A.P.M. Forrest. 1973. Plasma prolactin in breast cancer. *Eur. J. Cancer* 9:99.

Cole, E.N., P.C. England, R.A. Sellwood, and K. Griffiths. 1977. Serum prolactin concentrations throughout the menstrual cycle of normal women and patients with recent breast cancer. *Eur. J. Cancer* 13:677.

del Pozo, E. and J. Brownell. 1979. Prolactin I. Mechanism of control, peripheral actions and modifications by drugs. *Horm. Res.* 10:143.

Gray, G.E., M.C. Pike, T. Hirayama, J. Tellez, V. Gerkins, J. Brown, J.T. Casagrande, and B.E. Henderson. 1981a. Diet and hormone profiles in teenage girls in four countries at different risk to breast cancer. *Prev. Med.* (in press).

Gray, G.E., P. Williams, V. Gerkins, J. Brown, B. Armstrong, R. Phillips, J.T. Casagrande, M.C. Pike, and B.E. Henderson. 1981b. Diet and hormone levels in Seventh-Day Adventists teenage girls. *Prev. Med.* (in press).

Hayward, J.L., F.C. Greenwood, G. Glober, G. Stemmermann, R.D. Bulbrook, D.Y. Wang, and S. Kumaoka. 1978. Endocrine status in normal British, Japanese, and Hawaiian-Japanese women. *Eur. J. Cancer* 14:1221.

Henderson, B.E., V. Gerkins, I. Rosario, J. Casagrande, and M.C. Pike. 1975. Elevated serum levels of estrogen and prolactin in daughters of patients with breast cancer. *N. Engl. J. Med.* 293:790.

Hill, P. and E. Wynder. 1976. Diet and prolactin release. *Lancet* ii:806.

Hill, P., E.L. Wynder, H. Kumar, P. Helman, G. Rona, and K. Kuno. 1976. Prolactin levels in populations at risk for breast cancer. *Cancer Res.* 36:4102.

Hill, P., L. Garbaczewski, P. Helman, J. Huskisson, J. Sporangisa, and E.L. Wynder. 1980. Diet, lifestyle and menstrual activity. *Am. J. Clin. Nutr.* 33:1192.

Kagawa, Y. 1978. Impact of Westernization on the nutrition of Japanese: Changes in physique, cancer, longevity and centenarians. *Prev. Med.* 7:205.

Kwa, H.G., E. Engelsman, M. De Jong-Bakker, and F.J. Cleton. 1974. Plasma-prolactin in human breast cancer. *Lancet* i:433.

Kwa, H.G., F. Cleton, M. De Jong-Bakker, R.D. Bulbrook, J.L. Hayward, and D.Y. Wang. 1976. Plasma prolactin and its relationship to risk factors in human breast cancer. *Int. J. Cancer* 17:441.

Kwa, H.G., R.D. Bulbrook, F. Cleton, A.A. Verstraeten, J.L. Hayward, and D.Y. Wang. 1978. An abnormal early evening peak of plasma prolactin in nulliparous and obese post-menopausal women. *Int. J. Cancer* 22:691.

Mack, T.M., B.E. Henderson, V.R. Gerkins, M. Arthur, J. Baptista, and M.C. Pike. 1975. Reserpine and breast cancer in a retirement community. *N. Engl. J. Med.* 293:790.

MacMahon, B., P. Cole, and J. Brown. 1973. Etiology of human breast cancer: A review. *J. Natl. Cancer Inst.* 50:21.

Malarkey, W.B., L.L. Schroeder, V.C. Stevens, A.G. James, and R.R. Lanese. 1977. Disordered nocturnal prolactin regulation in women with breast cancer. *Cancer Res.* 37:4650.

McFayden, I.J., R.J. Prescott, G.V. Groom, A.P.M. Forrest, M.P. Golder, and D.R. Fahmy. 1976. Circulating hormone concentrations in women with breast cancer. *Lancet* i:1100.

Ohgo, S., Y. Kato, K. Chihara, and H. Imura. 1976. Plasma prolactin responses to thyrotropin-releasing hormone in patients with breast cancer. *Cancer* 37:1412.

Phillips, R.L. and J.W. Kuzma. 1977. Rationale and methods for an epidemiologic study of cancer among Seventh-Day Adventists. *Natl. Cancer Inst. Monogr.* 47:107.

Pike, M.C., J.T. Casagrande, J.B. Brown, V. Gerkins, and B.E. Henderson. 1977. Comparison of urinary and plasma hormone levels in daughters of breast cancer patients and controls. *J. Natl. Cancer Inst.* 59:1351.

Pike, M.C., V.R. Gerkins, J.T. Casagrande, G.E. Gray, J. Brown, and B.E. Henderson. 1979. The hormonal basis of breast cancer. *Natl. Cancer Inst. Monogr.* 53:187.

Sheth, N.A., K.J. Ranadive, J.N. Suraiya, and A.R. Sheth. 1975. Circulating levels of prolactin in human breast cancer. *Br. J. Cancer* 32:160.

Vekemans, M. and C. Robyn. 1975. Influence of age on serum prolactin levels in women and men. *Br. Med. J.* 2:738.

Yu, M.C., V.R. Gerkins, B.E. Henderson, J.B. Brown, and M.C. Pike. 1981. Elevated levels of prolactin in nulliparous women. *Br. J. Cancer* (in press).

COMMENTS

MOON: There has been considerable emphasis on prolactin and estrogen levels of the serum or blood, but what is the role of progesterone? Do you have any data on progesterone?

HENDERSON: We have tended to find that progesterone mean values were higher in the daughters of breast cancer patients than in the control daughters. We presume that this indicates that more of such high-risk women are having ovulatory cycles.

MOON: Did you run the progesterone levels for the nuns?

HENDERSON: No.

SEGALOFF: What about the relative risk in nuns? As I understand it, Mick [Bulbrook] and some of the others who worked with the Catholic nuns reported a greater risk than you would expect from the nuns just being nulliparous.

BULBROOK: Gordon Sarfaty did the experiment in Australia and found low androgens in nuns.

SEGALOFF: What is their risk?

HENDERSON: Their risk is elevated some twofold. Whether it is entirely explained by the known risk factors or not, I'm not sure.

MEITES: In connection with Dr. Henderson's talk on human prolactin I would just like to say that the situation in the rats is quite interesting and, after all, rats are what count. In aging rats, prolactin goes up (in both males and females, incidentally) and gonadotropins go down—just the opposite from women. The breast cancer incidence—spontaneous benign fibroadenomas that increase with age—go along together with the increase in prolactin. However, in carcinogen-induced mammary cancers in rats, there is no change. Nagasawa and I (Nagasawa et al. 1973) reported this a few years ago. These rats continued to cycle normally, both during the development of the cancers and after the cancers are established. Prolactin values do not change. Presumably, the estrogen and progesterone values do not change, because they continue to cycle normally.

However, in these carcinogen-induced breast cancers in rats, even though the values are normal, one can change very drastically the development and growth of these breast cancers by increasing or decreasing prolactin. So prolactin really is essential for development and growth of these breast cancers. By manipulating these levels, you can alter the development and growth of breast cancers, even though they normally develop and grow in the face of constant level.

So I would suppose prolactin may have a role even in women—although it may not increase significantly.

SIITERI: I just thought of something that goes with what Joe [Meites] just said, and also what I said. There is one paper in the literature by Hymer et al. (1976) where they looked at mammotrophs in about five women who had breast cancer. They found a very striking degree of hypertrophy as well as hyperplasia, suggesting that the pituitary was seeing a lot of estrogen.

SHELLABARGER: I want to ask Dr. Henderson two quick technical questions. Is the decline in prolactin in the morning after waking or after getting out of bed?

HENDERSON: Those are minutes from waking.

SHELLABARGER: And were those values on the same patient, so that you really know that each patient is going down, or were those just general averages?

HENDERSON· We collected two blood specimens from each female, one at approximately 8:30 AM and one at 10:30 AM. The 10:30 AM prolactin level was lower than the 8:30 AM value for most females, but there was considerable individual variation.

BULBROOK: Kwa, Wang, and I (Kwa et al. 1976) have data on the relation between plasma prolactin and age in a normal population of 4500 women. The fit is cubic and is very highly significant. If you take values for afternoon or for evening blood samples, you still get a significant cubic fit. The levels drop at the menopause and then rise again after age 60, up to age 80. If you ask the question, what 'sort of incidence curve would this generate if prolactin were a promotor, then it would be exactly the curve you find for the southwestern region of England.

The effect of parity on prolactin in these 4500 women is as follows. In premenopausal women, prolactin levels fall, from nulliparous levels to the lowest levels in para-5. But, in the latter, the levels rise again, perhaps 10 years after the multiparous have completed their families, to the levels found in nulliparous women.

From this, one deduces that the epidemiologists have got it wrong again because they don't seem to have studied intensity of reproduction. If prolactin is a carcinogen, then we ought to look at risk in spaced families and bunched ones.

COLE: Intensity of reproduction was one of the things that distinguished the Burmese and the Icelanders. They had extremely high parity over a relatively short period of time, intense reproduction if you will. Both groups have a strong parity effect and little or no age-at-first-birth effect; whereas in São Paulo you also had a high parity, but it was distributed over almost the total reproductive life-span. We wondered about those kinds of things, Mick [Bulbrook], but were never able to make anything more out of it than what I've just said.

PIKE: That's an interesting picture. It's true that we haven't looked at our data in that sort of way.

HENDERSON: We have looked at a number of births and prolactin levels and have found no further drop after the first birth. However, we had few females with more than three births.

References

Hymer, W.C., J. Snyder, W. Wilfinger, R. Bergland, B. Fisher, and O. Pearson. 1976. Characterization of mammotrophs separated from the human pituitary gland. *J. Natl. Cancer Inst.* **57**:995.

Kwa, H.G., F. Cleton, M. De Jong-Bakker, R.D. Bulbrook, J.L. Hayward, and D.Y. Wang. 1976. Plasma prolactin and its relationship to risk factors in human breast cancer. *Int. J. Cancer* **17**:441.

Nagasawa, H., C. Chen, and J. Meites. 1973. Relation between growth of carcinogen-induced mammary cancers and serum prolactin values in rats. *Proc. Soc. Exp. Biol. Med.* **142**:625.

A Prospective Study of the Relation between Thyroid Function and Subsequent Breast Cancer

RICHARD D. BULBROOK, BRIAN S. THOMAS, VERA E. FANTL,
AND JOHN L. HAYWARD
Department of Clinical Endocrinology
Imperial Cancer Research Fund
London, England WC2A 3PX

There is still considerable controversy over the role of the thyroid hormones in the etiology and clinical course of breast cancer. Both hypothyroidism (Repert 1952; Bogardus and Finley 1961) and administration of thyroid hormones (Kapdi and Wolfe 1976) have been claimed to enhance risk, but other workers have found no clear associations (Backwinkel and Jackson 1964; Humphrey and Swerdlow 1964). The confusion in the literature may be exemplified by citing Itoh and Maruchi (1975), who found that Hashimoto's thyroiditis was associated with an increased incidence of breast cancer, whereas Maruchi et al. (1976) did not.

During the past 18 years, we have measured various aspects of endocrine function in a population of 10,000 normal women living on the island of Guernsey (Bulbrook and Hayward 1967; Bulbrook et al. 1971). The population has been followed up, and 78 cases of breast cancer have occurred. It is now possible to examine whether abnormalities in thyroid function were present in these women before their cancer developed. In addition, thyroid function has been assessed in other high-risk groups—women with a family history of breast cancer and women whose estimated risk of developing breast cancer was calculated using the mathematical model described by Farewell (1977).

METHODS

The Population Studied

Guernsey prospective trial 1. Between 1961 and 1968, a single 24-hr urine specimen was collected from each of 5000 normal women aged 30 to 65 years. In 1500 of these women, urinary androsterone and etiocholanolone were measured. The ratio of these two steroids (the $5\alpha/5\beta$ ratio) is a sensitive index of thyroid function (Hellman et al. 1959). Breast cancer developed subsequently in 48 women (termed precancer cases).

Guernsey prospective trial 2. Between 1968 and 1975, a 50-ml sample of blood was obtained from a further 5000 normal Guernsey women. Plasma was separated and stored at −20°C. Triiodothyronine (T3), thyroxine (T4), and thyroid-stimulating hormone (TSH) were measured in various subsets of these women. Breast cancer developed in 30 women in this population.

Women with a family history of breast cancer. The occurrence of familiar disease in the Guernsey population was elicited by questionnaire, without further confirmation. Women who reported that their sisters or mothers had had breast cancer were included in family history groups.

Women with a calculated estimate of risk. The estimated probability of developing breast cancer was calculated using the method of Farewell (1977). This is based on age at menarche, age at first child, family history, and the excretion of etiocholanolone in the urine. Four broad risk groups (0, 1, 2, 3) can be delineated with an estimated probability of developing breast cancer of 0.010, 0.022, 0.051, 0.111, respectively. Plasma specimens were available for 377 women for whom a risk estimate had been computed.

Analytical Methods

Urinary androsterone (5α-androstane-3α-ol-17-one) and etiocholanolone (5β-androstane-3α-ol-17-one) were measured by the method of Thomas (1978, 1980).

Radioimmunoassay of plasma T3 and T4 was performed according to the methods recommended by Ratcliffe et al. (1974). Antisera against both hormones, raised in sheep, were purchased from Precision Assays Ltd. (Great Britain). TSH was measured by the method of Hall et al. (1971).

Oral contraceptives increased plasma T3 levels from the control mean of 1.58 to 2.13 nmoles/liter ($P < 0.001$) and T4 levels from 97.5 to 137.4 nmoles/liter ($P < 0.001$). Women taking oral contraceptives, therefore, were excluded from the study.

RESULTS

The 5α/5β Ratio in Precancer Cases and in Women with a Family History of Breast Cancer

The 5α/5β ratio for controls, precancer cases, and women whose mothers or sisters had breast cancer are shown in Figure 1, for subjects aged less than 36 years and for those aged 36-40 years. There are no differences in the ratios for the 3 groups of women: Both of the high-risk groups appear to be random samples from the normal population. Similar results were found for the 41-45-year-old women (data not shown). From this result we can conclude that up to the age of 45 years, thyroid dysfunction is not related to the enhanced risk carried by women with a positive family history of breast cancer, nor is it of etiological significance in the precancer group.

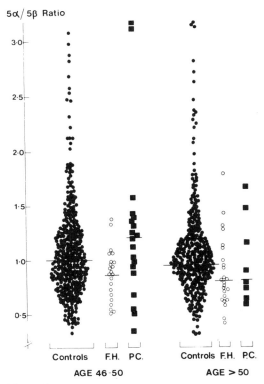

5α/5β Ratio

Controls   F.H.   P.C.

AGE 46-50

Controls F.H. P.C.

AGE > 50

Figure 1
The 5α/5β ratio in controls in women with a family history (F.H.) of breast cancer and in precancer (P.C.) cases. Age range 36-40 years. Horizontal bars show the medians.

Results for women aged 46-50, or more than 50 years, are shown in Figure 2. Once again, there are no significant differences between the 5α/5β ratios in the precancer cases and their normal controls, but the ratios for the family history groups are clearly at the lower end of the normal range. Of 46 such women, no less than 37 have values of the 5α/5β ratio below that for the median value of the 660 age-matched controls, a difference in distribution that is highly significant (χ^2 = 16.0; $P < 0.001$).

Precancer Cases with and without a Family History of Breast Cancer

If women aged over 45 years, at enhanced risk because of a positive family history, have low 5α/5β ratios, then the logical question to ask is whether the precancer cases (who by definition are a 100% risk group) show a similar relationship. Accordingly, the data for such women (shown in Figs. 1 and 2) were

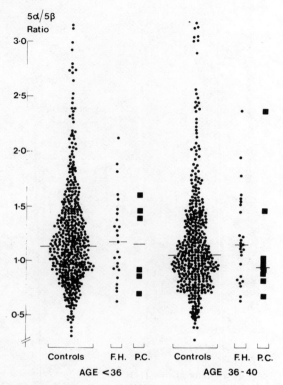

Figure 2

The $5\alpha/5\beta$ ratio in controls (●), women with a family history of breast cancer (○), and in precancer cases (□). Age range 45-50 years. Horizontal bars show the medians.

reanalyzed, and the ratios for precancer cases with a positive history were compared with those from precancer cases with no history of breast cancer within their family. The results are shown in Figure 3.

Although the numbers are small, it is quite apparent that the $5\alpha/5\beta$ ratio in precancer cases with a positive family history became increasingly subnormal with advancing age and that the results for this group are in harmony with those found for the family history group who have not yet developed breast cancer.

The $5\alpha/5\beta$ Ratio in Calculated High-risk Groups

The $5\alpha/5\beta$ ratio was measured in 337 women whose risk of breast cancer had been calculated by the method described by Farewell (1977). The results are shown in Table 1. There are no significant differences between the ratios in any of the risk groups, either in pre- or postmenopausal women.

Table 1

The 5α/5β Ratio in Women at Varying Degrees of Estimated Risk

	Risk group			
	0	1	2	3
Premenopausal	1.08 ± 0.37 (24)	1.14 ± 0.43 (84)	1.13 ± 0.37 (93)	1.21 ± 0.45 (36)
Postmenopausal	1.05 ± 0.23 (7)	1.05 ± 0.47 (41)	1.12 ± 0.48 (50)	1.06 ± 0.46 (42)

The means of the 5α/5β ratios are shown ± S.D.

Figures in brackets are numbers of women in each category. Risk groups calculated by combining age at menarche, age at first child, family history, and excretion of etiocholanolone (see Farewell 1977).

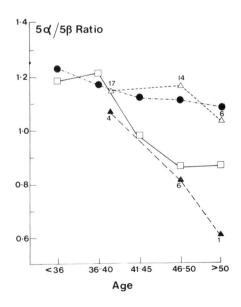

Figure 3

The 5α/5β ratio by age in controls (●) in women with a family history of breast cancer (□), in precancer cases with no family history (△), and in precancer cases with a positive family history (▲). The numbers above points on the curves show the number of subjects.

Plasma T3, T4, and TSH Levels in Precancer Cases and in Women with a Family History of Breast Cancer

The mean plasma level of T3 in 90 controls was 1.46 ± 0.25 (S.D.) nmoles/liter compared with 1.40 ± 0.24 (S.D.) nmoles/liter in 30 precancer cases. The difference is not significant. The comparable figures for T4 are 96.2 ± 22.2 (S.D.) nmoles/liter and 91.8 ± 16.9 (S.D.) nmoles/liter; again, the means do not differ. There are insufficient data for analyzing these results by age.

Plasma T3, T4, and TSH levels in matched controls and in normal women whose mothers or sisters had breast cancer are shown in Table 2.

There are no significant differences for any given comparison of means. These results disagree with those found for the $5\alpha/5\beta$ ratios where a trend towards hypothyroid ratios was found for women with a positive family history, provided that they were aged more than 45 years.

Precancer Cases, with or without a Family History of Breast Cancer

When plasma T3 levels in precancer cases with or without a family history of breast cancer were compared with those of controls (Fig. 4), it is apparent that

Table 2

Plasma T3, T4, and TSH, by Age, in Controls, and in Women with a Mother or Sister with Breast Cancer

Hormones	Age group	Controls	Mothers	Sisters
T3	30-39	1.46 ± 0.26 (21)	1.53 ± 0.25 (39)	1.35 ± 0.36 (9)
	40-49	1.48 ± 0.29 (20)	1.53 ± 0.26 (47)	1.64 ± 0.22 (14)
	50+	1.58 ± 0.28 (42)	1.55 ± 0.23 (61)	1.60 ± 0.22 (46)
T4	30-39	98.8 ± 21.1 (22)	94.2 ± 15.5 (39)	87.0 ± 17.7 (9)
	40-49	94.7 ± 13.6 (20)	97.4 ± 18.6 (47)	107.6 ± 23.8 (14)
	50+	101.0 ± 19.5 (42)	99.1 ± 18.7 (61)	96.7 ± 18.0 (46)
TSH	30-39	3.28 ± 1.74 (22)	3.31 ± 2.05 (33)	3.86 ± 5.00 (8)
	40-49	3.93 ± 2.58 (20)	4.09 ± 2.60 (38)	3.54 ± 1.95 (12)
	50+	4.22 ± 3.05 (42)	4.50 ± 2.55 (55)	4.65 ± 2.59 (38)

The means of the T3 and T4 plasma levels (in nmoles/liter) are shown $\pm$ S.D. Figures in parentheses are numbers of women in each group.

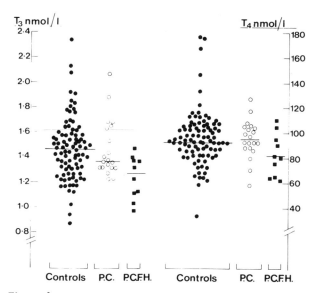

Figure 4

Plasma T3 and T4 values for controls (●), precancer cases with either no family history of breast cancer (○) or a positive history (■). Horizontal bars show the medians.

the precancer family history group has T3 values at the lower end of the normal range: All 10 cases are below the median of the control value. A similar but less marked trend was found for T4. These results are in striking agreement with those found for the $5\alpha/5\beta$ ratio in precancer cases with a positive family history (see Fig. 3).

Plasma T3, T4, and TSH in Calculated High-risk Groups

The plasma levels of T3 and T4 by calculated risk group are shown in Figures 5 and 6 for pre- and postmenopausal women. The complete absence of any variation in the levels of these hormones with increasing risk makes a statistical analysis superfluous.

DISCUSSION

Women in Guernsey who subsequently developed breast cancer and who had no family history of breast cancer appear to have no abnormalities in thyroid function in the decade before their disease is diagnosed. This conclusion is supported by the finding that no thyroid abnormalities were observed in women whose risk of breast cancer was calculated by the method of Farewell (1977). Because

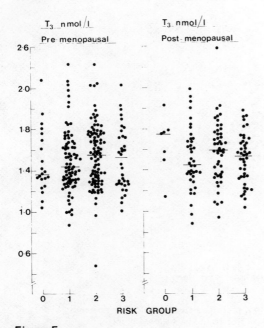

Figure 5
Plasma T3 values in relation to increasing estimated risk of breast cancer, in pre- and post-menopausal women. For definition of risk groups, see Methods section. Horizontal bars show the medians.

the majority of women who develop breast cancer have no history of the disease in their families, it can be concluded that thyroid dysfunction is not an important factor in the etiology of the disease in the generality of women.

There is, however, a substantial subgroup of women where the thyroid gland does appear to be involved. These are women whose $5\alpha/5\beta$ ratios and plasma T3 and T4 values indicate some degree of hypothyroidism and who also have a mother or a sister with breast cancer. The abnormality only appears in peri- and postmenopausal women.

A consistent finding has been that women with first-degree relatives with breast cancer are at two- or threefold risk. Anderson (1975) has pointed out that the disease is heterogenous in etiology and that very high risks are found in premenopausal women whose relatives also had premenopausal disease, especially if it was bilateral. Our results indicate the possibility of another genetic subset in that some thyroid abnormalities are inheritable (see Hutchinson and McGirr 1956). This would be in line with the suggestion by Bain et al. (1980) that part of the increased risk of breast cancer associated with a family history might be mediated through the inheritance of features associated with reproductive function, such as age at menarche.

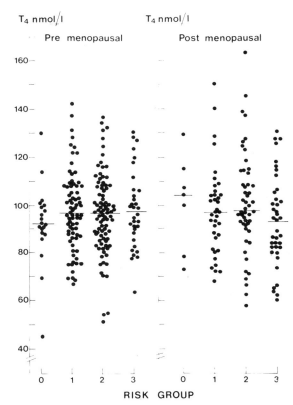

Figure 6

Plasma T4 values in relation to increasing estimated risk of breast cancer, in pre- and post-menopausal women.

Our data are not wholly consistent: Whereas $5\alpha/5\beta$ ratios were subnormal in women aged over 45 years with a family history of breast cancer, the plasma T3 and T4 levels were in the normal range. This raises the question of the feasibility of distinguishing small differences in thyroid function using the analytical methods described earlier. Of the two, it appears to us that the indirect assessment of thyroid function using the $5\alpha/5\beta$ ratio is to be preferred, because the ratio gives an end point of the biological activity of the thyroid hormones. The range of the ratio between frank hypothyroidism and hyper-thyroidism is wide (some tenfold), whereas, in our hands, the T3 and T4 measurements appear to be insensitive. It might be sensible to repeat the experiments using more sophisticated methods for the direct assessment of thyroid function.

Finally, our results do not resolve much of the existing confusion concerning the thyroid and breast cancer. They indicate that thyroid function may be important only in a limited group of women and that, for the majority of patients, it is unlikely that thyroid dysfunction is an important determinant of risk.

REFERENCES

Anderson, D.E. 1975. Familial susceptibility. In *Persons at high risk of cancer* (ed. J.F. Fraumeni), p. 39. Academic Press, New York and London.

Backwinkel, K. and A.S. Jackson. 1964. Some features of breast cancer and thyroid deficiency: Report of 280 cases. *Cancer* 17:1174.

Bain, C., F.E. Speizer, B. Rosner, C. Belanger, and C.H. Hennekens. 1980. Family history of breast cancer as a risk indicator for the disease. *Am. J. Epidemiol.* 111:301.

Bogardus, G.M. and J.W. Finley. 1961. Breast cancer and thyroid disease. *Surgery* 49:491.

Bulbrook, R.D. and J.L. Hayward. 1967. Abnormal urinary steroid excretion and subsequent breast cancer. *Lancet* i:519.

Bulbrook, R.D., J.L. Hayward, and C.C. Spicer. 1971. Relation between urinary androgen and corticosteroid excretion and subsequent breast cancer. *Lancet* ii:1971.

Farewell, V.T. 1977. The combined effect of breast cancer risk factors. *Cancer* 40:931.

Hall, R., J. Amos, and B.J. Ormston. 1971. Radioimmunoassay of human serum thyrotrophin. *Br. Med. J.* 1:582.

Hellman, L., H.L. Bradlow, B. Zumoff, D.K. Fukushima, and T.F. Gallagher. 1959. Thyroid-androgen interactions and the hypocholesteremic effect of androsterone. *J. Clin. Endocrinol. Metab.* 19:396.

Humphrey, L.J. and M. Swerdlow. 1964. The relationship of breast disease to thyroid disease. *Cancer* 17:1170.

Hutchinson, J.H. and F.M. McGirr. 1956. Sporadic nonendemic goitrous cretinism. Hereditary transmission. *Lancet* i:1035.

Itoh, K. and N. Maruchi. 1975. Breast cancer in patients with Hashimoto's thyroiditis. *Lancet* ii:1119.

Kapdi, C.C. and J.N. Wolfe. 1976. Breast cancer. Relation to thyroid supplements for hypothyroidism. *J. Am. Med. Assoc.* 236:1124.

Maruchi, N., J.F. Annegers, and L.T. Kurland. 1976. Hashimoto's thyroiditis and breast cancer. *Mayo Clin. Proc.* 51:263.

Ratcliffe, W.A., G.S. Ghalland, and J.G. Ratcliffe. 1974. A critical evaluation of separation methods in radioimmunoassays for total triiodothyronine and thyroxine in unextracted human serum. *Ann. Clin. Biochem.* 11:224.

Repert, R.W.J. 1952. Breast carcinoma study: Relation to thyroid disease and diabetes. *J. Mich. St. Med. Soc.* 51:1315.

Thomas, B.S. 1978. Subtle gas chromatography. In *Blood, drugs and other analytical challenges* (ed. E. Reid), p. 77. Ellis Horwood, Chicester, England.

————. 1980. Steroid analysis by gas chromatography with SCOT and widebore WCOT columns. *High Resolution Chromatography and Chromatography Communications* 3:241.

COMMENTS

LIPPMAN: Mick [Bulbrook], can you tell me something about androgen excretion in these Guernsey women as it might relate to either height or weight? Is that a linkage that exists or not? Is there a way of putting together those risk factors?

BULBROOK: The androgens are highly correlated with weight.

LIPPMAN: How about height independent of fat?

BULBROOK: I've not looked at it. But, as we don't believe that weight is a risk factor, we usually shrug that one off. It's very highly correlated with weight.

LIPPMAN: Well, how could you shrug it off if it's highly correlated with weight and your factor is highly correlated with risk? I don't see how you can do that from your own data.

BULBROOK: Fair criticism. I haven't got any answer, so the sensible thing to do is to answer some other question.

SIITERI: I would like to remind you of my summary slide showing that the $5\alpha/5\beta$ ratio is low—which really is the only thing Mick has published that I really believe. From Barney's [Zumoff] studies with Jack Fishman, a low $5\alpha/5\beta$ ratio can be correlated with hypothyroidism. That would fit perfectly well with the finding of low sex-hormone-binding globulin (SHBG) levels in cancer patients because thyroid hormones are a potent stimulus for SHBG. That's why I had TSH, T4, and T3 on that slide because in my mind it's the only way that I can make a link between the thyroid hormone status and estrogenicity through the binding globulin.

BULBROOK: Yes.

LIPPMAN: Obesity is there.

SIITERI: Well, if low thyroid increases estrogen availability, then the estrogen could chronically elevate prolactin.

LIPPMAN: It used to be popular to say that those people who were hypothyroid had high thyrotropin-releasing hormone (TRH) levels and high prolactin. But hypothyroid people do have higher prolactin.

KORENMAN: They do.

Abnormal Plasma Hormone Levels in Women with Breast Cancer

BARNETT ZUMOFF
Clinical Research Center
Institute for Steroid Research and the Department of Oncology
Montefiore Hospital and Medical Center
Bronx, New York 10467

Cancer of the breast is described as hormone-dependent on the basis of two facts: It arises from a tissue that normally is responsive to endogenous hormones, and its course often can be influenced, favorably or unfavorably, by administration of hormones or removal of hormones (by surgical or radiation ablation of endocrine glands or by administration of antihormones). Because of the therapeutic effects of iatrogenic alterations of the hormonal environment, there has been considerable interest in the possibility that the endogenous hormonal environment may be related either to the induction of breast cancer or to its untreated clinical course. We have studied this problem by measuring the 24-hr mean plasma concentration of 14 hormones or hormone metabolites in carefully selected breast cancer patients and healthy controls. We have found abnormalities in three areas: Thyroid hormones, adrenal androgens, and luteinizing hormone (LH).

PLASMA LEVELS OF THYROID HORMONES

There is considerable literature, going back nearly 30 years (Repert 1952), suggesting on epidemiological grounds that breast cancer in women is associated with abnormalities of thyroid function. Most frequently, it is suggested that the association is with hypothyroidism, because the incidence of breast cancer parallels that of endemic goiter due to iodine deficiency (Doll 1969; Stadel 1976), is decreased in hyperthyroid patients (Finley and Bogardus 1960; Humphrey and Swerdlow 1964), and is increased in patients who are receiving thyroid hormone therapy for the treatment of hypothroidism (Kapdi and Wolfe 1972). An occasional report (Wanebo et al. 1966) describes an association between hyperthyroidism and increased incidence of breast cancer. A careful study by Schottenfeld (1968) of his own patients (including measurement of protein-bound iodine [PBI] levels) and of the literature up to that time failed to confirm a relationship between hypothyroidism and breast cancer. The American Thyroid Association subsequently resummarized and commented upon the evidence for hypothyroidism in breast cancer in two editorial statements (Gorman et al. 1977a,b) and also found it unconvincing.

Only a few studies of the uptake and (or) conversion of radioactive iodide have been carried out in breast cancer. The first was by Edelstyn et al. (1958), who concluded that thyroid function was decreased; Reeve et al. (1961) found normal function; Lencioni et al. (1962) found slightly subnormal function; Stoll (1965) found normal function; and Bignazzi et al. (1965) found values compatible with hyperthyroidism, although there were no corresponding clinical signs.

Mittra and Hayward (1974), using the indirect approach of measuring thyroid-stimulating hormone (TSH) levels, found slightly increased basal and thyrotropin-releasing hormone (TRH)-stimulated TSH levels in women with breast cancer, which they interpreted as indicating ". . . the presence of relatively low levels of circulating thyroid hormones in breast cancer." Unaccountably, they did not report the levels of the plasma thyroid hormones themselves in their patients, even though these might have confirmed their hypothesis.

Prior to the availability of radioimmunoassay (RIA) methods for determining plasma thyroxine (T4) and triiodothyronine (T3) levels, six studies of plasma PBI levels (essentially equivalent to T4 levels) in women with breast cancer were reported. Carter et al. (1960) found a statistically significant elevation; Dargent et al. (1962) also found significantly elevated levels, Lencioni et al. (1962) found normal levels, Myhill et al. (1966) found elevated levels in metastatic breast cancer but not in localized disease, Schottenfeld (1968) reported normal levels, and Sicher and Waterhouse (1967) found normal levels.

Since RIA methods became available, there have been four published reports of plasma levels of thyroid hormones in women with breast cancer. Rose and Davis (1978) found normal levels of T4; they did, however, find slightly elevated TSH levels in a small percentage of their patients. In a subsequent paper (Rose and Davis 1979), these authors reported slightly subnormal levels of T3. Adami et al. (1978) found normal levels of T4, slightly subnormal levels of T3, and slightly elevated levels of TSH. MacFarlane et al. (1978), in contrast, found elevated levels of T4, with normal levels of T3 and TSH; they found similar elevations of T4 in women with benign breast disease, so that the abnormality was not specific for breast cancer.

Inasmuch as plasma T4 and T3 concentrations show considerable fluctuation throughout the 24-hr diurnal cycle (O'Connor et al. 1974; Balsam et al. 1975), as do those of many hormones (Weitzman et al. 1966; Takahashi et al. 1968; Hellman et al. 1970; Krieger and Glick 1971; Yen et al. 1972; Finkelstein et al. 1973; West et al. 1973; Boyar et al. 1973, 1974a,b), the concentration in a single spot sample may be unrepresentative and therefore misleading. For this reason, we initially measured the 24-hr mean plasma concentrations of T4 and T3 in a group of 27 normal control subjects and a group of 29 breast cancer patients rigorously selected to exclude any factors known or suspected to affect endocrine function (e.g., significant past or current disease, medications, and previous chemotherapy or endocrine therapy). Because we found elevated T4 levels in these breast cancer patients, we measured 8 AM spot plasma T4 levels in a second and larger group of 43 unselected breast cancer patients, a group of 22 women with other-than-breast cancer, and a group of 21 women with miscellaneous noncancerous illnesses, and we compared these levels with 8 AM spot levels from the original normal controls.

The group of selected breast cancer patients consisted of 21 women with localized disease (8 operable and 13 inoperable) and 8 with metastatic disease. The group of unselected breast cancer patients consisted of women with cancer in all stages. The group of patients with other-than-breast cancer consisted of 7 women with cancer of the ovary, 3 with cancer of the cervix, 3 with cancer of the lung, 2 with cancer of the kidney, 2 with cancer of the colon, and 1 each with cancer of the esophagus, stomach, rectum, endometrium, and liver. The diagnoses of the patients with miscellaneous noncancerous illnesses are listed in Table 1. The normal control group consisted of healthy women aged 21-75 (plasma T4 and T3 levels are age-invariant).

The patients' 24-hr mean plasma concentrations were determined by sampling venous blood every 20 min around the clock, pooling aliquots of the 72 specimens, and measuring the concentration of hormone in the pooled

Table 1
Clinical Data of the Women with Miscellaneous Noncancerous Illnesses

Subject	Age	Diagnosis
1	35	hyperprolactinemia
2	34	Stein-Leventhal syndrome
3	34	schizophrenia
4	32	Stein-Leventhal syndrome
5	97	postmenopausal bleeding
6	47	familial polyposis
7	42	reactive depression
8	64	insulinoma
9	32	galactorrhea of unknown origin
10	64	psychotic depression
11	50	diabetes mellitus
12	35	hyperprolactinemia
13	62	cerebello-pontine degeneration
14	49	chronic insomnia
15	47	diabetes mellitus
16	60	ulcer of the ankle
17	45	coronary heart disease
18	66	reactive depressive
19	32	premature ovarian failure
20	62	psychotic depression
21	57	mesenchymal tumor

sample; details of this technique have been described previously from this laboratory (Zumoff et al. 1980). T4 and T3 concentrations were determined by RIA.

We found no difference between the selected breast cancer patients and the normal controls with respect to the 24-hr mean T3 concentration (Fig. 1), but there was a marked and highly significant ($P < 0.001$) difference between the groups with respect to 24-hr mean T4 levels (Fig. 2). The normal women had a geometric mean value of 5.8 μg/dl[1], whereas that of the cancer patients was increased by 33% to 7.7 μg/dl; the mean values for patients with localized disease and patients with metastatic disease were both 7.7 μg/dl.

The 8 AM spot plasma T4 levels showed a similar elevation over normal in the breast cancer patients. The geometric mean level for the cancer patients was 8.8 μg/dl, 21% higher than the value of 7.3 μg/dl in the normal controls ($P < 0.005$) (Fig. 3). The fact that the breast cancer vs normal difference was slightly smaller percentagewise for spot samples than for 24-hr samples, with a

[1] 24-Hr mean values for plasma T4 are lower than spot morning values because of diurnal fluctuation, with lower T4 values in the afternoon and night.

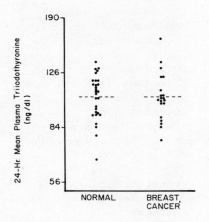

Figure 1
24-Hr mean plasma T3 concentration in normal women and selected women with breast cancer. P = N.S.

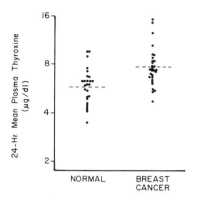

Figure 2
24-Hr mean plasma T4 concentration in normal women and selected women with breast cancer. $P < 0.001$.

correspondingly slightly lower significance of the difference, is due probably to the greater clinical heterogeneity of the patients in the spot group and the greater interindividual variation of spot than of 24-hr mean values.

The spot T4 values for the women with other than breast cancer and with miscellaneous noncancerous illnesses essentially were identical to those of the women with breast cancer (Fig. 4), i.e., significantly elevated above normal levels.

Our findings of normal plasma T3 levels and elevated plasma T4 levels in women with breast cancer agree with those of MacFarlane et al. (1978); the latter authors also found normal levels of TSH, which we did not measure. These two studies provide clear-cut evidence against the presence of the hypothyroidism in women with breast cancer. The other two groups that have

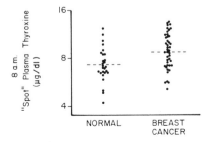

Figure 3
8 AM spot plasma T4 concentration in normal women and unselected women with breast cancer. $P < 0.005$.

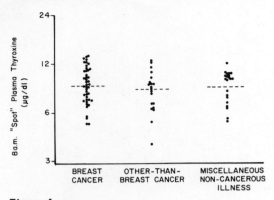

Figure 4

Comparison of 8 AM spot plasma T4 concentration in unselected women with breast cancer, women with other-than-breast cancer, and women with miscellaneous noncancerous illnesses. The means for all three groups are essentially identical and all are significantly higher than that of normal women.

reported plasma thyroid hormone levels in breast cancer (Rose and Davis 1978, 1979; Adami et al. 1978) both described normal T4 levels, slightly decreased T3 levels, and slightly increased TSH levels. This, too, is certainly not hypothyroidism in any usual sense; the findings are most nearly compatible with the nonspecific low-T3 syndrome (Bermudez et al. 1975), although TSH levels generally are not elevated in the latter (Maturlo et al. 1980).

What are we to make of the fact that two of the four studies that have been done found elevated T4 levels and three of the six studies that have been done found elevated PBI levels in women with breast cancer? Although it is obvious to experienced clinicians that women with breast cancer do not, as a group, have overt clinical hyperthyroidism, the possibility that they may have more subtle degrees of this dysfunction cannot be dismissed out of hand. To be sure, MacFarlane found that women with benign breast disease showed just as much elevation of T4 levels as women with breast cancer, and we found that women with other-than-breast cancer and women with miscellaneous noncancerous illnesses showed just as much T4 elevation as women with breast cancer; thus, increased T4 levels, if they are characteristic of women with breast cancer, are not specific to that disease. Indeed, it may well be that hyperthyroxinemia represents another nonspecific thyroid dysfunction in illness, in addition to the well-documented hypotriiodothyroninemia.

PLASMA LEVELS OF ADRENAL ANDROGENS

One of the first hormonal groups studied in breast cancer was the adrenal androgens. The earliest publication in this area was by Allen et al. (1957), who investigated the urinary excretion of various steroids prior to adrenalectomy or hypophysectomy for the treatment of breast cancer and found that the ratio of 11-deoxy-17-ketosteroids (derived from adrenal androgens) to 11-oxo-17-ketosteroids (derived from cortisol) was considerably lower in patients who did not respond to the operation. This approach was expanded and refined over the next few years, culminating in the formulation of the Bulbrook discriminant relating the urinary excretion of etiocholanolone to that of 17-hydroxycorticosteroids (Bulbrook et al. 1960); negative values of the discriminant (i.e., low levels of etiocholanolone) were associated with poor response to adrenalectomy or hypophysectomy, whereas positive values (i.e., normal levels of etiocholanolone) were associated with good response. Juret et al. (1964) and Kumaoka et al. (1968), while confirming the predictive value of the level of urinary androgen metabolite excretion in patients undergoing adrenalectomy or hypophysectomy, reported that the corticoid excretion values added no useful information and could be omitted.

Bulbrook et al. (1962) reported that women with primary operable breast cancer excreted subnormal amounts of 11-deoxy-17-ketosteroids in the urine prior to mastectomy and suggested that this abnormality might precede the clinical onset of the disease. To explore this possibility, these workers set up a large-scale study on the island of Guernsey, in which urines were collected from about 5000 healthy women who were then followed clinically for up to 9 years. At the end of that time, as subsequently reported (Bulbrook et al. 1971), 27 of the women had developed breast cancer, most or perhaps all of them at either premenopausal age or just beyond. The excretion of various metabolites in the urines collected initially (i.e., 5 months to 9 years before the clinical diagnosis of the cancer) was compared with that of 187 carefully matched controls from the same population who had not developed cancer, and it was found that the excretion of both etiocholanolone and androsterone (the two principal urinary metabolites of the adrenal androgens) was significantly lower in the women who had gone on to manifest breast cancer. These results appear to confirm that subnormal urinary excretion of adrenal androgen metabolites is present before clinical breast cancer develops. A follow-up paper from this group (Wang et al. 1975) suggests that this abnormality may be genetic in origin: It was found that a group of 52 unaffected sisters of the Guernsey study women who developed breast cancer likewise showed subnormal urinary excretion of androsterone and etiocholanolone.

More recently, with the development of suitable analytical methods, the attention of workers in this field has turned to the measurement of plasma adrenal androgen levels. Wang (1971) initially reported normal plasma levels of dehydroisoandrosterone sulfate (DHAS) and its metabolite androsterone sulfate in women with breast cancer, but after Brownsey et al. (1972) had reported subnormal DHAS levels in these women, Wang et al. (1974) confirmed this finding in a later restudy; they also found subnormal levels of androsterone sulfate. Šonká et al. (1973) reported subnormal plasma levels of "dehydroisoandrosterone" in breast cancer, but their method, employing solvolysis, measured both dehydroisoandrosterone (DHA) and DHAS, and because the latter is present at hundreds of times the concentration of the former, the data represent essentially the levels of DHAS. Rose et al. (1977) also reported that breast cancer patients had subnormal plasma levels of DHAS, and they added the information that plasma androstenedione levels were normal in these patients; Wang et al. (1977), however, reported subnormal levels of androstenedione. Thomas et al. (1976) appear to have published the only study of plasma DHA levels in women with breast cancer; they reported subnormal levels in these women.

We were prompted to restudy plasma DHA and DHAS levels in women with breast cancer for three reasons:

1. Reported plasma levels have been measured in spot samples, but studies from this and other laboratories have shown that the levels of many hormones, specifically including DHA (Rosenfeld et al. 1971), fluctuate markedly (up to several hundred percent) during a 24-hr cycle, so that spot values may be unrepresentative and therefore misleading. To avoid this problem, we measured the 24-hr mean plasma concentrations.

2. The groups of patients reported in most studies have been heterogeneous, sometimes complicated by other diseases and (or) medications, and sometimes poorly or not at all characterized by stage of disease. We have studied only well-characterized patients with primary operable breast cancer and normal controls, with both groups rigorously selected to exclude factors known or suspected to alter endocrine function.

3. The distinction between premenopausal and postmenopausal breast cancer often has not been taken into consideration, despite the fact that various lines of evidence point to the possibility that premenopausal and postmenopausal breast cancer may represent two biologically and epidemiologically distinct diseases (de Waard et al. 1960; de Waard 1979; Manton and Stallard 1980). In the present study, we considered the results for premenopausal and postmenopausal breast cancer patients separately and found different DHA and DHAS abnormalities in these two groups.

Since the 24-hr mean plasma levels of both DHA and DHAS normally show an inverse linear correlation with age (Zumoff et al. 1980), we studied enough healthy controls ($n = 37$) over the age range 21-75 to define the regression line adequately. The group of breast cancer patients consisted of 11 women, aged 31-78, with clinically operable stage 1 or 2 breast cancer studied preoperatively.

DHA was determined by RIA, as described by Rosenfeld et al. (1975), and DHAS was determined by RIA, as described by Nieschlag et al. (1972). To help define the mechanism of the abnormalities in DHA and DHAS levels that will be described, we also determined the 24-hr mean plasma concentration of androsterone in all patients and controls, using the RIA method of Kream et al. (1976).

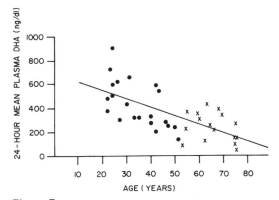

Figure 5
24-Hr mean plasma DHA concentration in normal women. (×) Postmenopausal; (●) pre-menopausal; $y = 696 - 7.2\times$; $r = -0.68$; $P < 0.001$.

We found that, in contrast to the marked and progressive decline of DHA and DHAS concentrations with age in normal women (Fig. 5 and 6), the concentrations of both steroids were age-invariant in the patients over the age range 32-78 (Fig. 7 and 8). When the regression lines of steroid concentration vs age in normal women and cancer patients were superimposed for DHA (Fig. 9) and DHAS (Fig. 10), a striking picture emerged: The two superimpositions resembled each other very closely—in each case, the regression line for cancer patients crossed that for normal women in the 45-50 age range, i.e., about at menopause; the farther in either direction from the crossover point, the greater the differ-

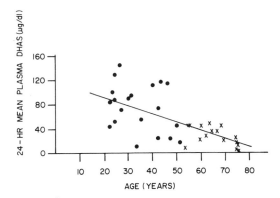

Figure 6
24-Hr mean plasma DHAS concentration in normal women. (×) Postmenopausal; (●) pre-menopausal; $y = 120 - 1.36\times$; $r = -0.63$; $P < 0.001$.

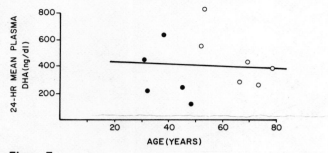

Figure 7

24-Hr mean plasma DHA concentration in women with operable breast cancer. The level is age-invariant. (●) Premenopausal; (○) postmenopausal; $y = 446 - 0.9x$; $r = -0.07$; P = N.S.

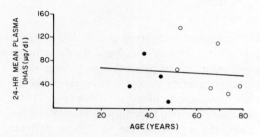

Figure 8

24-Hr mean plasma DHAS concentration in women with operable breast cancer. The level is age-invariant. (●) Premenopausal; (○) postmenopausal; $y = 72 - 0.2x$; $r = -0.08$; P = N.S.

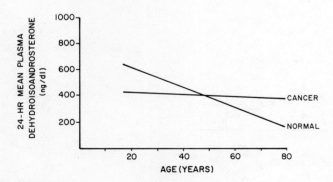

Figure 9

Superimposed regression lines of the 24-hr mean plasma DHA concentrations in normal women ($r = -0.65$; $P < 0.001$) and women with operable breast cancer. Note the crossover at about the age of menopause.

152

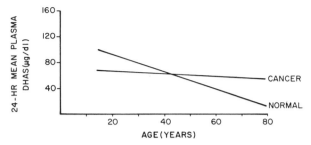

Figure 10
Superimposed regression lines of the 24-hr mean plasma DHAS concentrations in normal women ($r = 0.63; P < 0.001$) and women with operable breast cancer. Note the crossover at about the age of menopause.

ence between normals and patients. The direction of the DHA and DHAS abnormalities differed in premenopausal and postmenopausal patients—the levels of both steroids were subnormal in premenopausal patients and supranormal in postmenopausal patients (this is shown for DHA in a conventional scattergram in Fig. 11).

In premenopausal cancer patients, the DHA/androsterone ratio essentially was identical to that of premenopausal controls (Fig. 12). In postmenopausal

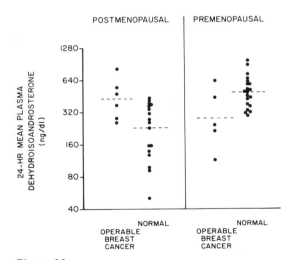

Figure 11
24-Hr mean plasma DHA levels in premenopausal operable breast cancer patients and normal controls ($P < 0.0005$) and in postmenopausal operable breast cancer patients and normal controls ($P < 0.025$). The premenopausal patients have significantly subnormal values and the postmenopausal patients have significantly supranormal values.

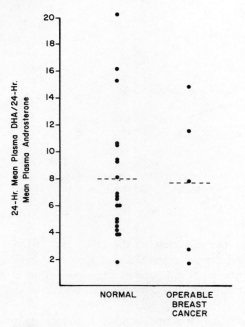

Figure 12
Ratio of 24-hr mean plasma DHA to 24-hr mean plasma androsterone in premenopausal operable breast cancer patients and normal controls. P = N.S.

patients, the ratio was significantly higher than that of postmenopausal controls (Fig. 13).

The explanation for the interesting crossover behavior of the plasma adrenal androgen levels in breast cancer patients and controls is not obvious. One possible explanation makes use of the fact that the curve of breast cancer incidence vs age in Western countries is bimodal (Fig. 14) and is a summation of two hypothetical unimodal distributions that cross at about age 50 and have peaks in the premenopausal and postmenopausal age ranges respectively (Fig. 15).[2] The probability that an individual patient belongs to one population or the other is a function of the distance of her age from the crossover age—at the crossover age, she has an equal probability of belonging to either population. Assuming that the DHA and DHAS levels in a pure premenopausal population

---

[2] These two populations commonly are referred to as premenopausal and postmenopausal. Actually, because premenopausal and postmenopausal groups each overlap onto the other side of menopause, and because the regression lines of DHA and DHAS vs age in normal women indicate that menopause is a nonevent with respect to these hormones, we should more properly speak of young and old, or perhaps Type-I and Type-II, breast cancer populations rather than premenopausal and postmenopausal. However, we will keep to the conventional terms here for historical continuity.

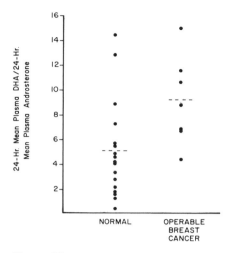

Figure 13
Ratio of 24-hr mean plasma DHAS to 24-hr mean plasma androsterone in postmenopausal operable breast cancer patients and normal controls. $P < 0.05$.

would be markedly subnormal and the levels in a pure postmenopausal population would be markedly supranormal, the observed levels at any given age of a patient would approach the expected pure population levels more and more closely as her age became increasingly distant from the crossover age. In other words, the deviation of patients' values from normal control values would increase as their ages moved away from the crossover age, as is observed. Though the observed values for the premenopausal and postmenopausal patients as

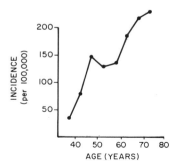

Figure 14
Age-incidence curve of female breast cancer in Holland, showing bimodality. (Data from de Waard 1975.)

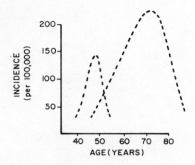

Figure 15
Theoretical unimodal age-incidence curves into which the bimodal curve of Fig. 14 can be resolved.

groups already differ significantly from normal (Fig. 11), the implication is that those of pure premenopausal or postmenopausal patients would differ even more from normal. Thus, studying only younger premenopausal patients (under age 40) and older postmenopausal patients (above age 60) should yield even greater deviations from normal plasma adrenal androgen levels.

The principal factors that could raise or lower plasma DHA and DHAS levels are changes in their production rate and (or) their metabolic removal rate. Since androsterone is a major plasma metabolite of DHA, we felt that examination of the plasma DHA/androsterone ratio could shed light on the role these factors play in the DHA (and presumably the DHAS) abnormalities. The fact that the DHA/androsterone ratio was normal in the premenopausal patients speaks against a significant role for increased metabolic removal rate as a factor, and therefore suggests by exclusion that the subnormal plasma DHA levels in these patients are due principally to diminished DHA production; this conclusion is compatible with the previous reports (Bulbrook et al. 1962, 1971) of subnormal amounts of adrenal androgen metabolites in the urine of premenopausal breast cancer patients. Conversely, the finding that the DHA/androsterone ratio was markedly elevated in the postmenopausal breast cancer patients suggests that the metabolic conversion of DHA to androsterone was slowed in these patients; this effect would probably be sufficient to account for the elevated plasma DHA levels in these patients without postulating any increase in DHA production (though the latter possibility cannot be excluded). If further studies should confirm that there are indeed two different mechanisms for the different plasma adrenal androgen abnormalities in premenopausal and postmenopausal breast cancer patients, namely decreased production in the former and slowed metabolic removal in the latter, a biochemical basis would have been provided for the two-disease distinction in breast cancer.

A very large amount of data accumulated over a 23-yr period, including the findings of our study, points to the existence of a deficiency of adrenal androgens in women with premenopausal breast cancer. Prospective studies and familial studies suggest that the deficiency antedates the clinical appearance of the disease and may well be a genetic marker. Of course, a genetic marker may be just that—a marker, with no implications for the pathophysiology, prevention, or treatment of the disease. However, the intriguing recent observation by Schwartz et al. (1979) that administration of DHA strongly inhibits the development of breast cancer in a strain of mice that is normally prone to the disease suggests that the subnormal levels of DHA in premenopausal breast cancer may indeed have pathophysiological significance, and even tempts one to consider the possibility of prophylactic trials of DHA, at least in high-risk young women.

PLASMA LEVELS OF LH

There have been a number of reports suggesting that chronic anovulation is a risk factor for breast cancer. Grattarola (1964) took endometrial biopsies of breast cancer patients just prior to menstruation and found that 83% of them showed proliferative rather than the expected secretory endometrium, indicating that the women had not ovulated that month; normal women biopsied at the same point in the menstrual cycle showed only a 32% incidence of proliferative endometrium. Earlier autopsy studies of women dying of breast cancer (Sommers 1955) had shown a high incidence of endometrial hyperplasia, evidence of a prolonged previous period of anovulatory cycling with the action of estrogen unopposed by that of progesterone. The fact that a high percentage of breast cancer patients complain of primary or secondary infertility (Gilliam 1951; Logan 1953; Grattarola 1964) can also be construed as evidence of a high incidence of chronic anovulation in these women. Sherman and Korenman (1974), trying to fit the role of various putative risk factors (late first pregnancy, nulliparity, early menarche, obesity, and late menopause) into a single comprehensive scheme, pointed out that an increased proportion of anovulatory cycles was common to all of them; therefore, they proposed that the presence of luteal inadequacy (i.e., insufficient production of progesterone) was the common physiological abnormality underlying a variety of high-risk conditions. Direct measurements of luteal-phase plasma progesterone or urinary progesterone metabolites in women with breast cancer have yielded differing findings: Swain et al. (1974), England et al. (1975), Malarkey et al. (1977), and Sherman et al. (1979) reported normal plasma progesterone levels. whereas Kodama et al. (1977) reported subnormal urinary pregnanediol excretion and Bulbrook (1979) reported subnormal plasma progesterone levels in both women with breast cancer and women at high familial risk for breast cancer (Bulbrook et al. 1978).

It seems reasonable that luteal-phase plasma levels of LH might also be abnormal in women with breast cancer if they are not ovulating. In the only published study on this topic, Malarkey et al. (1977) found normal 24-hr mean plasma levels of LH in premenopausal women with breast cancer. We too have measured 24-hr mean plasma LH levels in such patients, with very different results.

We studied 14 otherwise healthy, regularly cycling women with breast cancer, aged 31-52, who were screened rigorously to exclude factors known or suspected to alter endocrine function, and 13 healthy, regularly cycling control women, aged 22-51, and similarly screened. Seven of the patients and 9 of the controls were in the follicular phase (days 2-10 of their cycle), and 7 patients and 4 control women were in the luteal phase (days 15-26 of their cycle). Of the patients studied in the follicular phase, 6 had localized disease (3 operable and 3 inoperable) and 1 had metastatic disease; of the patients studied in the luteal phase, 5 had localized disease (2 operable and 3 inoperable) and 2 had metastatic disease.

Specimens of venous blood were taken from an indwelling catheter every 20 min for 24 hr. In all patients and controls, a 200 μl aliquot was taken from each of the samples, the aliquots were pooled, and the LH concentration of the pool (i.e., the 24-hr mean plasma concentration) was determined by RIA. In 1 of the control women and 5 of the 7 cancer patients studied during the luteal phase, the LH content of each of the 72 samples was determined to construct a 24-hr plasma concentration profile.

We found that the follicular-phase, 24-hr, mean plasma LH levels in the control women ranged from 10 mIU/ml to 23 mIU/ml; the geometric mean level was 17, with 95% confidence limits of 9.8-30 (Fig. 16). Of the 7 patients studied during the follicular phase, 5 had LH levels within this normal range,

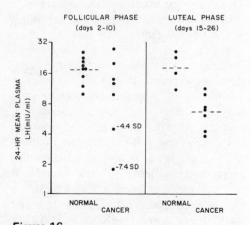

Figure 16

24-Hr mean plasma LH concentrations in normal women and women with breast cancer. Note that 2 of the 7 cancer patients studied in the follicular phase had markedly subnormal values, and all of the cancer patients studied in the luteal phase had values at or below the lower limit of normal ($P < 0.005$). The mean of the luteal-phase cancer group was about one-third the control mean.

but the other 2 had markedly subnormal levels: 4.4 S.D. and 7.4 S.D. below the normal mean.

The luteal-phase levels in the control women were quite similar to the normal follicular-phase levels: They ranged from 11 mIU/ml to 26 mIU/ml and the geometric mean was 18 mIU/ml, with 95% confidence limits of 8.4-39. One of the luteal-phase cancer patients had an LH level equal to the lowest normal value (11 mIU/ml); the other 6 had levels (3.5-9.6 mIU/ml) that were below the lowest normal value. The geometric mean of the cancer group was 6.3 mIU/ml, with 95% confidence limits of 2.7-15; the difference from the normal mean was highly significant ($P < 0.005$). The abnormality was independent of the stage of the disease, because it occurred in women with operable, localized but inoperable, or metastatic cancer (Table 2); however, we did not study patients who had been "cured" surgically—all our patients had cancerous tissue present at the time of study.

When detailed 24-hr profiles of plasma LH concentration were studied in 5 of the 7 luteal-phase cancer patients, it was found that all of them were abnormal in a pattern of immaturity. Boyar et al. (1974a) described a characteristic ontogeny of LH secretion in females, in which prepubertal girls show low plasma levels around the clock with little secretory activity, early pubertal girls show gradually increasing secretory activity while asleep and little secretory activity while awake, and older girls show increasing daytime secretory activity that gradually rises to match nocturnal activity as puberty progresses, finally

Table 2
Clinical and Hormonal Data of the Breast Cancer Patients

Subject	Age	Day of cycle	24-hr mean LH	Stage of breast cancer
		Follicular phase		
1	32	9	28	localized, operable
2	38	9	4.5[a]	localized, operable
3	31	9	10	localized, operable
4	51	8	1.8[a]	localized, inoperable
5	39	10	20	localized, inoperable
6	39	9	14	localized, inoperable
7	38	8	13	metastatic
		Luteal phase		
8	45	15	3.5[a]	localized, operable
9	48	20	5.8[a]	localized, operable
10	34	25	7.0[a]	localized, inoperable
11	38	26	3.9[a]	localized, inoperable
12	31	26	9.6[a]	localized, inoperable
13	48	22	6.7[a]	metastatic
14	52	17	11	metastatic

[a] Below the lowest normal value.

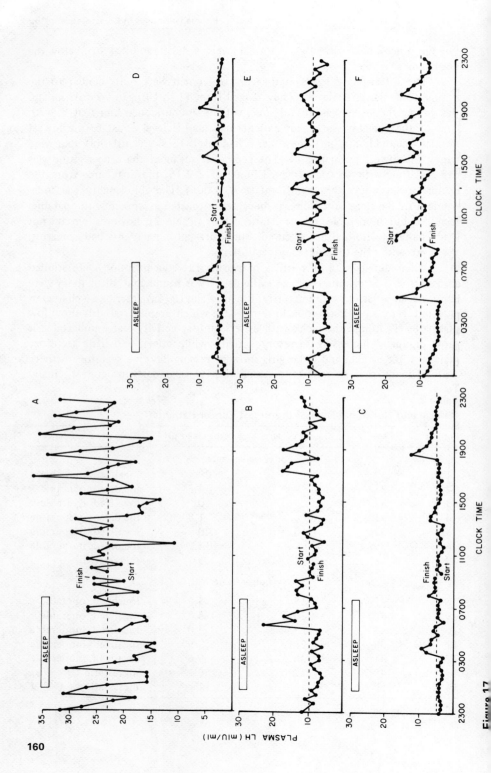

Figure 17

160

achieving the adult pattern of 15-20 clear-cut episodes of secretion at intervals of 1-1.5 hr throughout the day and night (Fig. 17A). In the light of this ontogeny, two of the cancer patients showed prepubertal LH profiles (Fig. 17,C and D), one showed an early pubertal pattern (Fig. 17B), and the other two showed less frequent and less intense secretory episodes than normal (Fig. 17,E and F). The degree of subnormality of the 24-hr mean LH level (represented by the dotted line in each panel of Fig. 17) was directly related to the degree of immaturity of the LH profile in that the more immature the profile the lower the mean level.

It seems reasonable to postulate that some type of hypothalamic dysfunction is responsible for the decreased and immature secretion of LH in these cancer patients, and that the more "regressive" the hypothalamic function the greater the disturbance of LH secretion. The mechanism of this dysfunction is not clear. The only other condition in which a similar immaturity of the LH secretory pattern has been described is anorexia nervosa (Boyar 1974b). This abnormality has been ascribed to subnormal estrogen levels that result in decreased responsiveness of the pituitary gonadotroph to stimulation by LH-releasing hormone (Frisch 1977) This however. cannot be the mechanism of the decreased LH secretion in breast cancer patients, in whom estrogen levels, in our experience and that of others (Hellman et al. 1971; Sherman et al. 1979), are normal or even elevated.

Other very important questions that are not answered by the present studies are whether subnormal LH levels are present before breast cancer becomes clinically manifest (as in the case with another hormonal abnormality seen in breast cancer, namely subnormal urinary androgen metabolite excretion [Bulbrook et al. 1971]) and whether they persist after cure of the cancer. Only carefully designed and extensive long-term studies can answer these questions.

ACKNOWLEDGMENTS

These studies were supported in part by Grants CA-07304 and CA-27795 from the National Cancer Institute and Grant RR-53 from the General Research Centers Branch, National Institutes of Health. I would also like to express my thanks for the outstanding technical assistance of Nathan Katz, Tonida Parker, and Ann Thalassinos (RIA), and William Greenhut, Joan Greenhut, Guillemet Barbet, Terri Levis, Susan Silverman, David Schessel, and Marc Schessel (24-hr blood-sampling studies).

REFERENCES

Adami, N.O., A. Rimsten, L. Thoren, J. Vegelius, and L. Wide. 1978. Thyroid disease and function in breast cancer patients and nonhospitalized controls evaluated by determination of TSH, T3, rT3, and TR levels on serum. *Acta Chir. Scand.* **144**:89.

Allen, B.J., J.L. Hayward, and W.H.H. Merivale. 1957. The excretion of 17-ketosteroids in the urine of patients with generalised carcinomatosis secondary to carcinoma of the breast. *Lancet* i:496.

Balsam, A., C.R. Dobbs, and E. Leppo. 1975. Circadian variations in plasma concentrations of thyroxine and triiodothyronine in man. *J. Appl. Physiol.* 39:297.

Bermudez, F., M.I. Surks, and J.H. Oppenheimer. 1975. High incidence of decreased serum triiodothyronine concentration in patients with non-thyroidal disease. *J. Clin. Endocrinol. Metab.* 41:27.

Bignazzi, A., P. d'Amico, and U. Veronesi. 1965. Thyroid function in patients with breast cancer. *Tumori* 51:199.

Boyar, R.M., J.W. Finkelstein, R. David, H. Roffwarg, S. Kapen, E.D. Weitzman, and L. Hellman. 1973. Twenty-four hour patterns of plasma luteinizing hormone and follicle-stimulating hormone in sexual precocity. *New Engl. J. Med.* 289:282.

Boyar, R.M., R.S. Rosenfeld, S. Kapen, J.W. Finkelstein, H.P. Roffwarg, E.D. Weitzman, and L. Hellman. 1974a. Human puberty: Simultaneous augmented secretion of luteinizing hormone and testosterone during sleep. *J. Clin. Invest.* 54:609.

Boyar, R.M., S. Kapen, J.W. Finkelstein, M. Perlow, J.F. Sassin, D.K. Fukushima, E.D. Weitzman, and L. Hellman. 1974b. Hypothalamic-pituitary function in diverse hyperprolactinemic states. *J. Clin. Invest.* 53: 1588.

Brownsey, B., E.H.D. Cameron, K. Griffiths, E.N. Gleave, A.P.M. Forrest, and H. Campbell. 1972. Plasma dehydroepiandrosterone sulphate levels in patients with benign and malignant breast disease. *Eur. J. Cancer* 8:131.

Bulbrook, R.D. 1979. Endocrine determinants of risk of breast cancer. Abstr. 9th Congr. Int. Study Group for Steroid Hormones, vii.

Bulbrook, R.D., F.C. Greenwood, and J.L. Hayward. 1960. Selection of breast-cancer patients for adrenalectomy or hypophysectomy by determination of urinary 17-hydroxycorticosteroids and aetiocholanolone. *Lancet* i: 1154.

Bulbrook, R.D., J.L. Hayward, and C.C. Spicer. 1971. Relation between urinary androgen and corticoid excretion and subsequent breast cancer. *Lancet* ii: 395.

Bulbrook, R.D., J.L. Hayward, C.C. Spicer, and B.S. Thomas. 1962. Abnormal excretion of urinary steroids by women with early breast cancer. *Lancet* ii:1238.

Bulbrook, R.D., J.W. Moore, G.M.G. Clark, D.Y. Wang, D. Tong, and J.L. Hayward. 1978. Plasma oestradiol and progesterone levels in women with varying degrees of risk of breast cancer. *Eur. J. Cancer* 14:1369.

Carter, A., E.B. Feldman, and H.L. Schwartz. 1960. Level of serum protein-bound iodine in patients with metastatic carcinoma of the breast. *J. Clin. Endocrinol. Metab.* 20:477.

Dargent, M., M. Berger, and B. Laheche. 1962. Thyroid function in patients with breast cancer. *Acta Unio Int. Contra Cancrum* 18:915.

de Waard, F. 1975. Breast cancer incidence and nutritional status with particular reference to body weight and height. *Cancer Res.* 35:3351.

_____. 1979. Premenopausal and postmenopausal breast cancer: One disease or two? *J. Natl. Cancer Inst.* 63:549.

de Waard, F., J.W.J. DeLaive, and E.A. Baanders-Van Halewijin. 1960. On the bimodal age distribution of mammary carcinoma. *Br. J. Cancer* 14: 437.

Doll, R. 1969. The geographical distribution of cancer. *Br. J. Cancer.* 23:1.

Edelstyn, G.A., A.R. Lyons, and R.B. Welbaum. 1958. Thyroid function in patients with mammary cancer. *Lancet* i:670.

• England, P.C., L.G. Skinner, K.M. Cottrell, and R.A. Sellwood. 1975. Sex hormones in breast disease. *Br. J. Surg.* 62:806.

Finkelstein, J.W., R.M. Boyar, H.P. Roffwarg, J. Kream, D.K. Fukushima, T.F. Gallagher, and L. Hellman. 1973. Growth hormone secretion in congenital adrenal hyperplasia. *J. Clin. Endocrinol. Metab.* 36:121.

Finley, J.W. and G.M. Bogardus. 1960. Breast cancer and thyroid disease. *Quart. Rev. Surg. Obstet. Gyn.* 17:139.

Frisch, R.E. 1977. Food intake, fatness, and reproductive ability. In *Anorexia nervosa* (ed. R. Vigersky), p. 149. Raven Press, New York.

Gilliam, A.G. 1951. Fertility and cancer of breast and of uterine cervix. Comparisons between rates of pregnancy in women with cancer at these and other sites. *J. Natl. Cancer Inst.* 12:287.

Gorman, C.A., D.V. Becker, F.S. Greenspan, P.P. Levy, J.H. Oppenheimer, R.S. Rivlin, J. Robbins, and W.P. Vanderlaan. 1977a. Breast cancer and thyroid therapy: Statement by the American Thyroid Association. *J. Am. Med. Assoc.* 237:1459.

_____. 1977b. American Thyroid Association Statement: Breast cancer and thyroid hormone therapy. *Ann. Intern. Med.* 86:502.

Grattarola, R. 1964. The premenstrual endometrial pattern of women with breast cancer: A study of progestational activity. *Cancer* 17:1119.

Hellman, L., F. Nakada, J. Curti, E.D. Weitzman, J. Kream, H. Roffwarg, S. Ellman, D.K. Fukushima, and T.F. Gallagher. 1970. Cortisol is secreted episodically by normal man. *J. Clin. Endocrinol. Metab.* 30:411.

• Hellman, L., B. Zumoff, J. Fishman, and T.F. Gallagher. 1971. Peripheral metabolism of ^{3}H-estradiol and the excretion of endogenous estrone and estriol glucosiduronate in women with breast cancer. *J. Clin. Endocrinol. Metab.* 33:138.

Humphrey, L.J. and M. Swerdlow. 1964. The relationship of breast disease to thyroid disease. *Cancer* 17:1170.

Juret, P., M. Hayem, and A. Flaisler. 1964. A propos de 150 implantations d'yttrium radio-actif intra-hypophysaires dan le traitement du sein à un stade avancé; technique; bilan clinique; indications. *J. Chir.* 87: 409.

Kapdi, C.C. and J.N. Wolfe. 1972. Breast cancer: Relationship to thyroid supplements for hypothyroidism. *J. Am. Med. Assoc.* 236:1127.

Kodama, M., T. Kodama, S. Miura, and M. Yoshida. 1977. Hormonal status of breast cancer. III. Further analysis of ovarian adrenal dysfunction. *J. Natl. Cancer Inst.* 59:49.

Kream, J., L. Hellman, and R.S. Rosenfeld. 1976. Radioimmunoassay of androsterone and androsterone-3-sulfate in plasma. *Steroids* 27:727.

Krieger, D.T. and S. Glick. 1971. Absent sleep peak of growth hormone release in blind subjects: Correlation with sleep EEG stages. *J. Clin. Endocrinol. Metab.* **33**:847.

Kumaoka, S., N. Sakauchi, O. Abe, M. Kusama, and O. Takatani. 1968. Urinary 17-ketosteroid excretion of women with advanced breast cancer. *J. Clin. Endocrinol. Metab.* **28**:667.

Lencioni, L.J., E. Richiger de Arranz, D. Davidovich, and J.J. Staffieri. 1962. A study of thyroid function in patients with breast cancer. *Medicina* **22**:215.

Logan, W.P.D. 1953. Marriage and childbearing in relation to cancer of breast and uterus. *Lancet* ii:1199.

MacFarlane, I.A., E.L. Robinson, H. Bush, P. Durning, J.M.T. Howat, C.G. Beardwell, and S.M. Shalet. 1978. Thyroid function in patients with benign and malignant breast disease. *Br. J. Cancer* **41**:478.

• Malarkey, W.B., L.L. Schroeder, V.C. Stevens, A.G. James, and R.R. Lanese. 1977. Twenty-four hour preoperative endocrine profiles in women with benign and malignant breast disease. *Cancer Res.* **37**:4655.

Manton, K.G. and E. Stallard. 1980. A two-disease model of female breast cancer: Mortality in 1969 among white females in the United States. *J. Natl. Cancer Inst.* **64**:9.

Maturlo, S.J., R.L. Rosenbaum, C. Panm, and A.J. Surks. 1980. Variable thyrotropin response to thyrotropin-releasing hormone after small decreases in plasma free thyroid hormone concentrations in patients with nonthyroidal diseases. *J. Clin. Invest.* **66**:451.

Mittra, I. and J.L. Hayward. 1974. Hypothalamic-pituitary-thyroid axis in breast cancer. *Lancet* i:885.

Myhill, J., T.S. Reeve, and I.B. Hales. 1966. Thyroid function in breast cancer. *Acta Endocrinol.* **51**:290.

Nieschlag, E., D.L. Loriaux, and M.B. Lipsett. 1972. Radioligand assay for Δ^5-3β-hydroxysteroids. I. 3β-hydroxy-5-androsten-17-one and its 3-sulfate. *Steroids* **19**:669.

O'Connor, J.F., G.Y. Wu, T.F. Gallagher, and L. Hellman. 1974. The 24-hour plasma thyroxine profile in normal man. *J. Clin. Endocrinol. Metab.* **39**:765.

Reeve, T.S., I.B. Hales, F.F. Rundle, J. Myhill, and M. Graydon. 1961. Thyroid function in the presence of breast cancer. *Lancet* i:632.

Repert, R.W. 1952. Breast carcinoma study: Relation of thyroid disease and diabetes. *J. Mich. St. Med. Soc.* **51**:1315.

Rose, D.P., P. Stauber, A. Thiel, J.J. Crowley, and J.R. Milbrath. 1977. Plasma dehydroepiandrosterone sulfate, androstenedione and cortisol, and urinary free cortisol excretion in breast cancer. *Eur. J. Cancer* **13**:43.

Rose, D.P. and T.E. Davis. 1978. Plasma thyroid-stimulating hormone and thyroxine concentrations in breast cancer. *Cancer* **41**:666.

———. 1979. Plasma triiodothyronine concentrations in breast cancer. *Cancer* **43**:1434.

Rosenfeld, R.S., L. Hellman, H. Roffwarg, E.D. Weitzman, D.K. Fukushima, and T.F. Gallagher. 1971. Dehydroisoandrosterone is secreted episodically and synchronously with cortisol by normal man. *J. Clin. Endocrinol. Metab.* **33**:87.

Rosenfeld, R.S., B.J. Rosenberg, D.K. Fukushima, and L. Hellman. 1975. 24-Hour secretory pattern of dehydroisoandrosterone and dehydroisoandrosterone sulfate. *J. Clin. Endocrinol. Metab.* **40**:850.

Schottenfeld, D. 1968. The relationship of breast cancer to thyroid disease. *J. Chronic Dis.* **21**:303.

Schwartz, A.G. 1979. Inhibition of spontaneous breast cancer formation in female C3H (Avy/a) mice by longterm treatment with dehydroepiandrosterone. *Cancer Res.* **39**:1129.

Sherman, B.M. and S.G. Korenman. 1974. Inadequate corpus luteum function: A pathophysiological interpretation of human breast cancer epidemiology. *Cancer* **33**:1306.

Sherman, B.M., R.B. Wallace, and P.R. Jochimsen. 1979. Hormonal regulation of the menstrual cycle in women with breast-cancer; effect of adjuvant chemotherapy. *Clin. Endocrinol.* **10**:287.

Sicher, K. and J.A.H. Waterhouse. 1967. Thyroid activity in relation to prognosis in mammary cancer. *Br. J. Cancer* **21**:512.

Sommers, S.C. 1955. Endocrine abnormalities in women with breast cancer. *Lab. Invest.* **4**:160.

Šonká. J., M. Vitková, I. Gregorová, Z. Tomsová, J. Hilgertová, and J. Staś. 1973. Plasma and urinary dehydroepiandrosterone in cancer. *Endokrinologie* **62**:61.

Stadel, B.V. 1976. Dietary iodine and risk of breast, endometrial, and ovarian cancer. *Lancet* i:890.

Stoll, B.A. 1965. Breast cancer and hypothyroidism. *Cancer* **18**:1431.

Swain, M.C., R.D. Bulbrook, and J.L. Hayward. 1974. Ovulatory failure in a normal population and in patients with breast cancer. *J. Obstet. Gynaecol. Br. Commonw.* **81**:640.

Takahashi, Y.D., D.M. Kipnis, and W.H. Daughaday. 1968. Growth hormone secretion during sleep. *J. Clin. Invest.* **47**:2079.

Thomas, B.S., P. Kirby, E.K. Symes, and D.Y. Wang. 1976. Plasma dehydroepiandrosterone concentration in normal women and in patients with benign and malignant breast disease. *Eur. J. Cancer* **12**:405.

Wanebo, H.J., R.J. Benua, and R.W. Rawson. 1966. Neoplastic disease and thyrotoxicosis. *Cancer* **19**:1523.

Wang, D.Y. 1971. Plasma androgens in breast cancer. In *Human adrenal gland and its relation to breast cancer. 1st Tenovus Workshop* (ed. K. Griffiths and E.H.D. Cameron), p. 71. Alpha Omega Alpha, Cardiff, Wales.

Wang, D.Y., R.D. Bulbrook, and J.L. Hayward. 1975. Urinary and plasma androgens and their relation to familial risk of breast cancer. *Eur. J. Cancer* **11**:873.

Wang, D.Y., R.D. Bulbrook, and J.L. Hayward. 1977. Plasma androstenedione levels in women with breast cancer. *Eur. J. Cancer* **13**:187.

Wang, D.Y., R.D. Bulbrook, M. Herian, and J.L. Hayward. 1974. Studies on the sulphate esters of dehydroepiandrosterone and androsterone in the blood of women with breast cancer. *Eur. J. Cancer* **10**:477.

Weitzman, E.D., H. Schaumburg, and W. Fishbein. 1966. Plasma 17-hydroxycorticosteroid levels during sleep in man. *J. Clin. Endocrinol. Metab.* **26**:121.

West, C.D., D.K. Mahajan, V.J. Chavre, C.J. Nabors, and F.H. Tyler. 1973. Simultaneous measurement of multiple plasma steroids by radioimmunoassay demonstrating episodic secretion. *J. Clin. Endocrinol. Metab.* **36**: 1230.

Yen, S.S.C., C.C. Tsai, F. Naftolin, G. Vandenberg, and L. Ajabor. 1972. Pulsatile patterns of gonadotropin release in subjects with and without ovarian function. *J. Clin. Endocrinol. Metab.* **34**:671.

Zumoff, B., R.S. Rosenfeld., G.W. Strain, J. Levin, and D.K. Fukushima. 1980. Sex differences in the 24-hour mean plasma concentrations of dehydroisoandrosterone (DHA) and dehydroisoandrosterone sulfate (DHAS) and the DHA to DHAS ratio in normal adults. *J. Clin. Endocrinol. Metab.* **51**: 330.

COMMENTS

KORENMAN: Could you tell us about some of the pertinent negatives for the sample? What were the TSHs, were there any prolactins, and so on?

ZUMOFF: We didn't do TSH, but the pertinent negatives that we did study were: Cortisol, testosterone, dihydrotestosterone, follicle-stimulating hormone, androsterone sulfate, and prolactin, all of which were unremarkable. Incidentally, we have some interesting observations about prolactin. We also find that it falls off with age; however, in our population, using 24-hr means, it doesn't fall off in that nice neat way that was shown if you plot age against 24-hr prolactin. We get a curve that looks almost like a square wave; it stays perfectly level with age, and then abruptly falls off at approximately age 60.

Interestingly enough, our preliminary data show that the nocturnal surge that Dr. Henderson showed, which of course everybody finds, is absent in these women over age 60. It disappears spontaneously, apparently. Anyway, there's no difference in the breast cancers.

We didn't do TSH, I'm sorry to say. We didn't do androstenedione, and we didn't do progesterone. Progesterones are in progress.

KORENMAN: Are all the breast cancer patients the same patients?

ZUMOFF: Yes.

KORENMAN: So that those people—for example, the ones with the poor LH curves—had normal prolactin compared to the controls?

ZUMOFF: That's correct.

HILF: While Dr. Zumoff is here, perhaps he can clarify a point that has me a bit confused. I presume that you showed some linear regression analyses for some of the urinary androgens, one that gave you a significant slope and the other that did not provide a significant slope. Now, what confuses me is how do you justify drawing a line for the latter? If I understand such an analysis, you simply have asked whether the coordinates of all the points taken together can fit a line. Since the confidence level achieved was so low, I must conclude that the data do not lend themselves to approximating a linear relationship.

ZUMOFF: It means that the line doesn't have a slope significantly different from zero. It doesn't mean there's no line.

HILF: But where do you position this? It could be up and down or all around (a circle). You've positioned it horizontally and then talked about a cross-over point. I just don't see how you justify where that purported line with no slope fits.

ZUMOFF: Well, I hope to go back to my statisticians to give me some help with that, but I have taken it at face value using the least mean squares and getting a computer-generated line, which doesn't differ significantly in its slope from zero.

SESSION 4:
In Vitro Studies
of Human Breast Tissue

Hormonal Regulation of
Human Breast Cancer Cells in Vitro

MARC LIPPMAN
Medical Breast Cancer Section
Medicine Branch
National Cancer Institute
Bethesda, Maryland 20205

The purpose of this chapter is to review briefly and in a general fashion some of the information that has accumulated concerning the hormonal regulation of human breast cancer cells in continuous tissue culture. Detailed reviews of this subject have been published (McGuire 1977; Monaco et al. 1979) and no effort will be made to review this subject exhaustively again. Rather, an attempt will be made to point out some of the complexities and pitfalls of studying hormonal dependency of human breast cancer in tissue culture as well as several of the unique advantages of such an approach. But before considering those hormonal effects that have been documented in vitro, it is worthwhile to examine some of the problems associated with such systems.

First, virtually all breast cell lines have been established from malignant effusions. As such, they represent a subset of the original tumor population, which has the ability to metastasize and grow in a specific environment completely unlike that of the primary tumor. Not only has this "natural selection" occurred, but, by the time the tumor sample is collected for culture, a number of therapies, such as irradiation, cytotoxic drugs, and hormonal manipulations, may have limited substantially the responses to many growth factors of the remaining cell population.

Second, conditions selected for initiation of culture may immediately lead to selection of cells capable of growth in the absence of factors omitted from the original medium. In addition, culture conditions almost invariably select against slower growing populations of cells. Since differentiation frequently is related inversely to growth rate, many populations of cells that may express those hormonal responses of greatest interest may be overgrown by hormone-independent cell populations before experiments can be undertaken.

Third, in an effort to provide some assurance of a homogenous population of cells, cloning may result in selection of a population of cells possessing a limited repertoire of the total responses of a given tumor.

Fourth, viral or mycoplasmic contamination of cultures can occur, leading to substantial alterations in expression of some phenotypic effects.

Fifth, cells grown in tissue culture are denied many factors that may be critical to the expression of a given response. Adherence to a basement membrane or substratum, a polarized orientation, additional supporting cell types, or growth factors may all be absolutely essential to the expression of any given response. Estrogen-induced hormones, such as putative estromedins discussed elsewhere in this volume, would represent a similar phenomenon.

Sixth, it is possible to misinterpret lack of responsiveness of a cell line because it is assumed incorrectly that the hormone is a mitogen or an inducer of a given measured product. For example, the MCF-7 cells will grow optimally in insulin and charcoal-treated calf serum in the absence of estradiol. If one adds estrogen to this system, no further stimulation of growth is observed and the cells might therefore be considered hormone independent. On the other hand, progesterone receptor is completely inducible under these same conditions. Vasopressin stimulates fatty acid synthesis, phospholipid turnover, and accumulation of protein within cells without having any mitogenic effect in a cell line derived from a rat breast cancer induced by 7,12-dimethylbenz[a]-anthracene (DMBA) (Monaco et al. 1978). Thus, failure to observe responses to a given hormone may be dependent on the phenomenon measured.

Finally, and most pernicious of all, a cell line may be thought to be unresponsive to a given factor because it is incorrectly assumed that this factor has been removed from the medium. Sera contain high concentrations of many growth factors, including steroids (Esber et al. 1973). We have shown that under certain conditions, up to 2 weeks may be required to remove physiologic concentrations of estradiol from cells in culture (Strobl and Lippman 1979; Strobl et al. 1980). Cells are capable of concentrating estrogens tenfold over the ambient medium concentration via a process not requiring receptor. Thus, any attempt to demonstrate responsiveness to this hormone that does not adequately control for this phenomenon would artefactually fail to demonstrate hormone responsiveness.

All of the above caveats make firm conclusions concerning the absence of a given hormonal response particularly difficult to interpret. On the other hand, positive experiments are substantially less ambiguous. Even in this setting, it is possible for mistakes to occur. For example it is well known that most DMBA-induced rat mammary tumors are prolactin dependent. Initial studies with a tissue culture cell line derived from one of these tumors suggested that it was prolactin dependent; but, careful, subsequent studies revealed that the response was due to contaminating vasopressin in the prolactin preparations (Monaco et al. 1980). Similarly, we reported that the MCF-7 human breast cancer cell line contained androgen receptor and responded to androgen administration (Lippman et al. 1976a). Subsequently, it has been suggested that the response to nonphysiologic concentrations of androgen was due to interaction of the androgen with the estrogen receptor and response system of these cells (Zava and McGuire 1978).

Despite these many difficulties, there are many advantages to the cell-culture approach to the study of hormonal interactions with human breast cancer. First, by using cells derived from a human neoplasm, many of the difficulties associated with species differences are eliminated. This may be a great advantage with such hormones as prolactin. Second, the use of a single, cloned cell type allows great confidence to be placed in what the primary responding cell type is, assuming an effect is seen. Thus, an unequivocal demonstration of an estrogen effect on a cloned cell type rules out the need for an intermediary effector system. Third, it recently has become possible to do many experiments in defined medium systems. In such situations, one can be certain that the hormonal effect studied is not mediated by some additional unknown factor in serum, etc. Fourth, cell-culture systems are particularly advantageous for the study of drug and hormone metabolism as tissue redistribution, plasma bindings, and nontarget tissue sites of metabolism and excretion can be eliminated. Finally, and most importantly, it is possible to develop drug- and hormone-resistant variant sublines derived from wild-type parental cell lines. With appropriate biochemical and genetic complementation techniques, it is possible to gain new insights into the mechanisms of hormonal dependency. Such an approach recently has been employed by selecting antiestrogen-independent human breast cancer cell variants and will briefly be described later.

With all of these considerations in mind, it is possible to enumerate those hormones now known to influence either growth or differentiated functions of human breast cancer cells. In addition, there is a shorter list of hormones for which specific receptors have been demonstrated but for which no response has as yet been shown.

ESTROGENS

For nearly a century, it has been known that removal of the ovaries would lead to objective improvement in some patients with metastatic breast cancer. Later, it was, of course, appreciated that many breast cancers in both humans and experimental animals were estrogen dependent. Nonetheless, it is only within the past 5 years that an estrogen-responsive cell system has been described. Following the initial description of the MCF-7 human breast cancer cell line (Soule et al. 1973), Brooks et al. (1973) demonstrated that these cells contained estrogen receptor (ER). Shortly thereafter, we showed that these cells showed a variety of growth responses to physiologically relevant concentrations of estrogen and inhibition of these cells by antiestrogen (Lippman et al. 1976a, 1977). A variety of specific products also have been shown to be under estrogenic control in these cells, including thymidine kinase (TK) (Bronzert et al. 1981), progesterone receptor (Horwitz and McGuire 1978), lactic dehydrogenase (LDH) isoenzymes (Burke et al. 1978), a secreted protein of unknown function (Westley and Rochefort 1980), plasminogen activator (Butler et al.

1979), and a cytoplasmic protein with a 26K m.w. (Edwards et al. 1980). In addition, we have characterized a second human breast cancer cell line (ZR-75-1), which also has ER (Engel et al. 1978). In defined medium, this cell line can be shown to be dependent on estrogen for its growth (Allegra and Lippman 1978), as well as having an estrogen-inducible secreted protein (Westley and Rochefort 1980). Several other groups have reported that estrogens can alter growth rate of human breast cancer cell lines (Weichselbaum et al. 1978; E.R. Jensen et al., pers. comm.), whereas others have failed to demonstrate growth responses to estrogen (Barnes and Sato 1979; Shafie 1980). The presence of antiestrogen inhibition, which is reversible by estrogen, and the presence of many functions that are estrogen inducible is, however, seemingly unequivocal. In many cases, the failure to demonstrate estrogenic effects seems clearly attributable to failure either to remove adequately endogenous hormone or failure to remove insulin from the medium, because insulin can serve as an alternative growth factor. In fact, when such efforts are made, it is possible to obtain estrogenic effects where previously they had been unobtainable (C. McGrath et al., pers. comm.). Recently, we have used a variety of novel probes for measuring DNA synthetic rates and pyrimidine biosynthesis (Aitken and Lippman 1980). These techniques reveal that some of the failure to obtain estrogenic responses is due to massive inhibition of the de novo pathway of pyrimidine biosynthesis by estrogen starvation, which can be partially overcome by thymidine administration. Under such circumstances in which the intracellular pool of de novo synthesized thymidine is low, thymidine administration alone can function as a growth factor. When true DNA synthetic rates are measured or quantification of the de novo pathway is accomplished, dramatic stimulation of DNA synthesis by estrogen is apparent. In addition, a variety of enzymes involved in DNA synthesis, including carbamyl phosphate synthetase, aspartate transcarbamylase, dihydroorotase, thymidylate synthetase, and dihydrofolate reductase (DHFR), all are induced.

By cloning hormone-responsive human breast cancer cells in soft agar in the presence of lethal concentrations of antiestrogens, we have been able to develop hormone-independent variants of MCF-7 cells with a variety of interesting phenotypes (in prep.). These include one variant which retains estrogen responsiveness with a complete loss of antiestrogenic response. In this cell line, activation of receptor in vitro is different from wild-type MCF-7 cells. In another variant that retains minimal antiestrogenic inhibition but has lost responsiveness to estrogens including progesterone receptor inducibility, the receptor has an abnormal chromatographic profile on DNA cellulose, eluting at a higher salt concentration. Thus, in both of these variants, the defect appears to be expressed at the level of receptor but at some site removed from the initial binding of ligand (estrogen or antiestrogen), which is entirely normal. We believe that such variants can add substantial insight into the mechanisms by which estrogens stimulate growth in human breast cancer.

GLUCOCORTICOIDS

It has long been appreciated that a small minority of patients with metastatic breast cancer will have beneficial although brief responses to exogenously administered glucocorticoids. Although several mechanisms may account for this effect, including modulation of the immune system or effects on supporting stroma, it is clear that direct inhibitory effects also are possible. In tissue culture, glucocorticoid hormones exert a variety of inhibitory effects on breast cell growth (Lippman et al. 1976d) as well as antagonizing the trophic effects of insulin (Osborne et al. 1979). These effects are mediated by glucocorticoid receptors found in these cells. Cell lines that lack high-affinity glucocorticoid receptors fail to respond to glucocorticoids. Although such receptors are found in about half of human breast cancer biopsies (Allegra et al. 1979), they do not appear to have significant associations with biological responses to classical endocrine therapies.

ANDROGENS

It has been observed empirically that some human breast cancers will improve with androgen therapy, although the basis for this response is unknown (Stoll 1972). In addition, about one-third of human breast cancers contain androgen receptors. Androgen dependence has been shown in at least one rodent breast cancer cell line (Smith and King 1972). Several human breast cancer cell lines contain androgen receptor which is readily distinguished from ER (Lippman et al. 1976b; Engel et al. 1978). We initially demonstrated that androgens could increase thymidine incorporation and protein synthesis in MCF-7 cells, but concentrations required were supraphysiologic and vastly in excess of those required to saturate androgen receptors (Lippman et al. 1976a). We also demonstrated that these cells could rapidly metabolize dihydrotestosterone (DHT) to androstanediols and more polar conjugates. We suggested that, because of this metabolism, nonphysiologic concentrations of androgen were required. Subsequently, it was shown that these high concentrations of androgen were capable of occupying and translocating the ER as well as antagonizing the inhibitory effects of antiestrogens (Zava and McGuire 1978). Thus, at the present time, there is no unequivocal demonstration of androgen responsiveness in a human breast cancer cell line and the mechanism of response of some human breast cancers to androgen administration remains mysterious.

IODOTHYRONINES

Although some epidemiologic evidence has suggested that derangements in thyroid function are associated with an altered rate of breast cancer incidence, an unequivocal association of therapeutic benefit for thyroid hormone replacement has not been demonstrated. Nonetheless, MCF-7 human breast cancer cells contain classical high-affinity nuclear receptors for thyroid hormone and have a growth response to physiological concentrations of thyroid hormones (Burke and McGuire 1978). The ZR-75-1 cell line has an absolute dependency on physiologic concentrations of triiodothyronine (T3) when grown in defined medium (Allegra and Lippman 1978). Working also in defined medium, Barnes and Sato (1979) have been able to demonstrate the thyroid hormone dependency of MCF-7 cells. Thus, human breast cancer cell lines appear to be an exciting system for the study of thyroid hormone interaction with human breast cancer.

INSULIN

Insulin is a critical hormone in the normal differentiation of the mammary gland and is required for normal lactogenesis in rodents. Major derangements in glucose homeostasis induced by surgical or chemical interference with pancreatic function are associated with altered tumor growth rates in several murine systems. An important regulatory role for insulin in human breast cancer has not been established. With this in mind, it was reasonable to study the effects of insulin on human breast cancer cell lines grown in tissue culture. In 1976, we reported that physiologic concentrations of insulin strongly stimulated the growth of both human (Osborne et al. 1976) and rodent mammary cancer cell lines (Monaco et al. 1978). In human cell lines, high-affinity, specific receptors for insulin readily are demonstrable and binding and biological effects are well correlated (Osborne et al. 1978). Mitogenic effects of insulin can be seen in defined medium for both the MCF-7 cell line (Barnes and Sato 1979) and the ZR-75-1 cell line (Allegra and Lippman 1978). Insulin also induces increases in fatty acid synthesis by increasing the activity of acetyl coenzymeA carboxylase (Monaco et al. 1980) as well as increasing the enzyme TK (Lippman et al. 1976e; Bronzert et al. 1981).

RETINOIDS

Vitamin A derivatives are required for normal epithelial differentiation and long have been known to have an antipromotional effect in a variety of carcinogenesis assays. The appearance of DMBA-induced breast cancers can be substantially decreased by the administration of vitamin A derivatives to rats (Moon et al. 1976). In addition, specific binding activities for vitamin A derivatives have been demonstrated in some human breast tumor cytosols (Ong et al. 1975). For these reasons, we decided to study the effects of retinoids on human breast cancer cell lines in tissue culture. We found that several lines of human breast cancer contained separable binding activities for retinol and retinoic acid (Lacroix and Lippman 1980). Vitamin A derivatives induced several effects on cell growth, depending on the cell lines studied. These included a slower growth rate but identical confluent density, slower growth rate to a lower confluent density, and cell death following a period of increasing growth inhibition. These effects were reversible by removal of retinoids. Although no direct evidence has been obtained proving that these binding activities serve as true receptors for retinoids, there is good agreement between relative binding affinity and biologic effectiveness. Clinical trials are underway at several institutions examining any activity of 13-*cis*-retinoic acid as an antineoplastic agent in breast cancer. Thus far, initial therapy trials at the National Cancer Institute have not been encouraging.

EPIDERMAL GROWTH FACTOR

Epidermal growth factor is a peptide first purified from the rodent submaxillary gland. It was later shown to have growth-promoting activity for several fibroblast and epithelial cell lines in culture. Its identification as a true hormone in humans has not been accomplished. Nonetheless, this peptide has been shown to function as a mitogen for MCF-7 human breast cancer cells (Osborne et al. 1980) and in defined medium as well (Barnes and Sato 1979). Other cell lines such as MDA-MB-231 were not stimulated by equivalent concentrations of hormone. Interestingly, an effect of epidermal growth factor could not be demonstrated in the presence of optimal concentrations of either serum or insulin. Whether epidermal growth factor is an important hormone in regulation of breast cancer cell growth or whether it is simply replacing promiscuously some other growth factor for mammary cancer cells will require further investigation.

VITAMIN D

A substantial body of data has suggested that, in many respects, the mechanism of action in vitamin D is highly analogous to that of the steroid hormones. Cytoplasmic receptor proteins have been described whose binding specificities closely parallel the known biological potencies of vitamin D analogs. Recently, vitamin D receptors have been described in human breast cancer tumor samples and the MCF-7 human breast cancer cell line (Eisman et al. 1980). These receptors are highly similar in both physical characteristics and binding properties to those described in intestinal mucosa. Human breast cancer has a remarkable propensity to metastasize to bone and to induce hypercalcemia. Whether some direct responsiveness of tumor cells to vitamin D is involved is conjectural but appealing as an hypothesis based on these binding studies.

PROGESTINS

Data derived from normal endometrial tissue have suggested that progesterone receptor activity is regulated by estrogens. Similar information has accumulated concerning human breast cancer. Both MCF-7 and ZR-75-1 human breast cancer cell lines contain progesterone receptor (Lippman et al. 1976d; Engel et al.

1978), and in both cases this receptor has been shown to be regulated by estrogens (Horwitz and McGuire 1978). However, in no breast cancer cell line has a direct action of progestins been identified.

PROLACTIN

The exact role of prolactin (if any) in human breast cancer is equivocal. No really substantial evidence has ever been presented proving prolactin dependence of human breast cancer. For example, the response rate to drugs such as ergoline derivatives and L-dopa are nil in patients with metastatic disease. Many of the patients who benefit from hypophysectomy can be shown to have higher plasma prolactin levels post therapy. For these reasons, it would be of great interest to define specific responses of human breast cancer cells to prolactin. Reports have appeared suggesting that prolactin may increase ER concentrations or growth rate (Shafie and Brooks 1977) in MCF-7 human breast cancer cells. Neither have been confirmed. Recently, specific prolactin receptors have been described in the MCF-7 cell line (Shiu 1979). These receptors have the usual binding affinity and specificities of other prolactin receptors and undergo internalization following occupancy by hormone (Shiu 1980). This important observation also awaits confirmation.

REFERENCES

Aitken, S.C. and M.E. Lippman. 1980. Hormonal regulation of net DNA synthesis in human breast cancer cell in tissue culture. In *Control mechanisms in animal cells* (ed. L. Jimenez de Asua et al.), p. 133. Raven Press, New York.

Allegra, J.C. and M.E. Lippman. 1978. Growth of a human breast cancer cell line in serum-free hormone-supplemented medium. *Cancer Res.* 38:3823.

Allegra, J.C., M.E. Lippman, E.B. Thompson, R. Simon, A. Barlock, L. Green, K. Huff, H.M.T. Do, S. Aitken, and R. Warren. 1979. Relationship between the progesterone, androgen and glucocorticoid receptor and response rate to endocrine therapy in metastatic breast cancer. *Cancer Res.* 39:1973.

Barnes, D. and G. Sato. 1979. Growth of a human mammary tumor cell line in a serum free medium. *Nature* 281:388.

Bronzert, D.A., M.E. Monaco, L. Pinkus, S. Aitken, and M.E. Lippman. 1981. Purification and properties of estrogen responsive of thymidine kinase from human breast cancer. *Cancer Res.* 41:604.

Brooks, S.C., E.R. Locke, and H. Soule. 1973. Estrogen receptor in a human receptor in a human cell line (MCF-7) from breast carcinoma. *J. Biol. Chem.* 248:6251.

Burke, R.E. and W.L. McGuire. 1978. Nuclear thyroid hormone receptors in a human breast cancer cell line. *Cancer Res.* 38:3769.

Burke, R.E., S.C. Harris, and W.L. McGuire. 1978. Lactate dehydrogenase in estrogen responsive human breast cancer cells. *Cancer Res.* 38:2773.

Butler, W.B., W.L. Kirkland, and T.l. Jorgenson. 1979. Induction of plasminogen activiation by estrogen in a human breast cancer cell line (MCF-7). *Biochem. Biophys. Res. Commun.* **90**:1328.

Edwards, D.P., D.J. Adams, N. Squage, and W.L. McGuire. 1980. Estrogen induced synthesis of specific proteins in human breast cancer cells. *Biochem. Biophys. Res. Commun.* **93**:804.

Eisman, J.A., T.J. Martin, I. MacIntyre, R.J. Framptin, J.M. Moseley, and R. Whitehead. 1980. 1,25-Dihydroxy vitamin D_3 receptor in a cultured human breast cancer cell line (MCF-7 cells). *Biochem. Biophys. Res. Commun.* **93**:9.

Engel, L.W., N.A. Young, T.S. Tralka, M.E. Lippman, S. O'Brien, and M.J. Joyce. 1978. Breast carcinoma cells in continuous culture: Establishment and characterization of three new cell lines. *Cancer Res.* **38**:3352.

Esber, H., I. Payne, and A. Bogden. 1973. Variability of hormone concentrations and ratios in commercial sera used for tissue culture. *J. Natl. Cancer Inst.* **50**:559.

Horwitz, K.B. and W.L. McGuire. 1978. Estrogen control of progesterone receptor in human breast cancer. *J. Biol. Chem.* **253**:2223.

Lacroix, A. and M.E. Lippman. 1980. Binding of retinoids to human breast cancer cell lines and their effects on cell growth. *J. Clin. Invest.* **65**: 586.

Lippman, M.E., G. Bolan, and K. Huff. 1976a. The effects of androgens and antiandrogens on hormone-responsive human breast cancer in long-term tissue culture. *Cancer Res.* **36**:4610.

————. 1976b. The effects of estrogens and antiestrogens on hormone-responsive human breast cancer in long-term tissue culture. *Cancer Res.* **36**:4595.

————. 1976c. Interactions of antiestrogens with human breast cancer in long term tissue culture. *Cancer Treat. Rep.* **60**:1421.

————. 1976d. The effects of glucocorticoids and progesterone on hormone-responsive human breast cancer in long-term tissue culture. *Cancer Res.* **36**:4602.

Lippman, M.E., M.E. Monaco, and G. Bolan. 1977. Effects of estrone, estradiol and estriol on hormone-responsive human breast cancer in long term tissue culture. *Cancer Res.* **37**:1901.

Lippman, M.E., G. Bolan, M.E.Monaco, L. Pinkus, and L. Engel. 1976e. Model systems for the study of estrogen action in tissue culture. *J. Steroid Biochem.* **7**:1045.

McGuire, W.L. 1977. Physiological principles underlying endocrine therapy of breast cancer. In *Breast cancer advances in research and treatment* (ed. W.L. McGuire), vol. 1, p. 217. Plenum Medical Book Co., New York.

Monaco, M.E., M.E. Lippman, R. Knazek, and W.R. Kidwell. 1978. Vasopressin stimulation of acetate incorporation into lipids in a dimethylbenz(a)-anthracene-induced rat mammary tumor cell line. *Cancer Res.* **38**:4101.

Monaco, M.E. J. Strobl, J.C. Allegra, and M.E. Lippman. 1979. Interactions of steroid hormones with human breast cancer in vitro. In *Steroid receptors and the management of cancer* (ed. E.B. Thompson and M.E. Lippman), vol. 2, p. 32. CRC Press, Cleveland.

Monaco, M.E., W.R. Kidwell, P.H. Kohn, J.S. Strobl, and M.E. Lippman. 1980. Neurohypophysial hormones and cancer. In *Hormones and cancer* (ed. S. Iacobelli et al.), p. 165. Raven Press, New York.

Monaco, M.E., C.K. Osborne, T.J. Bronzert, W.R. Kidwell, and M.E. Lippman. 1981. The mechanism of insulin regulation of lipid synthesis in MCF-7 human breast cancer cells. *Eur. J. Biochem.* (in press).

Moon, R.C., C.J. Grubbs, and M.B. Sporn. 1976. Inhibition of 7,12-dimethyl benz(a)anthracene-induced mammary carcinogenesis by retinyl acetate. *Cancer Res.* **36**:2626.

Ong, D.E., D.L. Page, and F. Chytil. Retinoic acid binding protein: Occurrence in human tumors. *Science* **190**:60.

Osborne, C.K., G. Bolan, M.E. Monaco, and M.E. Lippman. 1976. Hormone responsive human breast cancer in long term tissue culture: Effects of insulin. *Proc. Natl. Acad. Sci.* **73**:4536.

Osborne, C.K., M.E. Monaco, M.E. Lippman, and C.R. Kahn. 1978. Correlation among insulin binding, degradation, and biological activity in human breast cancer cells in long-term tissue culture. *Cancer Res.* **38**:94.

Osborne, C.K., M.E. Monaco, C.R. Kahn, and M.E. Lippman. 1979. Direct inhibition of growth and antagonism of insulin action by glucocorticoids in human breast cancer cells in culture. *Cancer Res.* **39**:2422.

Osborne, C.K., B. Hamilton, G. Titus, and R.B. Livingston. 1980. Epidermal growth factor stimulation of human breast cancer cells in culture. *Cancer Res.* **40**:2361.

Shafie, S.M. 1980. Estrogen and the growth of breast cancer: New evidence suggests indirect action. *Science* **209**:701.

Shafie, S. and S.C. Brooks. 1977. Effect of prolactin on growth and the estrogen receptor level of human breast cancer cells (MCF-7). *Cancer Res.* **37**:792.

Shiu, R.P.C. 1979. Prolactin receptors in human breast cancer cells in long term tissue culture. *Cancer Res.* **39**:4381.

_____. 1980. Processing of prolactin by human breast cancer cells in long term tissue culture. *J. Biol. Chem.* **255**:4278.

Smith, J.A. and R.J.B. King. 1972. Effects of steroids on growth of an androgen dependent mouse mammary carcinoma in cell culture. *Exp. Cell Res.* **73**:351.

Soule, H.D., J. Vazquez, A. Long, S. Albert, and M. Brennan. 1973. A human cell line from a pleural effusion derived from a breast carcinoma. *J. Natl. Cancer Inst.* **51**:1409.

Stoll, B.A. 1972. *Endocrine therapy in malignant disease*. W.H. Saunders Co., London.

Strobl, J.S. and M.E. Lippman. 1979. Prolonged retention of estradiol by human breast cancer cells in tissue culture. *Cancer Res.* **39**:3319.

Strobl, J.S., M.E. Monaco, and M.E. Lippman. 1980. The role of intracellular equilibria and the effect of antiestrogens on estrogen-receptor dissociation kinetics from perfused cultures of human breast cancer cells. *Endocrinology* **107**:450.

Weichselbaum, R.R., S. Hellman, A.J. Piro, J.J. Nove, and J.B. Little. 1978. Proliferation kinetics of a human breast cancer cell line in vitro following treatment with 17β-estradiol and 1-β-D-arabinofuranosylcytosine. *Cancer Res.* **38**:2339.

Westley, B. and H. Rochefort. 1980. A secreted glycoprotein induced by estrogen in human breast cancer cell lines. *Cell* **20**:353.

Zava, D.T. and W.L. McGuire. 1978. Human breast cancer: Androgen action mediated by estrogen receptor. *Science* **199**:787.

COMMENTS

MEITES: I would like to ask Marc [Lippman] to clarify something. You stated that you could get growth from breast cancer cells in vitro with estradiol (E_2), that is, an increase in DNA. Was that in absence of serum?

LIPPMAN: Yes.

MEITES: In other words, in the absence of pituitary hormone.

LIPPMAN: Yes. It is in the October 1978 *Cancer Research* (Allegra and Lippman 1978).

MEITES: Thus, you can get growth of human breast cancer cells with estrogen in the absence of pituitary hormone.

LIPPMAN: Right.

MEITES: How does that correlate with the results of Shiu (see Shiu, this volume)?

LIPPMAN: He is talking about normal mammary tissue.

WELSCH: I was talking about normal human breast explants—normal human breast maintained in the athymic nude mouse.

MEITES: Didn't you tell me that breast cancer tissue also doesn't respond unless you have a prolactin source?

WELSCH: Normal human breast tissue, not cancerous breast.

LIPPMAN: In a straightforward in vitro system, there never has been a demonstration of a growth hormone or a prolactin growth response.

ROSEN: Marc, there is one critical thing, though, that everybody is doing, and that is they are plating cells on a plastic dish and trying to look for response. I think the studies of Dr. Nandi (this volume) and other laboratories have shown clearly that even normal human mammary and rodent cells do not grow well on plastic and that, if you do the experiment that way, you set it up ahead of time so the cells are not going to respond to hormones even if they should.

LIPPMAN: I am not trying to make that case.

ROSEN: Okay, but you need to say that when you talk about the system, because I think it is important to realize that growing cells on a plastic dish is not the normal environment. The collagen gel matrix or some other substrate may be a critical variable. Regardless of how many hormones you isolate or find, you may need other factors in addition to just adding hormones to the cell.

LIPPMAN: No question.

SEGALOFF: Marc, what would happen if, instead of tamoxifen at 10^{-6}, you used E_2 at 10^{-6}?

LIPPMAN: Well, you recall that I showed you the basic response to high concentrations of E_2. When we first reported about the responses of these cells in 1976, we showed that very response—high concentrations of E_2 are inhibitory to growth.

We have never spent a lot of time working on that, because we think that it is most likely that the effects of high concentrations of E_2, as we see them in culture, are nonspecific; that is, we can inhibit at those concentrations cells that lack ER.

Although it is true that high concentrations of estrogen clearly work clinically in experimental animals and in women with breast cancer (as well as in men with breast cancer), that in no way implies that this is a direct action. No one, including ourselves, has presented the ways of getting around the nonspecific effects of these micromolar concentrations of steroids, which will load up lysosomes, etc. I just don't have any strong feeling that we are looking at a specific inhibition.

SEGALOFF: The other half of it is, what does tamoxifen do in the other cells without the receptor.

LIPPMAN: Tamoxifen at those concentrations has been shown by several other investigators reproducing our work not to have any inhibitory effects.

KORENMAN: Marc, in light of this morning's discussion, I wonder whether you can comment on a role for progesterone in cells, particularly with regard to the estrogen.

LIPPMAN: I am not aware, frankly, of any tissue culture system, except some short-term endometrial systems, that responds to progesterone, except occasionally, when it can be shown pretty clearly to be a promiscuous interaction with a glucocorticoid receptor.

KORENMAN: What about an effect on the ER?

LIPPMAN: We have done no experiments with it.

NANDI: Marc, has anybody looked at primary human tumors to see whether there is any effect of estrogen, in terms of growth?

LIPPMAN: I am not familiar with that. A lot of people have reported that, in many cases, they do get increased labeling indices with tumor explants, but much of that literature is poor.

NANDI: We cannot find any of that in the collagen gel system.

SIRBASKU: I just reviewed that for a review article going back through all the human tumor work. Marc and I are usually the protagonists at a meeting. But the position is that, in reviewing all the experiments that have been done with human mammary tumor explants, the labeling index of incorporation of [³H]thymine into DNA rests at 1.5 to maybe 2.0 increases at best, and usually in less than 50% of the samples. So it doesn't really look as though you can take those explants and easily establish that fact by that method.

That brings up a point that was made by Jeff [Rosen] that I disagree with in a sense. I reviewed a lot of the literature using organ explants, because the argument about substrate is very important here. It is not a trivial argument. But when you look at the facts, what happens is that organ explants maintain their structure better and have a better basement membrane than something we have synthesized ourselves and put into the medium. Even there you do not see the proper estrogen responses. It is low. The magnitude is 50% increase in [³H]thymine. If anybody accepts [³H]thymine as an example of growth, it is a very dangerous position, very dangerous.

References

Allegra, J.C. and M.E. Lippman. 1978. Growth of a human breast cancer cell line in serum free hormone-supplemented medium. *Cancer Res.* 38:3823.

Lippman, M.E., G. Bolan, and K. Huff. 1976. The effects of estrogens and antiestrogens on hormone responsive human breast cancer in long term tissue culture. *Cancer Res.* 36:4595.

Prolactin, Pituitary Hormones, and Breast Cancer

ROBERT P. C. SHIU
Department of Physiology, Faculty of Medicine
University of Manitoba
Winnipeg, Manitoba, Canada R3E OW3

One of the continuing goals in this laboratory is to elucidate the mechanism of action of prolactin in target cells. It is without doubt that at least four aspects of prolactin action are mediated by an initial binding of prolactin to cell surface receptor sites. These aspects are: the prolactin-induced casein synthesis and amino acid transport in the mammary tissue (Shiu and Friesen 1976); the prolactin-induced proliferation of Nb2 cells, a rat lymphoma cell line whose proliferation is dependent solely on prolactin (Gout et al. 1980; Tanaka et al. 1980; R.P.C. Shiu et al., in prep.); the prolactin-induced luteolysis in the rat (Bohnet et al. 1978); and the prolactin-stimulated water transport across the human amnion (Leontic and Tyson 1977). In view of these observations, it is rationalized that the study of prolactin receptors may provide some insight into the biological significance of prolactin in breast cancer.

A number of studies have indicated that specific prolactin binding sites, which have all the characteristics of prolactin receptors, are present in some human breast cancer biopsies (Holdaway and Friesen 1977; Morgan et al. 1977; Stagner et al. 1977). For obvious reasons, biopsy specimens are not suitable for long-term studies on the biological consequence of the interaction of prolactin with its receptors. Human breast cancer cells maintained in culture are, therefore, potentially useful for this purpose.

METHODS

Human breast cancer cell lines used in these studies were obtained from Dr. M. Rich (Michigan Cancer Foundation), Dr. E.Y. Lasfargues (Institute for Medical Research, Camden, N.J.), E.G. & G/Mason Research Institute, Rockville, Md., and J.F. Weaver (Cell Culture Department, Naval Biosciences Lab., Oakland, California). GH_3 rat pituitary tumor cells were obtained from the American Type Culture Association. Growth conditions for these cells have been described previously (Shiu 1979). Procedures used for the determinations of specific binding of ^{125}I-labeled human prolactin also have been described (Shiu 1979).

Immunocytochemical procedures similar to those employed by Sternberger (1979), have been detailed elsewhere (Salih et al. 1979; R.P.C. Shiu, H. Salih, and J.A. Paterson, in prep.). Detailed procedures for studying tumor growth in athymic nude mice have been described (Leung and Shiu 1981). Other details are described in the text and legends to Figures and Tables.

RESULTS AND DISCUSSION

A number of human breast cancer cell lines were assayed for prolactin receptors. The result of such a survey is illustrated in Table 1. Twelve cell lines tested contain varying degrees of prolactin-binding activity. The number of prolactin receptor sites per cell varies among cell lines: The values range from 26,000 for T-47D to about 1000 sites for DU 4475. HBL-100, a cell line derived from human milk, also contains a low level of prolactin receptors. Furthermore, the receptor sites have very high affinity for prolactin: The dissociation constant (K_D) ranges from 1-2.5×10^{-10} M.

The hormone specificity of the prolactin receptors in the breast cancer cells is illustrated in Figure 1. All lactogenic hormones, namely, human prolactin, human growth hormone (hGH), and human placental lactogen (hPL) compete with ^{125}I-labeled human prolactin for the receptor sites; hPL is about 1% as potent as are human prolactin and hGH. Sheep prolactin is almost as effective as is human prolactin, consistent with its biological activity, which was determined in organ culture experiments using human breast tumor biopsy

Table 1
Prolactin Receptors in Human Breast Cell Lines

Cell line	Number of prolactin receptors per cell
Tumor cells	
T-47D	25,800
MCF-7	8,310
MDA-MB-157	7,663
BT-20	6,435
BT-474	5,480
MDA-MB-231	3,760
ALAB 496	3,650
SK-BR-3	3,329
Hs0578T	2,260
Levine III	1,619
Du 4475	1,094
Normal cells	
HBL-100	1,700

Part of the results presented in this table are reprinted with permission, from Shiu (1979).

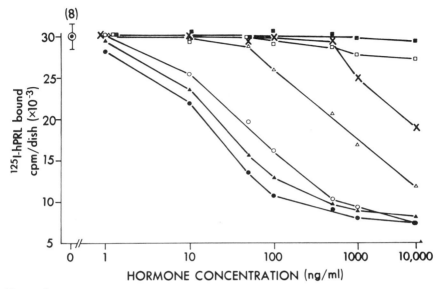

Figure 1
Hormone specificity of binding of ^{125}I-labeled human prolactin (hPRL) to human breast cancer cells (T-47D). Unlabeled hormones: (■) hLH; (□) hCG; (×) oGH; (△) hPL; (○) sheep prolactin; (▲) hGH; (●) human prolactin. (Reprinted, with permission, from Shiu 1979.)

specimens (Kleinberg 1975). Sheep growth hormone (oGH), which is not lactogenic, is ineffective as a competitor. Other human hormones fail to compete with ^{125}I-labeled human prolactin for the receptor sites. The same hormone specificity was reported for the prolactin binding sites in membrane preparations derived from human breast tumor biopsy specimens (Holdaway and Friesen 1977; Stagner et al. 1977). The characteristics of the receptor sites in these human breast cancer cells are identical to those of the classical prolactin receptors (Shiu et al. 1973). The observation that hGH shares the same receptor site for prolactin in human breast tumor cells raises the possibility that hGH may have prolactin-like effects. Indeed, studies using biopsy specimens maintained in organ culture support this notion (Salih et al. 1972; Kleinberg 1975; Welsch et al. 1976). Assuming that prolactin has a role in the etiology of human breast cancer, any attempts to induce tumor regression by the mere suppression of prolactin secretion (e.g., by bromocriptine) may not be enough. It may be essential to suppress hGH secretion as well.

The binding of prolactin to some human breast cancer cell lines has also been studied morphologically by using the technique of immunocytochemistry (Salih et al. 1979; R.P.C. Shiu, H. Salih, and J.A. Paterson, in prep.). This technique revealed one feature of prolactin binding that was not apparent from studies using the aforementioned biochemical techniques, namely, the prolactin binding within a human breast cancer cell line can be heterogeneous. Figure 2A illustrates the result after T-47D tumor cells were incubated with prolactin, fixed, reacted with an antiserum to the hormone, and the cell-bound prolactin visualized by the soluble peroxidase-antiperoxidase method of Sternberger (1979). It was observed that not all the cells are stained equally for prolactin (darker spots indicate staining), indicating heterogeneity of prolactin binding in this cell line. We do not yet know the reasons for this observation. It is possible that the heterogeneity in prolactin binding reflects cells in different phases of the cell cycle or cells representing distinct types. No staining was observed if the antiserum to prolactin was replaced by a nonimmune serum (Fig. 2B) and if cells not previously incubated with prolactin were reacted with antiprolactin serum (not shown).

Having established that human breast cancer cells maintained in tissue culture possess prolactin receptors, it is, therefore, essential to establish the

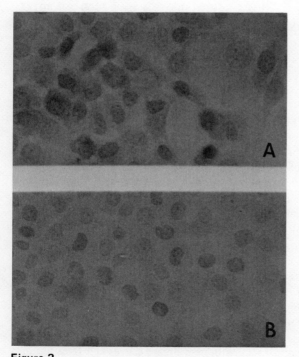

Figure 2

Immunocytochemical demonstration of binding of human prolactin to human breast cancer cells (T-47D). Monolayer cells were incubated for 1 hr at 37°C with 5 μg/ml human prolactin, followed by washing, fixation, reacted with rabbit anti-human prolactin serum (A) or nonimmune rabbit serum (B), and visualized by soluble peroxidase-antiperoxidase (see Sternberger 1979; and R.P.C. Shiu, H. Salih, and J.A. Paterson, in prep. for details).

biological significance of prolactin receptors and the biological responses that prolactin produces in these cells. There have been only limited studies on the effects of prolactin on human breast cancer cells in culture. Studies with human breast tumor biopsies maintained in organ culture suggested that some tumors responded to prolactin treatment with an increase in pentose pathway enzyme activity (Salih et al. 1972), in the production of α-lactalbumin (Kleinberg 1975), and in the uptake of [^{3}H]thymidine (Welsch et al. 1976). Furthermore, it has been reported that prolactin stimulates estrogen receptor (ER) activity (Shafie and Brooks 1977) and protein synthesis (Burke and Gaffney 1978) in a breast tumor cell line, MCF-7. One of the important questions that remains to be answered is, "Can prolactin affect the rate of proliferation (growth) of human breast tumor cells?" We, therefore, examined whether or not prolactin and other hormones are mitogenic in several human breast cancer cell lines that contain appreciable amounts of prolactin receptors. The data of several experiments are summarized in Table 2. Purified human prolactin and hGH (at concentrations of 10 ng/ml to 1 μg/ml) failed to affect the growth rate of T-47D and MCF-7 cells in vitro. In contrast, insulin and epidermal growth factor (EGF) stimulated the growth of both cell lines, whereas pituitary-derived fibroblast

Table 2

Effect of Hormones and Growth Factors on Growth of Human Breast Cancer Cells in Monolayer Cultures

| | Cell number ($\times 10^{-5}$) | | | |
| | T-47D | | MCF-7 | |
Additions	no serum	1% CFCS[a]	no serum	1% CFCS
None	0.4 ± 0.1	5.6 ± 0.2	0.8 ± 0.1	7.4 ± 0.1
Human prolactin	0.4 ± 0.1	5.5 ± 0.6	0.8 ± 0.2	7.2 ± 0.3
hGH	0.5 ± 0.1	—	0.9 ± 0.1	—
Insulin	$1.1 \pm 0.2*$[b]	$10.1 \pm 0.2*$	1.0 ± 0.2	$9.6 \pm 0.5*$
FGF	$1.6 \pm 0.4*$	$9.3 \pm 0.1*$	0.9 ± 0.2	7.0 ± 0.1
EGF	$0.8 \pm 0.1*$	—	$1.4 \pm 0.2*$	—
17β-E$_2$	—	6.3 ± 0.1	—	$11.0 \pm 0.3*$
Testosterone	—	5.4 ± 0.5	—	—
Dexamethasone	—	5.7 ± 0.4	—	$4.4 \pm 0.4*$
Progesterone	—	6.3 ± 0.4	—	7.6 ± 0.7
T3	—	$10.2 \pm 0.8*$	—	$9.6 \pm 0.4*$

Cell numbers were determined 7 days after the additions of hormones or growth factors. Each value represents mean of triplicate $\pm$ S.D.

The final concentrations of hormones and growth factors were: Human prolactin, 1 μg/ml; hGH, 1 μg/ml; insulin, 10 μg/ml; FGF, 10 ng/ml; EFG, 10 ng/ml; 17β-E$_2$, 10^{-8} M; testosterone, 10^{-8} M; dexamethasone, 10^{-7} M; progesterone, 10^{-7} M; T3, 5×10^{-7} M.

[a]Charcoal-treated fetal calf serum.

[b]Asterisks indicate values which are significantly different from the control (no addition) with $P < 0.05$.

growth factor (FGF) stimulated the growth of T-47D but not that of MCF-7 cells. For the steroids tested at low concentrations, 17β-estradiol (17β-E_2) was stimulatory in MCF-7 but had much less effect on T-47D cells. Dexamethasone was inhibitory in general, and progesterone and testosterone were without effect. High concentrations ($> 10^{-5}$ M) of all the steroids were inhibitory. The thyroid hormone, triiodothyroxine (T3), consistently stimulated the growth of both T-47D and MCF-7 cells. Furthermore, when tested in combination with several other hormones, prolactin did not produce any further stimulation over that observed for the other hormones alone (data not shown).

In short, so far we have been unable to demonstrate a growth-regulatory effect of prolactin in vitro. There are, of course, many possible reasons to explain why this is so. First, prolactin may play no role in the growth regulation of human breast cancer cells, although it affects other cellular functions such as ER activity and protein synthesis, as reported by others. Second, it is possible that our in vitro culture conditions are not appropriate and that human breast cancer cells grown in such artificial environments are unable to respond to prolactin. Third, other permissive factors, which are absent in in vitro situations, may be needed to render the cells responsive to prolactin, and fourth, prolactin may act in vivo through an intermediate pathway that is missing in our in vitro experiments.

To test some of these possibilities, we decided to examine whether pituitary hormones are capable of influencing the growth of the human breast cancer cells in vivo, i.e., in athymic nude mide (Leung and Shiu 1981).

Four groups of nude mice were used: T group was injected with 2×10^7 T-47D breast tumor cells. TE group was injected with T-47D cells and estradiol valerate (500 μg/2 wk). TG group was injected with T-47D and 4×10^5 GH$_3$ rat pituitary tumor cells. GH$_3$ rat pituitary tumor cells were used in the hypopituitary nude mice because the cells secrete prolactin and GH (Tashjian et al. 1970) and, being of pituitary origin, may produce other factors that are essential to the growth of breast cancer cells. TEG group was injected with T-47D, GH$_3$ cells, and estradiol valerate. Tumor cells were injected s.c. in the flanks of each animal: T-47D on the left and GH$_3$ on the right. Estradiol valerate was injected s.c. at the dorsal midline, caudal to the neck. The growth of T-47D human breast tumors in the four groups of mice was monitored. Figure 3 shows that T-47D breast cancer cells did not proliferate in female nude mice (T group), indicating that the hormonal milieu in these animals is not optimal for the growth of human breast cancer cells. Russo et al. (1976) reported similar findings for another breast cancer cell line, MCF-7. It is interesting to note that in mice bearing GH$_3$ pituitary tumors (TG group), there was no apparent growth of T-47D human breast tumor despite very high concentrations of prolactin and GH (437 ± 376 ng/ml and 1008 ± 204 ng/ml, respectively) in the blood of the animals. Thus, it seems that prolactin and GH alone are not sufficient to stimulate the proliferation of T-47D tumor. On the other hand, injection of estrogen alone (TE group) resulted only in a very moderate growth

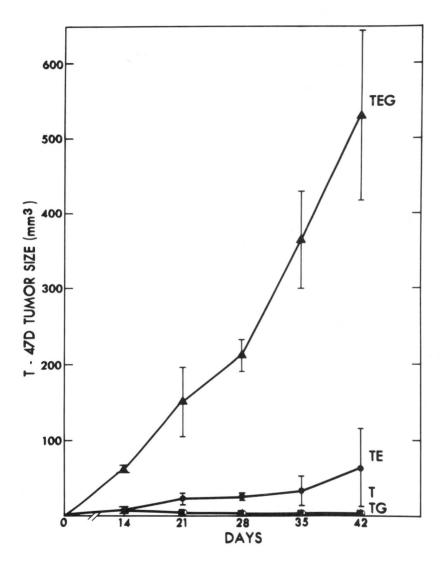

Figure 3
Growth of human breast cancer cells (T-47D) in athymic nude mice. Each point represents the mean ± S.D. from 4 animals. Tumor size, in mm^3, was the product of the three dimensions. T (○), mice injected with human breast cancer cells, T-47D, only; TG (■), mice injected with T-47D cells and GH$_3$ rat pituitary tumor cells; TE (●), mice injected with T-47D cells and estradiol valerate; TEG (▲), mice injected with T-47D and GH$_3$ cells and estradiol valerate. (Modified, with permission, from Leung and Shiu 1981).

of T-47D tumor, reaching a mean size of 63 ± 52 mm^3 (43 ± 11 mg) in 42 days. The simultaneous presence of estrogen, GH$_3$ tumor (i.e., TEG group), in contrast, induced rapid and sustained growth of T-47D tumors to a mean size of 528 ± 52 mm^3 (175 ± 26 mg). These values represent an eightfold increase in volume and about sixfold increase in weight over that of TE group, indicating that estrogen alone cannot produce maximal growth of the human breast cancer cells, T-47D. We have also observed that normal rat pituitaries implanted in estrogen-treated nude mice also induced very rapid proliferation of T-47D tumor cells (R.P.C. Shiu and C.K.H. Leung, unpubl.).

It is obvious from the in vivo studies that the human breast cancer cells are responsive to estrogen and pituitary hormones, even those hormones of another species. The magnitude of hormone response is quite dramatic, relative to what one sees when the same tumor cells were studied in vitro. The key questions from these studies are, therefore, What are the pituitary factors that stimulate the growth in vivo of human breast cancer cells? Could the principal active factor be prolactin or GH or some other unidentified factors? If it were prolactin, then why does it not stimulate the growth of breast cancer cells in vitro? It is possible that prolactin is only active when other permissive factors are present. These permissive factors would have been missing in in vitro culture conditions. These permissive factors could be estrogen, GH-induced intermediates (i.e., somatomedin-like substances), and other unrecognized substances. On the other hand, the active pituitary principle may belong to none of the "traditional" hormones. This notion is supported by the data of Ptashne et al. (1979) and Rudland et al. (1977, 1979), who demonstrated that mitogenic activity for breast cancer cells of rodents was present in plasma and the pituitary gland, respectively. Finally, the active pituitary factor could have been induced by estrogen. With regard to pituitary growth factors for mammary glands, Mittra (1980a,b) had recently identified a new form of prolactin which has a cleavage in its large disulfide loop and is synthesized and secreted by rat pituitary glands. This "cleaved" prolactin is made up of two chains; the two component polypeptides are separable into an N-terminal 16K-dalton fragment and a C-terminal 8K-dalton fragment by the reduction of the intervening disulfide bridge. The 16K-dalton N-terminal fragment was capable of stimulating mitosis of mammary epithelial cells, whereas the traditional prolactin was inactive. The author also suggested that the "cleaved" prolactin itself may be mitogenic as well. Moreover, the production of this "cleaved" prolactin was estrogen-dependent: It was not produced in pituitaries of ovariectomized rats but its production was resumed if ovariectomized rats were injected with estrogen. It would, therefore, be very interesting to see if the pituitary factor that stimulated the growth of the human breast cancer cells observed in our study is related to this "cleaved" form of prolactin.

No matter which one of the above possibilities turns out to be correct, the human breast cancer cell lines that possess prolactin, estrogen, and other hormone receptors should be useful models to elucidate the mechanism of interplay between ovarian steroids, pituitary hormones, and other yet to be characterized growth factors, in the control of proliferation of human breast cancer.

ACKNOWLEDGMENT

The work done in the author's laboratory was supported by the medical Research Council of Canada. The author is a Scholar of the Medical Research Council of Canada. The study on the immunocytochemical demonstration of prolactin binding was performed in collaboration with Dr. H. Salih, and the study on the growth of breast cancer cells in nude mice was carried out in collaboration with C.K.H. Leung. The author would also like to acknowledge Dr. E.Y. Lasfargues, Dr. M. Rich, Mr. C.V. Piczak, and Mr. J.F. Weaver for providing the cell lines used in his studies.

REFERENCES

Bohnet, H.G., R.P.C. Shiu, D. Grinwich, and H.G. Friesen. 1978. In vivo effects of antisera to prolactin receptors in female rats. *Endocrinology* **102**: 1657.

Burke, R.E. and E.V. Gaffney. 1978. Prolactin can stimulate general protein synthesis in human breast cancer cells (MCF-7) in long-term culture. *Life Sci.* **23**:901.

Gout, P.W., C.T. Beer, and R.L. Noble. 1980. Prolactin-stimulated growth of cell cultures established from malignant Nb rat lymphomas. *Cancer Res.* **40**:2433.

Holdaway, I.M. and H.G. Friesen. 1977. Hormone binding by human mammary carcinoma. *Cancer Res.* **37**:1946.

Kleinberg, D.L. 1975. Human α-lactalbumin: Measurement in serum and in breast cancer organ cultures by radioimmunoassay. *Science* **190**:276.

Leontic, E.A. and J.E. Tyson. 1977. Prolactin and fetal osmoregulation: Water transport across isolated human amnion. *Am. J. Physiol.* **232**:124.

Leung, C.K.H. and R.P.C. Shiu. 1981. Required presence of both estrogen and pituitary factors for the growth of human breast cancer cells in athymic nude mice. *Cancer Res.* **41**:546.

Mittra, I. 1980a. A novel "cleaved" prolactin in the rat pituitary: Part I. Biosynthesis, characterization and regulatory control. *Biochem. Biophys. Res. Commun.* **95**:1750.

————. 1980b. A novel "cleaved prolactin" in the rat pituitary: Part II. In vivo mammary mitogenic activity of its N-terminal 16k moiety. *Biochem. Biophys. Res. Commun.* **95**:1760.

Morgan, L., P.R. Raggatt, I. deSouza, H. Salih, and J.R. Hobbs. 1977. Prolactin receptors in human breast tumors. *J. Endocrinol.* **73**:17p.

Ptashne, K., H.W. Hseuh, and F.E. Stockdale. 1979. Partial purification and characterization of mammary stimulating factor, a protein which promotes proliferation of mammary epithelium. *Biochemistry* **18**:3533.

Rudland, P.S., D.C. Bennett, and M.J. Warburton. 1979. Hormonal control of growth and differentiation of cultured rat mammary gland epithelial cells. *Cold Spring Harbor Conf. Cell Proliferation* 6:677.

Rudland, P.S., P.C. Hallowes, H. Durbin, and D. Lewis. 1977. Mitogenic activity of pituitary hormones on cell cultures of normal and carcinogen-induced tumor epithelium from rat mammary glands. *J. Cell Biol.* 73:561.

Russo, J., C. McGrath, I.H. Russo, and M.A. Rich. 1976. Tumoral growth of human breast cancer cell line (MCF-7) in athymic mice. In *Prevention and detection of cancer* (ed. H.E. Nieburgs), vol. 1, p. 617. Marcel Dekker, Inc. New York and Basel.

Salih, H., K.W. Cheng, and R.P.C. Shiu. 1979. Immunocytochemical demonstration of prolactin binding to human breast cancer cells in long term tissue culture. In *Program and abstracts, 61st annual meeting, The Endocrine Society,* p. 151. (Abstr. 316)

Salih, H., H. Flax, W. Brander, and J.R. Hobbs. 1972. Prolactin dependence in human breast cancers. *Lancet* ii:1103.

Shafie, S. and S.C. Brooks. 1977. Effect of prolactin on growth and the estrogen receptor level of human breast cancer cells (MCF-7). *Cancer Res.* 37:792.

Shiu, R.P.C. 1979. Prolactin receptors in human breast cancer cells in long term tissue culture. *Cancer Res.* 39:4381.

Shiu, R.P.C. and H.G. Friesen. 1976. Blockade of prolactin action by an antiserum to its receptors. *Science* 192:259.

Shiu, R.P.C., P.A. Kelly, and H.G. Friesen. 1973. Radioreceptor assay for prolactin and other lactogenic hormones. *Science* 180:968.

Stagner, J.I., P.R. Jochimsen, and B.M. Sherman. 1977. Lactogenic hormone binding to human breast cancer: Correlation with estrogen receptor. *Clin. Res.* 25:320A.

Sternberger, L.A. 1979. *Immunocytochemistry* (2nd edition), p. 104. John Wiley & Sons, New York.

Tanaka, T., R.P.C. Shiu, P.W. Gout, C.T. Beer, R.L. Noble, and H.G. Friesen. 1980. A new sensitive and specific bioassay for lactogenic hormones: Measurement of prolactin and growth hormone in human serum. *J. Clin. Endocrinol. Metab.* 51:1058.

Tashjian, A.H., Jr., F.C. Bancroft, and L. Levine. 1970. Production of both prolactin and growth hormone by clonal strains of rat pituitary tumor cells. *J. Cell Biol.* 47:61.

Welsch, C.W., G. Calaf de Iturri, and M.J. Brennan. 1976. DNA synthesis of human, mouse and rat mammary carcinomas in vitro: Influence of insulin and prolactin. *Cancer* 38:1272.

COMMENTS

LIPPMAN: I am not sure I understand exactly why this isn't a GH receptor. You showed that hPL in competition was much less able to compete than human prolactin. I seem to remember that PL is usually as good as human prolactin in the other radioreceptor assays. Is this a GH receptor?

SHIU: Yes. I think, in general, that hPL is never as effective as a competitor for the prolactin site. hPL is never as biologically active in terms of the competition.

Second, these sites are not GH receptors, because if, for instance, you use radioactive oGH, it doesn't bind. On the other hand, if you use radioactive hGH, then it would bind.

LIPPMAN: Yes but oGH has no growth-promoting effects in humans, so you wouldn't expect it to bind to a hGH receptor. I don't understand why that experiment shows what you suggest. It is true that you can only use hGH to bring about a GH response in man. So why would you anticipate that oGH would bind to that receptor?

SHIU: Well, not in this case, I agree. oGH itself may not work.

LIPPMAN: So it shouldn't bind.

ROSEN: The reciprocal you showed in your competition experiment is ovine prolactin, and it does compete for binding. Is that not correct?

SHIU: That is right.

ROSEN: And ovine prolactin does not have GH activity.

LIPPMAN: Does it have anti-GH activity?

ROSEN: As far as I know, none. So that is the answer to your question. In a similar vein, when you did your injections to nude mice, you left out the ovine prolactin plus E_2 experiment. Have you done that?

SHIU: No.

ROSEN: You really can't answer whether you have prolactin-like receptors or GH receptors that are responding in the nude mice. The easiest way to test that is to add E_2 plus ovine prolactin and see if the cells grow in nude mice.

LIPPMAN: One more thing. Isn't your GH experiment with the GH_3 cells a kind of proof that the effect is not due to prolactin, because I didn't think rat prolactin interacted with human receptor?

SHIU: No. Actually, I haven't shown it here, but I think, if you use the comparable preparation, that is, a preparation which is comparable in terms of biologic activity in tissue, you would see displacement by rat prolactin. So this GH_3 experiment really doesn't rule out whether it is prolactin or not.

SIRBASKU: Along that line, we have been, I think, chasing exactly the same pituitary hormone. We have been getting it from $GH_3/C14$ pituitary tumor cell. Our activity promotes the growth of our mammary tumor cells. We have been using the antiserum against rat prolactin and rat GH to remove those two hormones. We cannot remove the mitogenic activity that way. On top of those experiments, we have shown about a 60K m.w. right now, which is heavier than the clipped form of prolactins. So at least right now we think, if it is a new hormone, that it is larger than known activities and it is not either GH or prolactin.

WELSCH: The athymic nude mouse experiment that Bob [Shiu] described is a simplistic study very similar to one that we have just completed. We will be reporting our data at the next cancer meeting (AACR, April 1981).

In our study, we transplanted normal human breast to the athymic nude mouse. During the past year or two, we have attempted to stimulate growth of this tissue by injecting estrogen or estrogen plus progesterone into the host animals. The transplanted tissue simply does not respond. We have transplanted a rat pituitary tumor, very much like the one described by Bob, to these animals bearing grafts of human breast tissue. The rat pituitary tumor alone did not stimulate growth of the human breast tissue. However, the combination of estrogen and the rat pituitary tumor markedly stimulated growth of the human breast tissue!

SIRBASKU: Is this normal tissue?

WELSCH: This is normal human breast tissue; the study was similar to what Bob described using the cancerous human breast cell line.

Estrogen Receptor Assays in Familial and Nonfamilial Breast Cancer

RUTH OTTMAN*
University of California
Department of Genetics
Berkeley, California 94720

PHILIP G. HOFFMAN AND PENTTI K. SIITERI
University of California
Department of Obstetrics, Gynecology and Reproductive Sciences
San Francisco, California 94143

An impressive amount of evidence has accumulated regarding the importance of estrogen receptor assays in the clinical management of breast cancer (McGuire 1978). In advanced breast cancer, high estrogen receptor levels are associated with positive response to endocrine therapy. In primary disease, patients whose malignant breast tissue contains large quantities of estrogen receptor have longer recurrence-free survival. However, the results of estrogen receptor assays are quite variable, and we still understand very little about why some breast tumors contain a large amount of receptor, and other contain almost none. It is possible that genetic differences among breast cancer patients influence the results of estrogen receptor assays in their malignant cells.

In some unusual families with extremely high incidence of breast cancer, high susceptibility may be explained by genetic inheritance (King et al. 1980). Nonfamilial breast cancer is less likely to have a genetic etiology (Anderson 1971). Risk for breast cancer is also influenced by ages at menarche, first pregnancy, and menopause, suggesting that reproductive hormones are involved in the etiology of the disease. Thus, differences in genetic susceptibility could be mediated by differences in estrogen stimulation. Further, estrogen receptor assays in breast cancer tissue might reflect subtle differences in estrogen production, transport, or metabolism that influence susceptibility. Because familial breast cancer is more likely than nonfamilial breast cancer to have a genetic etiology, we investigated the possibility that estrogen receptor assay results differ between familial and nonfamilial breast cancer. Specifically, we asked: Do familial and nonfamilial breast cancer differ in either the binding capacity (ER) or the dissociation constant (K_D) of the estrogen receptor?

*Present address: G.H. Sergievsky Center, Faculty of Medicine, Columbia University, 630 West 168 Street, New York, New York, 10032.

METHODS

Information Analyzed

The study population consisted of 2062 breast cancer patients from approximately 50 hospitals throughout California whose biopsy or mastectomy samples were assayed between 1976 and 1979. As described in detail elsewhere (Ottman et al., in prep.), the assay procedure involved Scatchard analysis (Scatchard 1949) of tumor cytosols, theoretically yielding estimates of ER and K_D for each tissue sample. In practice, K_D was difficult to estimate when ER was very low; hence, only 87.1% of all assays produced K_D estimates. Figure 1 compares the observed cumulative distribution of ER with that expected, assuming a log-normal distribution. The close correspondence between observed and expected indicated that it would not be useful to dichotomize assay results, as is frequently done. Instead, we viewed ER as a continuous variable with a log-normal distribution. As shown in Figure 2, the K_D values also fit a log-normal distribution. Thus, we were able to use the more powerful parametric statistics procedures in analyses involving both ER and K_D.

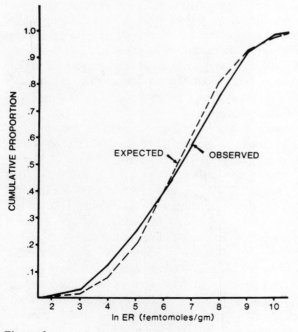

Figure 1

Distribution of ER. Observed cumulative proportion of cases with various *ln*ER values (———) compared with expected, assuming a normal distribution of *ln*ER values (————) (*N* = 2062).

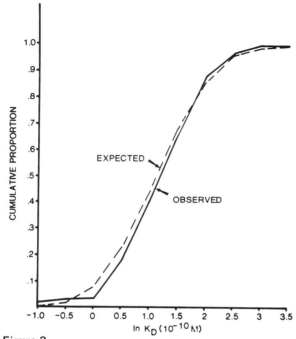

Figure 2

Distribution of K_D. Observed cumulative proportion of cases with various lnK_D values (———) compared with expected, assuming a normal distribution of lnK_D values (————) ($N = 1797$).

Information on family history of breast cancer came from discharge summaries submitted to the laboratory with samples by one hospital (67 cases) and from medical record reviews, which were possible at two hospitals (348 cases). Cases were considered to be familial if at least one first-degree relative (mother, sister, or daughter) was known to be affected with breast cancer. We were concerned that various clinical or epidemiologic characteristics might influence the assay and confound comparisons between familial and nonfamilial patients. Therefore, we also collected information on the variables listed in Table 1.

Statistical Approach

We were interested in the potential influences of the clinical and epidemiologic variables in Table 1 on each of the estimates produced by the assay (ER and K_D). Therefore, we did two separate statistical analyses, each using one of the

Table 1

Clinical and Epidemiologic Characteristics Analyzed in Relation to ER Assays

Clinical

Hormonal
- Menopausal status[a]
- Phase of menstrual cycle
- Current pregnancy
- History of bilateral oophorectomy
- Current (within 2 weeks) use of
  exogenous hormones
- History of cytotoxic or radiation therapy

Pathologic
- Specimen site
- Histological classification
- Stage
- Size of primary tumors
- Differentiation

Epidemiologic

Age
Race
History of contralateral primary breast cancer
First-degree family history of breast cancer

[a] Premenopausal, age less than 50 or last menses less than 1 yr before surgery; perimenopausal, age 50-55 or last menses 1-5 yr before surgery; postmenopausal, age greater than 55 or last menses more than 5 yr before surgery.

estimates as the dependent variable. Since the distributions of both variables were log normal, all analyses were in terms of $lnER$ or lnK_D.

The method used throughout the analysis was analysis of covariance, with lnK_D and age as the controlling variables in analysis of $lnER$ and with $lnER$ as the controlling variable in analysis of lnK_D (Ottman et al., in prep.). First, each clinical or epidemiologic characteristic was analyzed separately to select subgroups that appeared to define separate populations of $lnER$ or lnK_D, using a relaxed criterion of significance ($p < 0.1$). Then, all of the separate subgroups that emerged in this preliminary analysis were analyzed simultaneously. This multivariate approach afforded two advantages. It allowed us to evaluate the independent effect of each clinical or epidemiologic variable, controlling for associations that could create or obscure its influences on $lnER$ and lnK_D. It also allowed us to focus on the potential differences between familial and nonfamilial breast cancer, since it was a means for simultaneously controlling the effects of all of the other variables.

RESULTS

Binding Capacity

Figures 3 and 4 show the results of the final multivariate analysis of ER. These histograms represent the antilogarithm of the mean $lnER$ ($\pm$ S.E.), after controlling for all other variables in the analysis. As is generally observed,

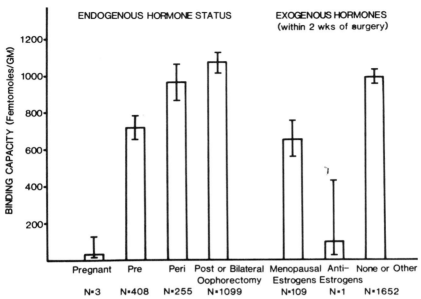

Figure 3

Hormonal characteristics that influenced ER. Comparisons of ER values in breast cancers from women with various endogenous and exogenous hormone characteristics. Histograms represent the antilogarithm of the mean lnER for each group (± S.E.), after controlling for all other variables that influenced ER (Figs. 3 and 4).

premenopausal cases had significantly lower ER than postmenopausal or oophorectomized cases. The ER values in three pregnant cases were also strikingly low. Two exogenous hormones also appeared to influence ER. Patients who had taken menopausal estrogens within 2 weeks of surgery had significantly lower ER values than those who were not known to have taken such hormones. Also, one patient who was taking antiestrogens had an extremely low ER.

Several pathologic characteristics also influenced ER (Fig. 5). When biopsy specimens from metastases to different tissues were compared, axillary nodal and liver metastases had unusually high ER values, and bone metastases had unusually low values. Medullary, scirrhous, and comedocarcinomas had lower ER values when compared with the remaining histologic types. Finally, well-differentiated tumors had higher ER values than those that were not known to be well-differentiated.

Dissociation Constants

Figure 5 shows the characteristics that influenced the K_D. First, breast cancers from cases who were in the luteal phase of the menstrual cycle (16-33 days

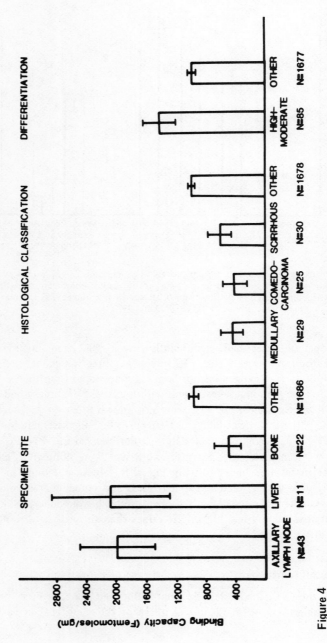

Figure 4

Pathologic characteristics that influenced ER. Comparison of ER values in breast cancers with various pathologic characteristics. Histograms represent the antilogarithm of the mean *ln*ER for each group (± S.E.), after controlling for all other variables that influence ER (Figs. 3 and 4).

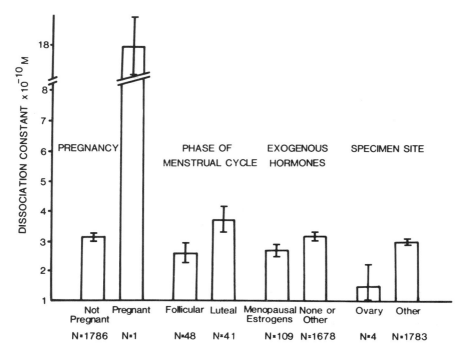

Figure 5

Clinical characteristics that influenced the K_D. Comparison of K_D values in breast cancers from women with various clinical characteristics. Histograms represent the antilogarithm of the mean lnK_D for each group (± S.E.), after controlling for all other variables that influenced K_D.

since last menses) had higher K_D values than those from cases who were in the follicular phase (0-12 days since last menses). Also the K_D in the sample from one pregnant case was elevated dramatically. Breast cancers from patients who had taken menopausal estrogens within 2 weeks of surgery had somewhat lower K_D values than those from patients who were not known to have taken such hormones. Finally, four ovarian specimens had lower K_D values than those from other tissue sites.

Family History

Figure 6 summarizes the comparison between familial and nonfamilial breast cancer, after controlling for all other variables that appeared to influence ER or K_D, respectively. K_D values were significantly higher in familial breast cancer than in nonfamilial breast cancer (two-tailed $p = 0.02$). ER was slightly lower in familial breast cancer than in nonfamilial breast cancer, but this difference was not significant (two-tailed $p = 0.24$).

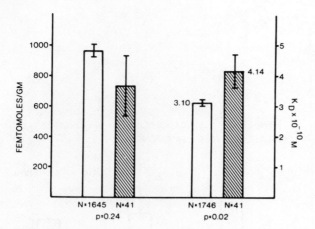

Figure 6

Comparison of familial and nonfamilial patients in ER and K_D. Patients with a first-degree family history (▨) are compared with those who are not known to have a family history (□). In analysis of binding capacity, ER, histograms represent the antilogarithm of the mean lnER (± S.E.), after controlling for all other variables that influenced ER. In analysis of K_Ds, histograms represent the antilogarithm of the mean $ln K_D$ (± S.E.), after controlling for all other variables that influenced K_D. P values pertain to two-tailed t test, comparing adjusted means of the two groups.

DISCUSSION

In our data, the ER content of breast cancer tissue was influenced by two types of variables. The first was related to the hormonal environment in which the tumor had grown. Patients with high circulating estrogen levels, whether endogenous or exogenous in origin, had tumors with relatively low ER values. Because our assay measures only unbound cytoplasmic receptor, high levels of circulating estrogen can reduce the observed ER values by (1) removing receptor from the cytoplasm through translocation to the nucleus and (2) binding to receptor that remains in the cytoplasm, making it unavailable for assay. Frequently, low ER levels in premenopausal breast cancer have been explained on this basis (McGuire et al. 1975), although other explanations are possible also (Saez et al. 1978).

The receptor content was also related to tumor pathology in our series. High ER levels in well-differentiated tumors have been observed previously (McGuire et al. 1975; Rosen et al. 1975). Recently, Silfversward et al. (1980) also reported low levels in medullary and comedocarcinoma. They attribute their finding to the low differentiation of these two histologic types.

When the epithelial cellularity of a tumor is low, the tissue sample removed from it often consists largely of stroma. In this situation, ER levels are likely to be low due to the low epithelial cellularity of the sample. Thus, as was suggested by Rosen et al. (1975), the low cellularity of scirrhous carcinoma could explain our observation of low ER content in this histologic type. Similarly, axillary lymph node and liver metastases, in which we found high ER levels, are likely to be highly cellular, and bone metastases, in which we found low ER levels, are likely to be acellular.

Our analysis of K_D values yielded several interesting findings, which stimulated consideration of the factors that could influence K_D estimation by Scatchard analysis. We found unusually high K_D values in pregnancy and in the luteal phase of the menstrual cycle, when estrogen production rates are high. In our assay procedure, unbound endogenous estrogens and other steroids are not removed from the tissue preparations before adding radiolabeled estradiol (E_2). Therefore, the unbound endogenous estrogens could compete with labeled E_2 for unoccupied receptor binding sites. This competition leads to a reduction of the tracer binding to receptor, causing an underestimate of the bound fraction which is used in the calculation of the Scatchard plot. The estimate of ER is not affected, because competition is insignificant when the amount of added tracer is at saturating concentrations. However, the slope of the Scatchard plot is decreased, leading to an elevation of the K_D estimate. The magnitude of the effect on the K_D is proportional to the amount of endogenous estrogen in the tissue sample which competes with the tracer for receptor binding.

The unusually higher K_D values that we observed in familial breast cancer could be due to a decreased binding affinity of the estrogen receptor molecule in some familial patients. However, the influence of endogenous estrogens on the K_D estimates suggests an alternative interpretation: Tissue estrogen concentrations may be higher in familial than in nonfamilial breast cancer.

Breast cancer affects approximately 1 in every 14 women at some time in her life (Zdeb 1977). Therefore, 2 women within the same family may often be affected with breast cancer due simply to the chance co-occurrence of a common disease. This means that a first-degree family history of breast cancer is not necessarily an indication of increased susceptibility within the family as a whole. Furthermore, even among families with exceptionally high incidence of breast cancer, only a minority appear to have a genetic predisposition to the disease (King et al. 1980). This implies that a very small proportion of familial breast cancer patients carries an allele increasing susceptibility to breast cancer. In our comparison of estrogen receptor assays in familial and nonfamilial breast cancer, we postulated that some of the variation in ER and K_D was explained by genetically determined differences in endocrine factors that are related to breast cancer susceptibility. Because only a minority of familial patients are genetically predisposed to breast cancer, these endocrine differences must be very large to appear in this type of comparison. In view of this, our finding of higher K_D values in familial than in nonfamilial breast cancer is particularly dramatic. If the difference is due to altered expression of susceptibility genes in some familial patients, it must be an underestimate of the effect on the K_D. Those patients who are members of families with extremely high susceptibility may have K_D values that are elevated far above average, while other familial patients have only average values.

Women in high-risk families have been found to have reduced excretion of estrogen glucuronides (Fishman et al. 1978a), although their circulating estrogen levels were no different from those of control women (Fishman et al. 1978b). This reduced excretion could result from increased uptake and retention of estrogens in target tissues, such as the breast. If this condition persisted after development of breast cancer, tissue samples removed from some familial patients would contain elevated quantities of estrogen, leading to elevated K_D values in estrogen receptor assays. Recently, we have found that some women with breast cancer have an abnormality in serum binding, such that the percentage of free E_2 is greater than normal (Siiteri et al., this volume). If some unaffected women in high-risk families also have this abnormality, the availability of estrogens to their tissues would be increased, possibly explaining their increased risk for breast cancer.

Thus, the elevated K_D values that we observed in familial breast cancer may reflect an underlying endocrine abnormality which led to development of the disease. Prospective studies will be critical in testing this hypothesis. We need to confirm that women in high-risk families who eventually develop breast cancer have unusually high tissue estrogen levels before they develop the disease.

ACKNOWLEDGMENTS

This research was supported in part by NIH-NRSA GM07127. Mary-Claire King and Steve Selvin made helpful suggestions during all phases of the research. Mary Davis and Robbie Franklin provided laboratory assistance.

REFERENCES

Anderson, D.E. 1971. Some characteristics of familial breast cancer. *Cancer* 28:1500.

Fishman, J., D. Fukushima, J. O'Connor, and H.T. Lynch. 1978a. Low urinary estrogen glucuronides in women at risk for familial breast cancer. *Science* 204:1089.

Fishman, J., D. Fukushima, J. O'Connor, R.S. Rosenfeld, H.T. Lynch, J.F. Lynch, H. Guirgis, and K. Maloney. 1978b. Plasma hormone profiles of young women at risk for familial breast cancer. *Cancer Res.* 38:4006.

King, M-C., R.C.P. Go, R.C. Elston, H.T. Lynch, and N.L. Petrakis. 1980. An allele increasing susceptibility to human breast cancer may be linked to the glutamate-pyruvate transaminase locus. *Science* 208:406.

McGuire, W.L. 1978. Steroid receptors in human B.C. *Cancer Res.* 38:4289.

McGuire, W.L., P.P. Carbone, M.E. Sears, and G.C. Escher. 1975. Human breast cancer: An overview. In *Estrogen receptors in human breast cancer* (ed. W.L. McGuire et al.), p. 1. Raven Press, New York.

Rosen, P.P., C.J. Menendez-Botet, J.S. Nisselbaum, J.A. Urban, V. Mike, A. Fracchia, and M.K. Schwartz. 1975. Pathological review of breast lesions analyzed for estrogen receptor protein. *Cancer Res.* 35:3187.

Saez, S., P.M. Martin, and C.D. Chouvet. 1978. Estradiol and progesterone receptor levels in human breast adenocarcinoma in relation to plasma estrogen and progesterone levels. *Cancer Res.* 38:3468.

Scatchard, G. 1949. The attraction of proteins for small molecules and ions. *Ann. N.Y. Acad. Sci.* 51:660.

Silfversward, C., J-A. Gustafsson, S.A. Gustafsson, S. Humla, B. Nordenskjold, A. Wallgren, and O. Wrange. 1980. Estrogen receptor concentrations in 269 cases of histologically classified human B.C. *Cancer* 45:2001.

Zdeb, M.S. 1977. The probability of developing cancer. *Am. J. Epidemiol.* 106:6.

COMMENTS

SIITERI: Ruth brought these data to me and asked, "What can we make out of these differences?" Obviously the differences in titers have been published previously by others. In my reading of the literature and looking at data, there are rather wide variations in values for the K_D. It is all over the lot, and everybody assumes that is the way life is.

But that one number, the one tumor from a pregnant woman, said that we had better look at this again. I recalled that the presence of endogenous hormones produces artefactual estimates of K_D. When receptor assays are analyzed by Scatchard plots, unbound hormone present in cytosol competes with the added radiolabeled estradiol (E_2) for binding with the unoccupied receptor.

Our assay is run at $2°C$ and uses a Sephadex gel filtration minicolumn to separate bound and free hormone. We do not remove endogenous hormones by charcoal extraction prior to incubation with labeled E_2. When I set it up 4 or 5 years ago, I decided to do as little as possible to the cytosol before running the assay, because many times you don't get a second chance.

Figure A illustrates a typical assay. The solid line shows the results obtained on cytosol from a breast tumor specimen. To other aliquots of the cytosol, we added nonlabeled E_2 (1 pM/g of tissue) or progesterone (10 pM/g of tissue) and repeated the assay. As can be seen from Figure A, progesterone addition had no effect on the slope of the plot whereas E_2 depressed the slope dramatically and increased the K_D from 1.5×10^{-10} M to 8.6×10^{-10} M.

If one assumes the existence of a single, true value of K_D for the ER binding of E_2, then the presence of endogenous hormone shifts the slope of the Scatchard plot downward and results in a higher apparent K_D. The difference between the apparent and the true K_D is the tissue concentration of estrogen (E) as shown by the simple relationship K_D (app.) $= K_D + E$.

So it occurred to me that perhaps we were actually doing a kind of crazy radioimmunoassay for total tissue "estrogens" defined only by their ability to bind the receptor.

To illustrate the point further, I have plotted the calculated breast tumor "estrogen" concentration against values for K_D that Ruth showed you (Fig. B). I had to assign some value for the true K_D, and I chose a value of 0.2 nM. As can be seen, the values for follicular- and luteal-phase tumors or nonfamilial and familial tumors differ by about 1 pM/g tissue. The value for the pregnancy sample is much higher (about 15 pM/g). I obviously cannot be too certain about the absolute values, but they are not totally unreasonable, i.e., 0.5 pM or 180 pg/g of tissue of total steroid

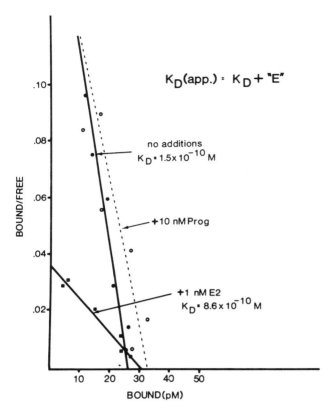

Figure A
Typical receptor assay

that competes for available receptor in the follicular phase of the menstrual cycle.

I see my friends Stanley [Korenman] and Marc [Lippman] shaking their heads in disbelief. They don't believe a word of this, but I thought it would be of interest to show these results to you anyway. I think you would agree that if these differences in K_D are due to the tissue estrogen, then the results certainly are consistent with what I said this morning (see Siiteri et al., this volume) concerning the greater availability of estrogen from the circulation to the tissues in some women with breast cancer.

I want to hear your reaction, Stanley.

KORENMAN: Yes. You know, in 1970, when we published a paper on the estrogen receptor assay (Korenman and Dukes 1970), we measured the estrogens in the cytosol.

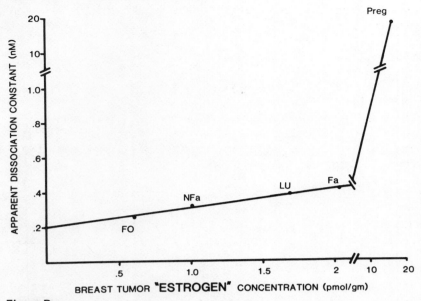

Figure B
Calculated breast tumor estrogen concentration vs K_D values. (FO) Follicular, (NFa) non-familial, (LU) luteal, and (Fa) familial tumors; (Preg) pregnancy.

SIITERI: I know you did.

KORENMAN: We didn't find very much. We found no significant E_2, and we found very little estrone (E_1).

SIITERI: If I remember the numbers correctly, they were about 50-100 pg E_1/g tissue, and about half of that for E_2.

KORENMAN: No. The E_2 was the blank of the technique, of the method.

SIITERI: That is not what your paper says.

KORENMAN: There was no significant E_2 above the blank of the method. The method is not as good as the current methods, and it would be nice to do it again. We would be happy to take a few samples and do them for you, if you would like. But I think that that is the way to get that information.

SIITERI: How many steroids do you want me to measure? Which radio-immunoassay do you want me to set up? This estimate, and to be sure it is rather imprecise, is essentially a receptor assay for anything that is in the tissue that competes with E_2. It doesn't make any difference what steroid it is.

KORENMAN: Use a radioreceptor assay.

SIITERI: That is what it is.

KORENMAN: That is not. This is a calculation, an indirect calculation.

SIITERI: I know that, but the principle is exactly the same as a radioreceptor assay.

KORENMAN: No.

SIITERI: Well, sure it is. If I add steroid and I predictably show you what the effect on the K_D or the slope of the Scatchard plot is, isn't that a radioreceptor assay?

OTTMAN: Stan, you are objecting to the assignment of numbers. You are not saying that endogenous steroids do not influence the K_D estimates through competition with the tracer for the receptor binding.

References

Korenman, S.G. and B.A. Dukes. 1970. Specific estrogen binding by the cytoplasm of human breast carcinoma. *J. Clin. Endocrinol. Metab.* **30**:639.

SESSION 5:
Exogenous Hormones and Breast Cancer

Epidemiological Studies of the Role of Exogenous Estrogens in the Etiology of Breast Cancer

JENNIFER L. KELSEY
Department of Epidemiology and Public Health
Yale University School of Medicine
New Haven, Connecticut 06510

Over the past decade, results of several epidemiological studies have been reported in which the relationships between use of oral contraceptives (OC) and of estrogen replacement therapy to the development of breast cancer have been examined. Nevertheless, we are still uncertain as to whether use of these compounds alters the risk for breast cancer in the general population of women or in any subgroups of women. All the major epidemiological studies published to date concerned with OC have found no overall association, either positive or negative, between use of OC and breast cancer. However, it is only around the present time that OC have been in use for long enough that a change in risk is likely to be detected, if it is assumed that a latent period of 15 years or more is necessary. Also, a few investigators have reported elevations in risk among certain subgroups of OC users, such as those with a history of biopsy-confirmed benign breast disease. Accordingly, it is agreed that more attention needs to be given to the risk of breast cancer among various subgroups of women who may react differently from the population as a whole. In respect to estrogen replacement therapy, there are studies that have reported increased risks, decreased risks, and no alteration in risk. Although methodological limitations of certain of these studies raise serious questions about the validity of their results, it will be seen that even the studies with better methodology still do not yet allow us to reach a firm conclusion as to whether use of estrogen replacement therapy affects the risk of breast cancer.

ORAL CONTRACEPTIVES

The results of the major case-control studies of breast cancer and OC are summarized in Table 1. It may be seen that, taken as a whole, these studies give little indication of either an increase or decrease in risk for breast cancer among the general population of women. An elevated risk for breast cancer found in one study among women who had used OC for 2-4 years originally was hypothesized to be due either to chance or to a cancer-promoting effect of OC on

215

Table 1
Case-Control Studies of OC and Breast Cancer

Investigator and year	Age range	Number of cases	Year begun	Odds ratio: ever used/ never used	Trend with length of use?
1. Sartwell et al. (1977)[a] Arthes et al. (1971)	15-74	284	1969	0.9	no
2. Boston Collaborative Drug Surveillance Program (1973)	20-44	23	1972	0.6	not reported
3. Vessey et al. (1979)[a] Vessey et al. (1975) Vessey et al. (1972)	16-50	707	1968	1.0	no
4. Stravraky and Emmons (1974)	premenopausal	95	1967	1.0	no
5. Henderson et al. (1974)	<65	308	1971	0.7	not reported
6. Fasal and Paffenbarger (1975)	<50	452	1970	1.1	elevated risk if used 2-4 years
7. Kelsey et al. (1978)	20-44	99	1971	1.3	no
8. Lees et al. (1978)	30-49	590	1971	0.9	possibly elevated risk if used 1-5 years
9. Brinton et al. (1979)	premenopausal naturally post- menopausal	126 160	1973	0.8 1.7	no increase in risk with greater time since first used
	surgically post- menopausal	110		0.9	no
10. Ravnihar et al. (1979)	20-49	190	1972	0.9	no

[a] In studies with publications describing different phases of the same study, data are presented from the most recent publication.

existing preclinical breast cancer (Fasal and Paffenbarger 1975). In fact, most other investigators have not found this trend, and it appears likely to be due to an unusually small number of women in the control group who had used OC for 2-4 years (Gross 1978). Results from cohort studies, all of which are based on small numbers of cases, are summarized in Table 2. These studies so far confirm the results of the case-control investigations that there is no evidence of an increase in risk for breast cancer among the general population of women who have used OC.

However, elevations of risk in certain subgroups· of women have been reported in case-control studies. Three studies (Paffenbarger et al. 1977; Lees et al. 1978; Brinton et al. 1979) have found an increased risk for breast cancer among women who have used OC for relatively long periods of time and who have a history of biopsy-confirmed benign breast disease. In one of the studies showing this trend (Fasal and Paffenbarger 1977), the elevation in risk was noted only in the one subgroup of women who had used OC for more than 6 years; otherwise, there was no trend towards increasing risk with greater length of use. In the second study (Brinton et al. 1979), numbers of women who had used OC and who had biopsy-confirmed breast disease were quite small. In the third study (Lees et al. 1978), not only were numbers small, but the comparison group was not appropriate. Moreover, other studies (Vessey et al. 1979) have not found elevations in risk among women who have used OC and who have a history of benign breast disease. Although the validity of this finding that OC increase the risk for breast cancer in women with biopsy-confirmed benign breast disease is thus uncertain, possible explanations will be considered later.

An increased risk for breast cancer has also been reported among women who have used OC before the birth of their first child (Fasal and Paffenbarger 1977). Because this is probably a period of life when the breasts may be particularly susceptible to the effects of carcinogenic agents, this finding needs to be evaluated further. Although no other studies published to date have reported this association, none has included large enough numbers of women who have used OC before their first birth to have much power to detect such an effect.

Table 2
Cohort Studies of OC and Breast Cancer

Investigator and year	Age range	Number of cases	Year begun	Relative risk	Trend with length of use?
Royal College of General Practitioners (1974)	15-49	31	1968	1.1	no
Ory et al. (1976)	25-49	137	1970	0.7	no
Vessey et al. (1976)	25-39	16	1968	0.4	no

Of some relevance to the question of whether use of OC increases the risk for breast cancer is the relationship between use of OC and benign breast diseases, because fibrocystic disease and probably fibroadenoma are associated with an increased risk for breast cancer (Donnelly et al. 1975; Monson et al. 1976; Haagensen 1977; Kodlin et al. 1977). A number of studies, both case-control (Vessey et al. 1972; Boston Collaborative Drug Surveillance Program 1973; Sartwell et al. 1973; Kelsey et al. 1974; Fasal and Paffenbarger 1975; Lees et al. 1978; Ravnihar et al. 1979) and cohort (Royal College of General Practitioners 1974; Ory et al. 1976; Vessey et al. 1976) have shown that women who have used OC for 2-4 years or more have a decreased frequency of benign breast diseases, including both fibrocystic disease and fibroadenoma. Typical are the findings from the cohort study of the Royal College of General Practitioners (1974). Table 3 shows that in that cohort the greater the length of time OC were used, the lower the risk for benign breast diseases. It is still unclear whether or not the reduced risk for benign breast diseases is limited to current users (Vessey et al. 1972; Royal College of General Practitioners 1974; Fasal and Paffenbarger 1975; Ory et al. 1976).

There is evidence that various forms of fibrocystic disease have different relationships to the development of breast cancer (McLaughlin et al. 1961; Black and Chabon 1969; Black et al. 1972; Haagensen 1977; Kodlin et al. 1977), and it was hypothesized by Cole et al. (1978) that the types of benign breast disease against which OC appear to protect may be different from the forms associated with a high risk for breast cancer. It was subsequently reported from one case-control study (LiVolsi et al. 1978) that when the slides from fibrocystic disease cases were classified according to the degree of epithelial atypia, long-term OC use was negatively associated only with fibrocystic disease with no or minimal epithelial atypia, a form that has been found not to be strongly associated with breast cancer (Black et al. 1972; Kodlin et al. 1977). However, this finding was not confirmed in a larger study by the same group (Pastides 1980). Thus, on the basis of current evidence it appears that: Long-term use of OC is associated with a lower-than-average risk of benign breast diseases;

Table 3
Relative Risk for Benign Breast Diseases According to Length of Use of OC

Length of use (years)	Relative risk
0	1.0
<1	0.9
1-	0.9
2-	0.8
3-	0.6
≥4	0.5

Data from Royal College of General Practitioners (1974).

benign breast diseases predispose to breast cancer; but use of OC does not substantially alter the risk for breast cancer. In fact, as was mentioned above, there is some evidence that use of OC by women with biopsy-confirmed benign breast disease may increase their risk for breast cancer. This suggests that the mechanism by which long-term use of OC is associated with a decrease in risk for benign breast diseases is independent of the mechanism responsible for the association between benign breast diseases and breast cancer.

Before leaving the topic of OC, it should be noted that in the one study in which the specific constituents of some of the OC used by the study population were considered (Royal College of General Practitioners 1977), it was found that the progestogen content appeared to be responsible for the decrease in risk for benign breast diseases. Specifically, the frequency of occurrence of benign breast diseases was related inversely to the amount of norethisterone in compounds containing the same amount of ethinylestradiol. Constituents and dosages have not been considered adequately in relation to breast cancer risk and more attention should be paid to this, particularly in studies reporting positive results in certain subgroups of women.

ESTROGEN REPLACEMENT THERAPY

A variety of approaches has been employed to address the question of whether use of estrogen replacement therapy alters tne risk for breast cancer. Earlier retrospective cohort studies generally indicated either no association or a protective effect (Wallach and Henneman 1959; Wilson 1962; Burch and Byrd 1971; Burch et al. 1974), but tnese studies were limited seriously by short-term follow-up of the cohort, the inclusion of relatively small numbers of women exposed to estrogen replacement therapy, or use of inadequate comparison groups. Unless a relatively large cohort is followed, one would expect few cases of breast cancer to occur. Unless enough years are allowed for a latent period to elapse, no association is likely to be detected. And, unless a comparison group is used that takes into account that many of the women exposed to estrogen replacement therapy were given this drug because their ovaries had been removed, a deficit of cases in the estrogen-exposed group would be expected because oophorectomy is known to protect against breast cancer.

Thus, other, more recent studies need to be considered. The results of three case-control studies, one using neighborhood controls (Casagrande et al. 1976), another hospital controls (Sartwell et al. 1977), and a third using cases and controls from a group of women participating in a breast cancer screening program (Brinton et al. 1979), were consistent with the hypothesis that estrogen replacement therapy does not increase the risk for breast cancer. Two other studies, however, have suggested a slight positive association between use of estrogen replacement therapy and breast cancer. One by Hoover and colleagues (1976) was a follow-up study of 1891 women given conjugated estrogens "for the menopause" for at least 6 months. On the average, these women were followed for 12 years. In Table 4 it may be seen that, overall, there were only slight elevations in risk for breast cancer among women who had used estrogen replacement therapy compared to the expected risk based on incidence rates in the general population. Among those who were followed for at least 15 years, however, the ratio of observed to expected numbers of cases was 1.8 in women with intact ovaries and 1.7 in women with ovaries removed. It may be noted that the trend towards higher risk with increasing number of years of follow-up was somewhat stronger in women with ovaries removed than in those with ovaries intact. A particularly high risk was reported among women who developed benign breast disease which was histologically confirmed after they had started using the estrogens, although numbers of women in this category were small. This study is, thus, somewhat indicative of a positive association between use of estrogen replacement therapy and breast cancer. However, the trends toward increasing risk for breast cancer with increasing length of follow-up were rather modest; the expected numbers were based on general population rates, and it might have been expected that the risk for breast cancer would have been more strongly related to the accumulated number of years estrogen replacement therapy was used rather than just to the years since follow-up.

A second study showing positive results was a case-control investigation undertaken by Ross et al. (1980). In all, 138 cases of breast cancer among residents younger than 75 years of age in a retirement community were compared with age- and race-matched community controls. The measure of exposure used was the total milligram accumulated dose of conjugated estrogen. Table 5 shows that among women with ovaries intact, the higher the accumulated dose, the greater the risk for breast cancer. For women with ovaries removed, however, there was no particular trend. There was again a suggestion, based on small numbers, that, for women with intact ovaries, conjugated estrogens had the greatest effect on women with biopsy-demonstrated benign breast disease.

Thus, the published evidence to date at most suggests a modest elevation in risk for breast cancer among women who use high-dose estrogen replacement compounds for long periods of time or who started using them many years ago. However, other studies do not show this trend and further investigation is needed.

Table 4

Ratio of Observed to Expected Numbers of Cases of Breast Cancer According to Ovarian Status and Duration of Follow-up

	Duration of follow-up (years)				
Ovarian status	<5	5-9	10-14	15+	total
Intact (N = 906)	1.0	0.7	0.9	1.8	1.1
Removed (N = 1028)	0.7	1.6	1.6	1.7	1.3

Data from Hoover et al. (1976).

Table 5

Estimated Risk Ratio for Breast Cancer According to Total Accumulated Dose
of Conjugated Estrogen by Ovarian Status

	Total accumulated dose (mg)		
Ovarian status	0	1-1499	≥ 1500
Ovaries intact (99 cases, 182 controls)	1.0	0.9	2.5
Ovaries removed (26 cases, 65 controls)	1.0	0.9	0.7

Data from Ross et al. (1980).

DIETHYLSTILBESTROL

It should also be mentioned that the possibility was raised by Bibbo et al. (1978) that women who had used diethylstilbestrol (DES) during pregnancy were themselves at increased risk for the subsequent development of breast cancer. Although their study had the advantage that women had been assigned at random to receive or not to receive DES, both the numbers of subjects and the difference in incidence and mortality rates from breast cancer were too small for definitive conclusions to be reached. Another study (Brian et al. 1980), which had a larger number of subjects but no randomization, did not find an excess of cases among those exposed to DES.

EXOGENOUS ESTROGENS AND RISK FOR BREAST CANCER IN WOMEN WITH HISTOLOGICALLY CONFIRMED BENIGN BREAST DISEASE

It may be noted that all the studies to date that have reported any type of positive association between use of either OC or estrogen replacement therapy and breast cancer have noted a particularly high risk among women who also have a history of histologically confirmed benign breast disease. All of these studies, however, have had relatively small numbers of women who used both exogenous estrogens and who had a history of biopsy-demonstrated benign breast disease; and some of the studies have methodological limitations. Also, other investigators have not found this association. Nevertheless, enough studies have reported this trend that explanations need at least to be considered. One is that exogenous estrogens accelerate the conversion of benign lesions with malignant potential to breast malignancies. However, because it is known that malignancies do not arise necessarily at the site where the benign lesion was identified (Donnelly et al. 1975), it is unlikely that the specific lesion in the area from which the biopsy was taken was converted to cancer. Rather, the lesion identified at biopsy would most likely be part of a more generalized disease process, part of which could conceivably be converted to cancer from exposure to exogenous estrogens. A second explanation would be that the presence of benign breast disease indicates that a woman's breasts are susceptible to effects of estrogens, including exogenous estrogens. In other words, benign breast disease could be a marker of susceptibility. Third, perhaps there is some bias related to the consideration in these studies of only the relatively small proportion of women with benign breast disease who have undergone biopsy. In autopsy studies (Frantz et al. 1951; Sloss et al. 1957), it has been found that more than 50% of women have fibrocystic breast disease, whereas most case-control studies indicate that perhaps 10% of the population has biopsy-confirmed benign breast disease. Therefore, if all women with fibrocystic breast disease were put at an increased risk for breast cancer by using OC, one would expect to see a much greater increase in risk for breast cancer among OC users in the population as a whole. Thus, an elevation in risk among women who have used OC and who have a history of biopsy-demonstrated benign breast disease would have to be explained either by the particular characteristics of women who have biopsies or by the specific types of benign breast disease that are likely to be biopsied. Also, if exogenous estrogens suppressed the recognition of some types of benign breast disease but not others, and if it were the former types that had less malignant potential, then an elevation in risk for breast cancer might be noted only among women with diagnosed benign disease. Thus, it is apparent that there are many possible explanations for the association between use of exogenous estrogens and breast cancer in women with benign breast disease, if this association is found to hold up in other studies.

CONCLUSION

It has been estimated (World Health Organization 1978) that about 80 million women in the world have used OC. In the United States in 1974 alone, about five million new prescriptions were issued for the most popular type of estrogen replacement therapy (Mack et al. 1976). Thus, determination of any increase or decrease in risk for breast cancer associated with use of these compounds is important, both because of the large numbers of women who have used them and because knowledge of effects of exogenous hormones could add to our understanding of effects of endogenous hormones. There is a need both for studies large enough to be able to detect effects in subgroups that may be particularly affected by OC or estrogen replacement therapy and for studies of more modest size that focus specifically on such subgroups.

REFERENCES

Arthes, F.G., P.E. Sartwell, and E.F. Lewison. 1971. The pill, estrogens, and the breast. Epidemiologic aspects. *Cancer* 28:1391.

Bibbo, M., W.M. Haenszel, G.L. Wied, M. Hubby, and A.L. Herbst. 1978. A twenty-five year follow-up study of women exposed to diethylstilbestrol during pregnancy. *N. Engl. J. Med.* 298:763.

Black, M.M. and A.B. Chabon. 1969. *In situ* carcinoma of the breast. *Pathol. Annu.* 4:185.

Black, M.M., T.H.C. Barclay, S.J. Cutler, B.F. Hankey, and A.J. Asire. 1972. Association of atypical characteristics of benign breast lesions with subsequent risk of breast cancer. *Cancer* 29:338.

Boston Collaborative Drug Surveillance Program. 1973. Oral contraceptives and venous thromboembolic disease, surgically confirmed gallbladder disease, and breast tumours. *Lancet* i:1399.

Brian, D.B., B.C. Tilley, D.R. Labarthe, W.M. O'Fallon, K.L. Noller, and L.T. Kurland. 1980. Breast cancer in DES-exposed mothers. Absence of association. *Mayo Clin. Proc.* 55:89.

Brinton, L.A., R.R. Williams, R.N. Hoover, N.L. Stegens, M. Feinleib, and J.F. Fraumeni, Jr. 1979. Breast cancer risk factors among screening program participants. *J. Natl. Cancer Inst.* 62:37.

Burch, J.C. and B.F. Byrd, Jr. 1971. Effects of long-term administration of estrogen in the occurrence of mammary cancer in women. *Ann. Surg.* 174:414.

Burch, J.C., B.F. Byrd, Jr., and W.K. Vaughn. 1974. The effects of long-term estrogen on hysterectomized women. *Am. J. Obstet. Gynecol.* 118:778.

Casagrande, J., V. Gerkins, B.E. Henderson, T. Mack, and M.C. Pike. 1976. Exogenous estrogens and breast cancer in women with natural menopause. *J. Natl. Cancer Inst.* 56:839.

Cole, P., J.M. Elwood, and S.D. Kaplan. 1978. Incidence rates and risk factors of benign breast neoplasms. *Am. J. Epidemiol.* 108:112.

Donnelly, P.K., K.W. Baker, J.A. Carney, and W.M. O'Fallon. 1975. Benign breast lesions and subsequent breast carcinoma in Rochester, Minnesota. *Mayo Clin. Proc.* 50:650.

Fasal, E. and R.S. Paffenbarger, Jr. 1975. Oral contraceptives as related to cancer and benign lesion of the breast. *J. Natl. Cancer Inst.* 55:767.

Frantz, V.K., J.W. Pickren, G.W. Melcher, and H. Auchincloss, Jr. 1951. Incidence of chronic cystic disease in so-called "normal breasts": A study based on 225 postmortem examinations. *Cancer* 4:762.

Gross, C. 1978. The analysis of matched triples and pooling results: An extension and an application of a multivariate method for the analysis of matched case-control studies. Ph.D. dissertation, Yale University.

Haagensen, C.D. 1977. The relationship of gross cystic disease of the breast and carcinoma. *Ann. Surg.* 185:375.

Henderson, B.E., D. Powell, I. Rosario, C. Keys, R. Hanisch, M. Young, J. Casagrande, V. Gerkins, and M.C. Pike. 1974. An epidemiologic study of breast cancer. *J. Natl. Cancer Inst.* 53:609.

Hoover, R., L.W. Gray, Sr., P. Cole, and B. MacMahon. 1976. Menopausal estrogens and breast cancer. *N. Engl. J. Med.* 295:401.

Kelsey, J.L., K.K. Lindfors, and C. White. 1974. A case-control study of the epidemiology of benign breast diseases with reference to oral contraceptive use. *Int. J. Epidemiol.* 3:33.

Kelsey, J.L., T.R. Holford, C. White, E.S. Mayer, S.E. Kilty, and R.M. Acheson. 1978. Oral contraceptives and breast disease: An epidemiological study. *Am. J. Epidemiol.* 107:236.

Kodlin, D., E.E. Winger, N.L. Morgenstern, and U. Chen. 1977. Chronic mastopathy and breast cancer. A follow-up study. *Cancer* 39:2603.

Lees, A.W., P.E. Burns, and M. Grace. 1978. Oral contraceptives and breast disease in postmenopausal Northern Alberton women. *Int. J. Cancer* 22:700.

LiVolsi, V.A., B.V. Stadel, J.L. Kelsey, T.R. Holford, and C. White. 1978. Fibrocystic breast disease in oral contraceptive users: A histopathologic evaluation of epithelial atypia. *N. Engl. J. Med.* 299:381.

Mack, T.M., M.C. Pike, B.E. Henderson, R.I. Pfeiffer, V.R. Gerkins, M. Arthur, and S.E. Brown. 1976. Estrogens and endometrial cancer in a retirement community. *N. Engl. J. Med.* 294:1262.

McLaughlin, C.W., J.R. Schenken, and J.X. Tampisica. 1961. A study of pre-cancerous epithelial hyperplasia and noninvasive papillary carcinoma of the breast. *Ann. Surg.* 153:735.

Monson, R.R., S. Yen, B. MacMahon, and S. Warren. 1976. Chronic mastitis and carcinoma of the breast. *Lancet* ii:224.

Ory, H., P. Cole, B. MacMahon, and R. Hoover. 1976. Oral contraceptives and reduced risk of benign breast diseases. *N. Engl. J. Med.* 294:419.

Paffenbarger, R.S., E. Fasal, M.E. Simmons, and J.B. Kampert. 1977. Cancer risk as related to use of oral contraceptives during fertile years. *Cancer* (Suppl.) 39:1887.

Pastides, H. 1980. The epidemiology of fibrocystic breast disease with special reference to its histopathology. Ph.D. thesis, Yale University.

Ravnihar, B., D.G. Seigel, and J. Lindtner. 1979. An epidemiologic study of breast cancer and benign breast neoplasms in relation to the oral contraceptive and estrogen use. *Eur. J. Cancer* 15:395.

Ross, R.K., A. Paganini-Hill, V.R. Gerkins, T.M. Mack, R. Pfeffer, M. Arthur, and B.E. Henderson. 1980. A case-control study of menopausal estrogen therapy and breast cancer. *J. Am. Med. Assoc.* 243:1635.

Royal College of General Practitioners. 1974. *Oral contraceptives and health.* Pitman, New York.

_____. 1977. Oral contraceptive study: Effect on hypertension and benign breast disease of progestagen component in combined oral contraceptives. *Lancet* i:624.

Sartwell, P.E., F.G. Arthes, and J.A. Tonascia. 1973. Epidemiology of benign breast lesions. Lack of associations with oral contraceptive use. *N. Engl. J. Med.* 288:551.

_____. 1977. Exogenous hormones, reproductive history, and breast cancer. *J. Natl. Cancer Inst.* 59:1589.

Sloss, P.T., W.A. Bennett, and O.T. Clagett. 1957. Incidence in normal breasts of features associated with chronic cystic mastitis. *Am. J. Pathol.* 33:1181.

Stavraky, K. and S. Emmons. 1974. Breast cancer in premenopausal and post-menopausal women. *J. Natl. Cancer Inst.* 53:647.

Vessey, M.P., R. Doll, and P.M. Sutton. 1972. Oral contraceptives and breast neoplasia: A retrospective study. *Br. Med. J.* 3:719.

Vessey, M.P., R. Doll, and K. Jones. 1975. Oral contraceptives and breast cancer. *Lancet* i:941.

Vessey, M.P., R. Doll, R. Peto, and B. Johnson. 1976. A long-term follow-up study of women using different methods of contraception—An interim report. *J. Biosoc. Sci.* 8:373.

Vessey, M.P., R. Doll, K. Jones, K. McPherson, and P. Yeates. 1979. An epidemiological study of oral contraceptives and breast cancer. *Br. Med. J.* 1:1757.

Wallach, S. and P.H. Henneman. 1959. Prolonged estrogen therapy in postmenopausal women. *J. Am. Med. Assoc.* 171:1637.

WHO Technical Report Series 619. 1978. *Steroid contraception and the risk of neoplasia.* Geneva.

Wilson, R.A. 1962. The roles of estrogen and progesterone in breast and genital cancer. *J. Am. Med. Assoc.* 182:327.

COMMENTS

BULBROOK: I have a question for Dr. Kelsey and also for Dr. Pike. Over and over again, we hear the epidemiologists say "the numbers are too small," even with the 80 million women using OC and 25 million using hormone replacement therapy. If you are dealing with relative risks of, say, 1.8, are you doing the right experiments?

　　If you look at the reserpine story, you find a mini-industry with some 20 papers published, but we still don't know whether the drug increases cancer incidence. So, I repeat, are you doing the right experiment?

KELSEY: It is not just a matter of numbers. I think that what both Malcolm [Pike] and I like to see is consistent patterns in several studies, despite the different methodologies used. With OC, so far there has been a fair degree of consistency in the results of various studies when the overall risk for breast cancer is considered. With respect to estrogen replacement therapy, it frequently is difficult in epidemiological studies to differentiate between low but real increases in risk and no increase in risk at all, because small methodological biases could account for slight increases in risk or for failure to detect slight increases in risk. I find it hard to suggest exactly what type of study is needed, however, to provide more definitive evidence on the estrogen replacement therapy question. Results of more studies will be published soon which, I believe, will provide some additional evidence that there is a positive association between use of estrogen replacement therapy and risk for breast cancer.

KORENMAN: Jennifer [Kelsey], one of the things that interested me about this is the distinction in the people who have their ovaries and people who don't have their ovaries, and why they got the estrogen replacement and what age they were. In the case of postmenopausal women who get the replacement therapy, it may not be relevant whether or not they have their ovaries, if they are given the estrogen replacement for menopausal symptoms or something like that.

　　First, if premenopausal women have their ovaries removed surgically, it is for a reason. Second, there is a negative feedback control system that no longer works in the group of postmenopausal women. That is, the situation in postmenopausal women, in terms of the control group, is different from premenopausal women. What is the control group for premenopausal women on estrogen therapy? It is very hard for me to understand what that is. Certainly premenopausal women with ovaries aren't the control group and premenopausal women without ovaries aren't a control group for premenopausal women on estrogen replacement therapy. I think it is very hard to know what an appropriate control group is. Third, estrogen replacement therapy is not physiological, and therefore you can't use unreplaced people often as a control group.

I find that I don't know what the "compared to what" is, and certainly you must distinguish between why they are getting the replacement therapy and at what age. Are there any studies in which this distinction is made?

KELSEY: We have some unpublished data that partially address the question. We made some effort to find out why the women were using estrogen replacement therapy, but the reasons for use did not alter our findings, which actually showed no increase in risk for breast cancer among women who had used estrogen replacement therapy anyway. The other part of your question was —

KORENMAN: What is the appropriate control group?

KELSEY: That is an important question in epidemiological studies, and I think different people have different views on that. There actually have been a lot of approaches to the selection of control groups. Maybe you are not satisfied with any of them.

KORENMAN: I probably am not aware of any of them.

KELSEY: In the case-control studies I have described, controls have been selected from a variety of different sources, including neighborhoods, hospitals, and other sources. I think you would like more detailed information about the comparability of cases and controls, such as whether they were comparable in respect to physiological variables rather than whether they were from the same hospital or the same neighborhood. Of course, some studies took a different approach and started with people exposed to estrogens and other people not exposed, and followed up on them.
Thus, there have been a variety of different methodologies. It may be hard, in practice, to get controls as tightly stratified as you would like them.

SIITERI: I don't understand what the problem is, Stanley [Korenman]. It doesn't make any difference if you have a postmenopausal woman that does or does not have ovaries as far as estrogen production is concerned. The only real question is whether she is taking the medication or not taking the medication.

KORENMAN: Well, let me make the point specifically, then. The Lexington, Kentucky, study that Hoover reported (Hoover et al. 1976) talked about the duration of therapy, but it did not talk about an age and initiation therapy. It did not discuss the rationale for therapy. So you did not know, for example, whether the women, the average woman, who had therapy initiated 15 years ago, was 35 years of age, in which case she would normally have had 10 years of progesterone, of progestational agent exposure. If she had not been put on an estrogen, she would have had no hormone exposure. But she was put on a hyperphysiologic dose of estrogen without any progestational agent for 10 years before she was due to be menopausal. Is that the group of women who have an increased risk of breast cancer when they are treated? Or is it the group of women who are postmenopausal at the initiation of estrogen therapy? It is never indicated in that paper.

SIITERI: But how many people were put on therapy 10 years before the menopause?

KORENMAN: Every one who is castrated.

HENDERSON: Dr. Kelsey referred to a paper of ours (Pike et al. 1981) which will be published soon and which shows an elevated risk to breast cancer in women aged 32 or under who have 4 years or more of use of OC prior to the first full-term pregnancy. The reason that we could do such a study was that we have access to all breast cancer cases in the whole of Los Angeles county.

A second point is that there are two studies that have shown an elevated risk for breast cancer in women who are taking the pill during the menopausal period. A possible explanation for this observation would be that by taking the pill during the menopausal period such women are artificially prolonging their menstrual life. They cannot experience menopause with its associated decrease in breast cancer risk while they are on the pill.

KORENMAN: What was the control group for your first study?

HENDERSON: Neighborhood controls.

KORENMAN: Are they matched for age at first pregnancy?

HENDERSON: There is no effect of age at first pregnancy in this young age group.

References

Hoover, R., L.W. Gray, Sr., P. Cole, and B. MacMahon. 1976. Menopausal estrogens and breast cancer. *N. Engl. J. Med.* 295:401.

Pike, M.C., B.E. Henderson, J.T. Casagrande, I. Rosario, and G.E. Gray. 1981. Oral contraceptive use and early abortion as risk factors for breast cancers in young women. *Br. J. Cancer* 43 (1).

Hormone Therapy of Breast Cancer

ALBERT SEGALOFF
Department of Medicine
Ochsner Medical Institutions
New Orleans, Louisiana 70121

I am disturbed that I am unaware of any study utilizing today's knowledge and methodology that would enable me to give you a concrete concept of how good modern hormonal therapy is in comparison with the multiple-agent cytotoxic chemotherapy for the treatment of breast cancer. I am unable to do this in terms of objective regression, or subjective advantages, penalties, or survival. I will try to tell you why this is true and attempt to put into focus what we can say about comparative efficacy.

Our scientific community has not completely learned the very hard lesson that historical controls can be a deadly trap. They also haven't learned that the use of probability statistics requires the true random entry of patients and the use of a concurrent, randomly entered control group. The worst trap, besides the changing patterns of the patients that come to us, is changing the rules of entry of patients as well as of evaluation of results and then using historical reference groups in whom the same criteria were not employed. Patients with breast cancer, as we see them, have changed continually over the years. Currently, patients are bombarded by the news media, who seem to believe that early diagnosis of breast cancer has proven survival advantage. I know of no unequivocal scientific evidence that this is true. In addition patients have heard through the media that adjuvant polyagent chemotherapy can cure them of their invasive breast cancer, even if they already have involved axillary nodes. Unfortunately, whether it is because of excessive newspaper publicity or inadequacy of the reporting to and by the scientific community, some patients are inappropriately and vigorously treated with adjuvant therapy. This may do nothing but create toxicity, loss of hair, bone marrow depression, and eliminate what I would consider a free period. If "cure" is really at the end of the rainbow of prolonged adjuvant chemotherapy, it might be different, but we do not know this.

Let me make it very clear that I am distinguishing between entering patients into carefully designed, prospective, randomized trials and treating them with any one of a large number of free-hand combinations that will not be given to enough patients for their comparative efficacy to be known. I think that it is also mandatory that adjuvant studies be devised and supported long enough to obtain meaningful survival data.

I would commend for your perusal Dr. Meyer's careful analysis of curing breast cancer by Halsted's operation (Meyer 1967). Halsted (1894) defined cure as preventing local recurrence of breast cancer. His mortality figures emphasize that his patients died of their distant disease. As a result of that operation, there was a tremendous change in the stage of the disease at which patients presented themselves. Now, as the result of mammography and screening for early tumors, we are having patients present with minute cancers. We are giving them the label of breast cancer and its associated terror for a longer period of time. I would point out to you that the average time it takes a .5-cm tumor to grow to 3.5-4 cm, the size so often found without screening or breast self-examination, is 5 years. Thus, finding them early may only add to our impression that we have a greater 5-year survival rate. All we have really done is made a 5-year-earlier diagnosis. Lead time needs evaluation and must be taken into account in our analyses.

The first study of systemic adjuvant therapy used testosterone propionate (Prudente 1945), and favorable results were reported. Although it is not realistic to think that we can ethically propose an untreated control group in node-positive patients who are premenopausal, comparative studies should be done. These studies should compare our best chemotherapy program, castration, and administered hormone therapy. In postmenopausal patients, a control group is feasible. These programs should be stratified according to the levels of estrogen receptor (ER) in the tumors as well as node status, etc.

The other influence on patient selection, both self-selection and by physicians, which is changing substantially the kind of patients we see is the question of whether or not the cancer contains ERs. A surprising number of breast cancer patients, because of their reading, patronizing "hotlines" for breast cancer patients, information gleaned from their physicians, or from casual talk from house staff, feel that they know all about receptors. I wish I could join them and feel that I knew all about receptors.

The determination is complex; break points used for deciding on positives and negatives differ all over the world; and possibilities for both false-positives and false-negatives are legion. To the best of my knowledge, the correlation of ERs and objective response to various hormonal manipulations in advanced breast cancer correlates best with the level of receptor and not with whether it has some arbitrarily chosen positivity or negativity (McGuire et al. 1977). There is the additional question of whether the presence of both estrogen and progesterone receptors is more predictive than either alone. Finally, although there is some difference in the interpretation of the various studies, there seems to be an increasing swell of papers indicating that ER-positive (ER$^+$) tumors endow the tumor-host relationship with a longer free period and a longer survival independent of other parameters (Knight et al. 1977). This may simply be an index that the ER positivity is really primarily an index of either differentiation or growth rate or both.

We are aware that patients whose tumors respond favorably to hormonal changes are more likely to respond to further hormonal therapy. Because the ER positivity of tumors also appears to select for response to hormonal manipulation using more than one means, we expect these two groups of patients to be essentially congruent. However, we are unable to say whether the lack of ERs selects for or against response to chemotherapy, since there are studies on all sides of this question (Kiang et al. 1978; Lippman et al. 1978; Manni et al. 1980). Whatever the final solutions of these dilemmas are, it remains that this is what is happening. Modern studies reporting our best techniques must take all of these factors into account. Any adequate study done in breast cancer today must not only take into account receptor levels in the tumors but it also must take into account the individual receptors and their levels. They must have sufficient patients so that differences, if they exist, are significant. The excuses that studies cutting across these lines should be done because they are feasible and that using such strict criteria makes the cells for randomization too small is an admission that I dislike, because it means that we are giving up good science for expedience.

The current fashionable, apparently well-bolstered and fortunately well-tolerated, administrative hormonal therapy is tamoxifen, an estrogen antagonist. It burst upon the scene shortly after the explosion of receptor determinations. It is, fortunately, well tolerated and, of course, has been given more frequently to patients who are host to ER$^+$ tumors than those with ER$^-$ tumors. I am aware of a prospective, open, cross-over study against fluoxymesterone. Though the study is small, ER$^+$ patients were equal in both arms and the objective response rate, even for osseous disease, was the same in both arms. The results have been evaluated according to recommendations by the UICC Committee on Advanced Breast Cancer. The tamoxifen groups experienced longer remissions and better survival (Wasterberg 1980).

Using such classic indices of estrogen activity as its ability to cornify the vaginal smear in castrates or postmenopausal women, I believe that tamoxifen is really a low-voltage estrogen with antiestrogen activity.

This does not mean that we should ignore what we have previously established with hormonal agents. I would like to point out that, in all the studies of which I am aware, at least an adequate evaluation of patients, including extramural peer review of the studies, was done; ER$^-$ patients have had at least 9-11% objective regression rates and ER$^+$ patients around 50%. In light of our current patient population, perhaps we should look into administrative hormonal therapy again to establish both efficacy and toxicity.

The first demonstration of efficacy of hormonal therapy in advanced breast cancer was by surgical castration. The dramatic effects of the castration of menstruating women with advanced breast cancer are well-recognized and documented. The possible exception is that the percentage of such regression varies with the observer and criteria for response. It is of interest that Beatson (1896) administered the then newly popular thyroid hormone to most of his patients and that this was thought possibly responsible for the favorable results. O'Bryan et al. (1974) finally showed that this was not the case.

The logical extension of the removal of growth-stimulating hormones by organ extirpation was made many years ago. Both adrenalectomy and hypophysectomy have become widely employed procedures. It is hard to be sure how comparable the results are, both because of the difficulties of setting up comparative studies—indeed some studies are impossible—and because we, thus, truly cannot evaluate the effects of major surgical intervention. Nonetheless, such ablative procedures produce objective regressions in patients who are known to respond to additive hormonal therapy or to castration in a higher percentage than those who have failed in these previous procedures. Gordan (1967) has pointed out that objective regressions can be produced by the administration of low-dose corticoid and thyroactive materials, such as those employed for replacement therapy in patients with the major endocrine ablative procedures. Such replacement therapy may be responsible for some favorable effects credited to the ablation. The widespread practice of simultaneous castration and adrenalectomy and crediting the good results to adrenalectomy alone also confounds efforts at evaluation. In today's receptorology terms, the response rates are also greater among patients who have ER^+ tumors.

What types of objective response are seen with ablative therapy? None of these appears to have a particular predilection for a particular metastatic site, and regression of osseous, local, and visceral lesions are seen. It should be recalled, however, that many patients with major visceral lesions are deprived of this maneuver because they are considered inoperable, and, therefore, would not be entered into any of the ablative series.

The early and striking effects of administered hormones were first seen with the administration of estrogen. It is interesting that the original group (Haddow et al. 1944) that predicted that they would work reported striking regression of malignant ulcerated local lesions. On the other hand, there are others who thought that the administered estrogen would accelerate the growth of the breast cancer and make it more sensitive to radiation therapy; they were favorably impressed by the striking objective regressions seen in some of the patients.

As far as we know, estrogens act solely through their estrogenicity. The most striking effects are seen with estrogens in elderly postmenopausal patients, particularly those with local disease. Such patients also tend to have a higher percentage of ER^+ tumors. Depending upon the site of visceral disease, lung lesions frequently are very responsive and hepatic lesions generally are unresponsive. However, objective regressions seen in osseous lesions are fewer than those seen with the use of androgens.

It is difficult to refer to the effects of hormonal administration as "side effects" because, except in rare instances, these are the result of the expected physiologic activity of the administered hormonal agent. For example, when you get withdrawal bleeding from the cyclic administration of estrogens to a castrated woman with an intact uterus, this is the expected effect, not a side effect. This effect, as well as the sodium retention so characteristic of estrogens, follows a dosage-response curve, as does the induced nausea and vomiting. This latter effect disappears with time and can often be prevented by gradual escalation in dosage or the administration of entire daily dose in the evening together with a long-acting antinauseant. The antinauseant can generally be discontinued after the first month of therapy without the return of the debilitating nausea and vomiting.

One of the really distressing results of estrogen therapy is stress incontinence. As many of you know, this is also seen in pregnancy. Interestingly enough, this does not appear to follow a dosage-response curve and is seen at about the same level in all patients given effective amounts of estrogen (Carter et al. 1977). We occasionally have seen women who have such substantial increases in cervical and vaginal secretions that it requires the wearing of sanitary napkins.

The other fascinating thing about objective regressions seen on estrogen therapy is that, as far as we know, such patients having objective regression have a greater possibility of getting a secondary objective regression, often long lasting, upon stopping the estrogen therapy when the disease progresses. This phenomenon, first described by Escher (1949), is also seen to a lesser degree when other forms of administered hormonal therapy are stopped.

The classic androgen, testosterone, has been employed and produces substantially the same proportion of objective responses as ablative therapy. Unfortunately, the physiologic effect of the administration of testosterone propionate is virilization and the concomitant change in appearance. In view of this, a search was made for androgens of less virilizing potential and 2-α-methyl dihydrotestosterone propionate was tested. Blackburn (1962) introduced this for clinical use. The objective regression rate appears to be congruent with that of testosterone propionate, but with a significantly less potential for virilization. It should be recognized that virilization has both a dose component and a time component; the longer one uses even a steroid of low androgenic potency, the more inevitable virilization becomes.

As far as we know, all of the active androgens produce objective regression in advancing breast cancer when given in adequate amounts. The regression rates are greatest in women who are the greatest distance postmenopausal, and androgens produce better regression in osseous disease than do other administered hormonal agents.

The superpotent androgen that has been tested adequately by prospective double-blind studies is 7-α-methyl-19-nortestosterone acetate, and it yielded a dosage-response curve with the greater objective regression rate seen with the highest dosage (Talley et al. 1973). Unfortunately, because of the disenchantment with the rapid virilization, this compound has never been brought to market and is not available.

The androgens mentioned so far have the disadvantage of having to be administered parenterally; therefore, studies of orally administered androgens were undertaken. Methyltestosterone was found early to be an effective androgen, but it has the unfortunate side effect of producing cholestatic jaundice. This is a side effect that correlates with the introduction of the 17-α alkyl radical to increase oral potency. As for the parenteral androgen, exploration of lesser virilizing androgens was undertaken with the careful prospective investigation of fluoxymesterone. This has been shown to be less virilizing than methyltestosterone, and it is quite free of the production of cholestatic juandice (Segaloff 1966).

Unfortunately, the superandrogenic androgens that have been available for oral trial have had a disproportionate increase in their toxicity over their efficacy, such that Halden et al. (1970) described a methyltrienolone syndrome with profound central nervous system difficulty, as well as cholestatic jaundice, which was also seen with 7-α-17, dimethyl-19-nortestosterone in my hands in unpublished data.

Antagonists to estrogen and androgens have been made. To my knowledge none of the androgen antagonists have had adequate clinical trials in advanced breast cancer, but estrogen antagonists have become very widely used. I believe they are better described as mixed agonists-antagonists. Some of them have distressing side effects such as photosensitivity, but the most widely used one, tamoxifen, has few side effects and a low enough level of estrogenic activity to be free of estrogenic effects.

Early results of progesterone therapy in advanced breast cancer were disappointing but the later availability and clinical trials of the more potent progestational agents has demonstrated greater objective and subjective response rates.

We introduced the use of Δ^1-testolactone (Teslac) at a time when we were unable to demonstrate any hormonal effects in the administration of this material. Our interest in the first arose from the belief that the D-ring lactones were normal metabolites of estrogens and androgens. This was later shown to be wrong, the effect being caused by contamination of the ether used to extract urinary steroids. Δ^1-testolactone was used for clinical trials because it was made available for our use after the observation by Dr. J. Fried that it could be easily prepared by incubation methods from progesterone. Although it produced regression in breast cancer, it was not until later that we came to understand its probable mechanism of action because it is a highly effective inhibitor of aromatization and therefore inhibits endogenous production of estrogen.

Corticoids have been widely employed for their subjective effects in advanced cancer and also as an aid in managing the hypercalcemia seen in so many patients with advanced breast cancer. However, from the available studies, it would appear that, by themselves, they are not as effective in producing objective regressions as when they are given in conjunction with thyroactive substances.

Hormonal manipulation and cytotoxic chemotherapy both produce objective regression in breast cancers. Those patients experiencing the regressions live longer than those who fail to respond. This "vacation from death" seems to be longer in the hormonal responders than in the chemotherapy responders. However, until we have truly comparable studies, there is no way to be sure which is the better choice for an individual.

REFERENCES

Beatson, G.W. 1896. On the treatment of inoperable cases of carcinoma of the mamma—suggestions for a new method of treatment with illustrative cases. *Lancet* ii:104, 162.

Blackburn, C.M. 1962. Use of 2-alpha-methyl dihydrotestosterone propionate in treatment of advanced cancer of the breast. *Cancer Chemother. Rep.* 16:279.

Carter, A.C., N. Hedransk, R.M. Kelley, F.J. Ansfield, R.G. Ravdin, R.W. Talley, and N.R. Potter. 1977. Diethylstilbestrol: Recommended dosages for different categories of breast cancer patients. *J. Am. Med. Assoc.* 237: 2079.

Escher, G.C. 1949. Clinical improvement of inoperable breast carcinoma under steroid treatment. In *Proceedings of the First Conference on Hormones in Mammary Cancer,* p. 92. Therapeutics Trial Committee of the Council on Pharmacy and Chemistry of the American Medical Association, Chicago.

Gordan, G.S. 1967. Why are the reported results of hypophysectomy for breast cancer so variable? In *Current concepts of breast cancer* (ed. A. Segaloff et al.), p. 342. Williams and Wilkins, Baltimore.

Haddow, A., J.M. Watkinson, and E. Patterson. 1944. Influence of synthetic oestrogens upon advanced malignant disease. *Br. Med. J.* 2:393.

Halden, A., R.M. Walter, and G.S. Gordan. 1970. Antitumor efficacy and toxicity of methyltrienolone (N.S.C.-92858) in advanced breast cancer. *Cancer Chemother. Rep.* 54:453.

Halsted, W.S. 1894. The results of operations for the cure of cancer of the breast performed at the Johns Hopkins Hospital from June 1889 to January 1894. *Ann. Surg.* 20:497.

Kiang, D.T., D.H. Frenning, A.I. Goldman, V.F. Ascensao, and B.J. Kennedy. 1978. Estrogen receptors and responses to chemotherapy and hormonal therapy in advanced breast cancer. *N. Engl. J. Med.* 299:1330.

Knight, W.A., III, R.B. Livingston, E.J. Gregory, and W.L. McGuire. 1977. Estrogen receptor as an independent prognostic factor for early recurrence in breast cancer. *Cancer Res.* 37:4669.

Lippman, M.E., J.C. Allegra, E.B. Thompson, R. Simon, A. Barlock, L. Green, K.K. Huff, H.M.T. Do, S.C. Aitken, and R. Warren. 1978. The relation between estrogen receptors and response rate to cytotoxic chemotherapy in metastatic breast cancer. *N. Engl. J. Med.* 298:1233.

Manni, A., J.E. Trujillo, and O.H. Pearson. 1980. Sequential use of endocrine therapy and chemotherapy in metastatic breast cancer: Effects on survival. *Cancer Treat. Rep.* 64:111.

McGuire, W.L., K.D. Horowitz, O.H. Pearson, and A. Segaloff. 1977. Current status of estrogen and progesterone receptors in breast cancer. *Cancer* 39:2934.

Meyer, K.K. 1967. The "cure" of cancer of the breast. In *Current concepts in cancer* (ed. A. Segaloff et al.), p. 3. Williams and Wilkins, Baltimore.

O'Bryan, R.M., G.S. Gordon, R.M. Kelley, R.G. Ravdin, A. Segaloff, and S.G. Taylor, III. 1974. Does thyroid substance improve response of breast cancer surgical castration? *Cancer* 33:1082.

Prudente, A. 1945. Postoperative prophylaxis of recurrent mammary cancer with testosterone propionate. *Surg. Gynecol. Obstet.* 80:575.

Segaloff, A., B.N. Horwitt, R.A. Carabasi, P.J. Murison, and J.V. Schlosser. 1953. Hormonal therapy in cancer of the breast. V. The effect of methyltestosterone on clinical course and hormonal excretion. *Cancer* 6:483.

Segaloff, A. 1966. Hormones and breast cancer. *Recent Prog. Horm. Res.* 22:351.

Talley, R.W., C.R. Haines, M.N. Walters, I.S. Goldenberg, K.B. Olson, and H.F. Bisel. 1973. A dose-response evaluation of androgens in the treatment of metastatic breast cancer. *Cancer* 32:315.

Wasterberg, H. 1980. Tamoxifen and fluoxymesterone in advanced breast cancer: A controlled clinical trial. *Cancer Treat. Rep.* 64:117.

COMMENTS

SIRBASKU: What is the proposed mechanism by which high estrogens induce inhibition of tumor growth?

SEGALOFF: I don't have any idea. You can do it with phenol, but phenol has a low therapeutic index even though it is estrogenic. Every estrogenic compound that I know of works; if you get in enough estrogenic activity, you get regressions in breast cancer. You can do it in tissue cultures, you can do it in intact animals, and you can do it in patients.

SIRBASKU: I am asking this question because we asked this question in a rat about 1978. We carried out the high-estrogen-dose experiment to inhibit mammary tumors in the rat. It is beautifully inhibitory in the intact female, but when we castrated the female and gave back exactly the same dose, it exaggerated tumor growth by eightfold over a normal female. So it appeared to be mediated, at least in part, by the ovary. I wonder if that is the case in the human as well.

SEGALOFF: You are talking about carcinogenesis as opposed to treatment.

SIRBASKU: No. I am talking about tumor promotion, i.e., the growth of pre-existing tumors.

MEITES: I can tell you why high doses of estrogen inhibit mammary tumor growth in rats. We published this in several papers, including *Cancer Research*, and showed that high doses of estrogen interfered with the peripheral action of prolactin on the mammary cancer tissue. Furthermore, we showed that high doses of estrogen decreased prolactin receptors in mammary cancers. McGuire confirmed it.

We also did the same thing with high doses of androgen. They inhibited prolactin action on mammary tumor growth.

SIRBASKU: But the line you were using is not prolactin dependent. I have read it.

MEITES: Well perhaps you were using the wrong line of rat. The carcinogen-induced mammary cancer in the Sprague-Dawley rat we used is prolactin dependent.

SEGALOFF: That is the problem. This is strain dependent.

MEITES: And it may work the same way in humans.

SEGALOFF: It is strain dependent. You can get any effect you want by picking the strain of rat and tumor line you want. That is the answer.

MEITES: Well, we were working with a hormone-dependent tumor in the Sprague-Dawley rat.

COLE: Al [Segaloff] made a very fundamental statement when he began, and it was the one incorrect statement that he made, that is, there is no evidence that the treatment that we have to offer women today for breast cancer is effective. He then went on to tell us a large number of truths, with which I am only too sad to have to agree.

SEGALOFF: My opening statement was that we had no proof that there is a survival advantage to the early detection of breast cancer.

COLE: That is it. Then, what do you make of the HIP study? Did it not show that there was a permanent survival advantage—a reduction in mortality rate—consequent to being randomized into the group to be screened as opposed to the unscreened group?

SEGALOFF: This brings up one of the problems that I have thought about the HIP study since it was done. (As you know, I was on the committee that set it up.) The fact is that there are an awful lot of patients that disappeared, and they disappeared disproportionately in the groups.

COLE: All I know is that the mortality rate, which is based on the total denominator, is less in the screened group than in the unscreened. Is the follow-up less complete in the screened group?

SEGALOFF: Yes.

PETRAKIS: Not much. It is only a couple percent difference, about 82-85%.

SEGALOFF: But the whole mortality difference is less than that.

COLE: It is almost 40% difference in the mortality rate.

SEGALOFF: Wait a minute. The 2% applies to the 30,000 and the 40% difference applies to a couple of hundred. You are talking about the same order of magnitude of numbers. Talking in percentages doesn't change the fact that the error is in the difference.

COLE: I am not trying to change it. But it is quite unlikely, isn't it, that the 2-3% that got lost were the same 2-3% who died from breast cancer?

SEGALOFF: I don't know whether it is unlikely or not. That is the whole point; you have got to find them. If the missing ones are as big as the difference, as far as I am concerned, every one of the missing ones died.

COLE: From breast cancer?

SEGALOFF: I don't care what they died from. Until you can show me where they are, I want to assume they died from breast cancer. And I don't know of anything that tells me differently.

SESSION 6:
Other Exogenous Factors and Breast Cancer

Epidemiologic Studies of Mutagenicity of Breast Fluids—Relevance to Breast Cancer Risk

NICHOLAS L. PETRAKIS
Department of Epidemiology and International Health
University of California
San Francisco, California 94143

During the past few years my colleagues and I have conducted interdisciplinary research on the genetic epidemiology of breast cancer and benign breast disease. Employing a nipple aspiration device, we have been able to sample breast-duct fluid from the mature nonlactating breast and to examine many aspects of its biochemical and cytologic composition (Petrakis et al. 1975, 1977a). Our findings indicate that the adult nonlactating breast secretes and reabsorbs fluid containing a variety of chemical substances, as well as exfoliated epithelial cells (King et al. 1975a,b). We have found that chemical substances of exogenous and endogenous origin are secreted and concentrated by the epithelia of the non-lactating adult breast. These include immunoglobulins, fatty acids, cholesterol and cholesterol metabolites, nicotine, lactose, caffeine, estrone, and other substances (Petrakis et al. 1977a,b, 1978, 1980). The breast is unique among secretory glands in that its secretions may be retained for variable periods of time before being reabsorbed. We have proposed the hypothesis that the secretion and accumulation by the breast of certain chemical substances might result in initiating and promoting actions on the mammary epithelium that could play an etiologic role in the pathogenesis of benign and malignant breast disease (Petrakis 1977b). These considerations are depicted in Figure 1.

At puberty, the breast buds of the preadolescent girl are activated into development by the endocrine system, at which time the rudimentary ductal system begins to proliferate to form the alveolar-lobular structure of the mature breast, leading to the onset of endogenous metabolic and secretory activity. It is at this time that exposure and initiation of the breast epithelia to mutagenic and cocarcinogenic substances of endogenous and exogenous origin might occur. Mechanisms are likely to be present to repair the DNA damage caused by these substances. Continued exposure of the initiated cells in the genetically susceptible subject to secreted cocarcinogens, hormones, and other promoting factors might alter the epithelial cells of the breast, leading through a progression of cytologic changes to benign disease and malignancy. Initiation could also occur in the rudimentary breast of the newborn infant, as histopathologic studies indicate that secretory activity transiently occurs at this time.

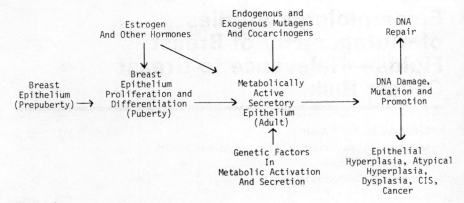

Figure 1
Interaction of multiple factors in the pathogenesis of the breast

In this presentation, I will describe some of our recent findings that offer support for this hypothesis. These include the detection of presumptive mutagens in breast fluid as determined by the Ames test, the detection of cholesterol 5-6 epoxide in the breast secretions of many women, and some recent data, which suggest an association between breast cancer risk factors, cerumen type, and epithelial dysplasia.

BREAST FLUID COLLECTION

The technique of breast fluid collection has been described previously (Petrakis et al. 1975). Briefly, this involves the use of a modified breast pump consisting of a suction cup placed over the nipple that is attached to a 10-cc syringe. On retraction of the syringe, breast fluid can be obtained in approximately 70% of white and 30% of Asian women. Approximately 5-50 μl of fluid is obtained from each breast by this technique. The breast fluid is collected in capillary tubes. For cytologic studies the fluid is prepared according to the method of King et al. (1975 a,b). Fluid for biochemical studies is deep frozen until analysis.

AMES TESTS OF BREAST FLUID FOR SECRETED MUTAGENS

In all, 557 breast fluid samples from 456 women were tested for mutagenic activity with the Ames *Salmonella* mutagenicity test (Ames et al. 1975). Tester strain TA1538 was employed because of its sensitivity to frameshift mutations and its low rate of spontaneous revertants. Due to the small amount of breast fluid, only one test was made per breast fluid sample. A "positive" Ames test was recorded if the number of revertant colonies induced by breast fluid and S-9 microsomal homogenate was at least 2 or more S.D. above the mean number of spontaneous revertants of control plates containing only S-9. Approximately 6.7% (31 of 456) of breast fluid samples we tested had revertant colony levels significantly elevated above the controls, as seen in Table 1 (Petrakis et al. 1980).

These results suggest that putative mutagenic substances are present in breast fluids of a significant number of women. The nature of the substance or substances giving the positive Ames tests is unknown. We believe that it is possible that the substances responsible for many of the positive Ames tests to be of endogenous origin, such as steroid oxidation products or peroxidated lipids. Exogenous sources might be medications, products of tobacco combustion, substances in food, etc. Exogenously derived mutagens have been demonstrated to gain access to the body through ingestion, inhalation, and through the skin (Feldmann and Maibach 1970; Bruce et al. 1977; Guerrero et al. 1979). It is likely that many of these mutagens would also be secreted by the breast epithelia. Breast fluids with strongly positive Ames tests had been collected from two women who were under medication with a chlorinated phenothiazine tranquilizer (Eskatrol®), which has been shown to cause positive Ames tests in vivo when exposed to UV radiation (Jose 1979). Interestingly, in one other woman, we observed a strong positive test in a breast fluid sample obtained 15 min following chemotherapy with IV thiotepa. Tester strain TA100 was used in this assay. Breast fluids from women receiving antimetabolite chemotherapy failed to give positive tests.

CHOLESTEROL EPOXIDE IN BREAST FLUIDS

Recently. we have investigated the cholesterol and cholesterol epoxide content of breast fluids (Petrakis et al. 1981). Cholesterol epoxide is probably formed from cholesterol by the action of epoxidases and destroyed by hydrases present in most tissues (Kadis 1978). Our findings indicate considerable variation of cholesterol concentration in breast fluid compared with plasma, ranging from traces of cholesterol to levels of over 10,000 mg/dl. When grouped into 10-year age groups, a significant increase in mean levels of breast fluid cholesterol occurs with advancing age (Table 2). Recently, Gray et al. (1971) identified cholesterol

Table 1
Ames Test Results on Nipple Aspirates of Breast Fluids in 456 Women

Source of fluid	Number of positive/number of women	Percent positive
Both right and left breasts	4/152	2.6
Right breast only	18/147	12.2
Left breast only	9/157	5.7
Total	31/456	6.7

(Reprinted, with permission, from Petrakis et al. 1980.)

Table 2
Total Cholesterol Concentration in Breast Fluid and Plasma by Age

Age	Breast fluid			Plasma		
	X ±	S.D.	N	X ±	S.D.	N
20-29	187 ±	182	8	196.6 ±	39.2	7
30-39	1957 ±	1488	22	185.7 ±	62.7	13
40-49	3554 ±	2073	31	240.2 ±	37.1	11
50+	2100 ±	1796	11	220.4 ±	46.7	5

α-epoxide in human serum, where increases in concentration of the epoxide occurred in direct proportion to serum concentration of cholesterol. The report stimulated us to investigate cholesterol-containing breast fluids for the presence of cholesterol epoxides. Employing deuterium-labeled cholesterol derivatives, gas-liquid chromatographic and mass spectrometric techniques, my colleagues and I have detected significant concentration of cholesterol epoxide in about 50% of fluids studied.

In 17 of 37 breast fluid samples we found cholesterol epoxide to be present. In six, the levels exceeded 1000 μg/dl, with the highest being 16,500 μg/dl. These findings may have considerable significance in view of earlier reports that cholesterol epoxides produced sarcomas following subcutaneous and intratesticular injection in animals (Bischoff 1969). More recently, cholesterol α-epoxide was reported to be as highly potent a transforming substance in the embryo hamster transformation system as the known carcinogen 3-methylcholanthrene (Kelsey and Pienta 1979). Cholesterol epoxide has also been found to produce chromosome damage and to stimulate DNA repair synthesis in human fibroblast cultures (Parsons and Goss 1978). Recent studies indicate that oxygenated sterols and some of their possible precursors, if given intravenously to experimental animals, can cause toxic damage to vascular endothelial cells (Imai et al. 1980). It is possible that high concentrations of cholesterol epoxides as well as other metabolic products of steroidal compounds in breast fluids might have similar damaging effects on the breast epithelia of certain women. Cholesterol epoxides are not mutagenic in the Ames test system, but preliminary studies in our laboratory indicate that they may induce sister chromatid exchanges in cell culture. Whether or not elevated cholesterol epoxide levels are associated with morphologic changes in breast epithelial cells is uncertain. However, a preliminary evaluation of cholesterol level and epithelial dysplasia in breast fluids suggests that dysplasia of epithelial cells occurs more frequently in fluids with markedly elevated levels of cholesterol (Table 3). Further studies are in progress to determine if a relationship exists between cholesterol epoxide levels and dysplasia.

Table 3
Correlation of Breast Fluid Epithelial Dysplasia and Cholesterol Level

Breast fluid cholesterol (mg/dl)	Number dysplasia/total	Percent dysplasia
≤199	4/26	15.3
200-4999	17/81	20.9
>5000	8/17	47.0

EPITHELIAL DYSPLASIA IN NIPPLE ASPIRATES OF BREAST FLUID: ASSOCIATION WITH BREAST CANCER RISK FACTORS

As noted earlier, breast fluids contain epithelial cells which desquamate from the alveolar-ductal epithelium of the breast. Studies by a number of pathologists (Black et al. 1972; Kodlin et al. 1977; Hutchison et al. 1980) indicate that cytologic atypical hyperplasia and dysplasia occur in association with breast cancer and are likely to reflect precursor glandular lesions. The progression of cytologic epithelial abnormalities in breast fluid from normal to hyperplasia and to dysplasia have been described by King et al. (1980). Recent studies on over 3800 women who underwent nipple aspiration indicate that 64% of patients with breast cancer, 31% with benign breast disease, and 21% of unbiopsied asymptomatic women had epithelial dysplasia. Based on these results we have investigated the possible association of dysplasia and breast cancer risk factors. These findings have been submitted for publication elsewhere but a brief account of the findings can be given here. Statistically significant associations were found only for first-degree family history of breast cancer (Table 4).

Table 4
Cytologic Dysplasia in Nipple Aspirates: Association with Breast Cancer Risk Factors (White women <50 years of age)

Risk factors	RR[a] (odds ratio)	90% CI[a]
Menarche: <12 vs >13 years	.943	.71-1.25
Parity: Nulliparous vs parous	1.04	.72-1.50
Age at first pregnancy: >26 vs <25 years	1.26	.90-1.80
Nursing: Never vs ever	.71	.52- .98[b]
Clinical fibrocystic disease: Present vs absent	1.21	.89-1.63
Family history of breast cancer (primary):		
Positive vs negative	1.60	1.10-2.37[b]
OC use: Ever vs never	1.21	.88-1.68
Menopausal estrogen use: Ever vs never	.72	.51- .96
Smoking: Current vs never	1.00	.69-1.44

[a] Age-adjusted.
[b] 90% CI does not overlap 1.00.

Women with a first-degree family history of breast cancer, compared to those without a history, were found to have a relative risk (RR) of 1.60 (confidence interval [CI], 1.10-2.32). A slightly elevated, but statistically nonsignificant, RR (1.20) of dysplasia was found for clinical fibrocystic disease (CI, .89-1.63).

The relationship of epithelial dysplasia and various risk factors for breast cancer in terms of potential genetic-environmental interactions, we believe, would warrant examination. Genes could influence susceptibility to breast cancer through their regulation of hormonal stimuli or by influencing the response of breast epithelium to these stimuli, as well as by regulating the metabolic response to carcinogens of endogenous and exogenous origin. In these studies, we analyzed the risk of dysplasia in terms of the classic nature-nurture model, whereby genes plus environment equals phenotype. A first-degree history of breast cancer arbitrarily was designated as entirely genetic, and the other risk factors were designated as entirely environmentally related. This is an obvious oversimplification, as both family history and the other risk factors probably have environmental and genetic components, respectively. It is well recognized that women with a first-degree family history of breast cancer are likely to have an increased risk of developing breast cancer during the premenopausal age. This suggests that such women may possess a gene or genes that increase the susceptibility and metabolic responsiveness of their breast epithelium to environmental factors. We suggest that an outcome of such a genetic-environmental interaction might be detectable as epithelial dysplasia.

Table 5 shows the RR of cytologic dysplasia in nipple aspirates associated with various combinations of family history and fibrocystic disease. The risk is elevated in the presence of either factor alone (1.29 and 1.63) and further elevated (to 1.91) in women who have both a positive family history of breast cancer and clinical fibrocystic disease. From these data, we conclude that first-degree family history of breast cancer and clinical fibrocystic disease act synergistically to increase the risk of dysplasia of epithelial cells in breast fluid aspirates. We believe that this may represent an example of genetic-environmental interaction in which environmental factors such as mutagens, toxins, and

Table 5

RR of Cytologic Dysplasia in Breast Nipple Aspirates Associated with Family History of Fibrocystic Disease (White women <50 years of age)

Family history	Clinical fibrocystic disease	RR (odds ratio)[a]	CI[a]
–	–	1.00	
–	+	1.29	.99–1.72
+	–	1.63	1.04–2.58[b]
+	+	1.91	1.09–3.25[b]

[a] Age-adjusted.
[b] 90% CI does not overlap 1.00.

nutritional components interact with the epithelium of the genetically susceptible host to produce cytopathologic changes in the epithelium. Evidence that benign disease has a large environmental component is suggested by studies of Japanese women in Hawaii and Japan, where proliferative breast lesions were markedly more common among the Japanese women residing in Hawaii (Sasano et al. 1978).

EPITHELIAL DYSPLASIA IN NIPPLE ASPIRATES OF BREAST FLUID: ASSOCIATION WITH CERUMEN TYPE

Several years ago, we reported a possible association between a genetically determined trait—wet cerumen—and breast cancer (Petrakis 1971). The hypothesis was developed from an observed correlation in several countries of the frequency of the dominant wet allele and mortality from breast cancer and was biologically based on the apocrine nature of the breast and ceruminous glands. A twofold increased RR of breast cancer was found among Japanese women of the wet cerumen phenotype as compared to those of the dry (homozygous recessive) phenotype. However, we were unable to confirm these findings in a larger study in Hong Kong (Ing et al. 1973). Subsequent studies demonstrated that a higher proportion of Asian and Caucasian women with wet-type cerumen yield breast fluid by the breast pump than do women with dry-type cerumen, suggesting that an apocrine-related genetic factor is associated with the occurrence and amount of secretory activity of the breast as determined by nipple aspiration (Petrakis et al. 1975, 1980). We proposed that this genetic factor might explain the differential risk of breast cancer of Western and of Asian women, in that the low breast secretory activity in women with dry-type apocrine glands might minimize the contact of the breast epithelium with endogenous or exogenous mutagens and carcinogens.

In our current studies of breast fluid cytology, we have sought to ascertain the proportion of dysplasia among women of the wet and dry cerumen type. The women were volunteers examined at the breast clinic at the University of California, San Francisco. Cerumen type and breast fluid cytologic examination were available from 1148 women (1097 white and 51 Asian women). Among white women, 697 were premenopausal and 400 postmenopausal. All Asian women were premenopausal.

Significant differences in the proportion of women with cytologic dysplasia were found in premenopausal white women where only a small proportion with dry cerumen had dysplastic cells compared to those with wet cerumen (Fig. 2). Dysplasia occurred in 20.1% of premenopausal women with wet cerumen and in 3.9% with dry cerumen (Table 6). A highly significant increased RR of dysplasia (7.2) was associated with the wet cerumen genetic marker. A similar elevated RR (3.2) was found in Asian women with wet cerumen, but did not reach statistical significance because of the small number of subjects. After menopause, no significant difference in dysplasia between wet and dry

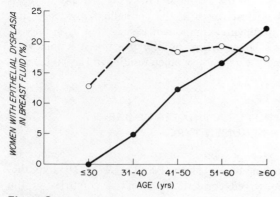

Figure 2
Cytologic dysplasia in premenopausal white women with wet (– – – –) and dry (———)
cerumen.

phenotypes was found. We believe that these findings provide support for our
hypothesis that a genetic apocrine factor affecting breast secretion may minimize exposure of breast epithelium to potential environmental carcinogens as
indicated by low frequency of cytologic dysplasia in premenopausal women with
dry cerumen. Further investigations will be needed to confirm these findings.

DISCUSSION

The causes of breast cancer in human populations remain obscure. Current
models of carcinogenesis, the transformation of normal to malignant cells, call
for at least two phases: Initiation and promotion (Brooks 1980). The primary
event, initiation, is considered to be due to a somatic genetic mutation of DNA
by a carcinogen. Recent studies suggest that a comutagenic or epigenetic
mechanism may also lead to permanent cell change predisposing to malignancy.

Table 6
Proportion of Women with Epithelial Dysplasia by Cerumen Type among
Premenopausal White Women

	Cytology[a]		
	dysplasia	normal	Percent dysplasia
Cerumen phenotype			
Wet	130	516	20.1
Dry	2	49	3.9

[a] Age-adjusted odds ratio 7.2 (CI, 1.81-22.3); $P < .005$.

In the latter mechanism, two nonmutagenic agents may interact at a critical time in cell development to alter permanently gene expression that could lead to malignancy.

We have demonstrated that a wide variety of chemical substances are secreted by the breast epithelium, including mutagenic, transforming, and carcinogenic chemicals, which might induce somatic mutations in breast epithelia. In addition, high concentrations of hormones, such as estrone and prolactin as well as dehydroepiandrosterone sulfate (DHAS)-like material, have been found in breast fluids which could act as promoting factors (Wynder and Hill 1977; Miller et al. 1977). These findings support our contention that both initiating and promoting substances do reach the breast epithelium; however, it remains to be determined if these factors actually affect the breast epithelium and, if so, why some women develop cytologic dysplasia whereas others do not.

Considerable experimental data indicate that genetic factors are involved in the activation and metabolism of carcinogens. It is likely that similar genetic factors control the metabolism of carcinogens and DNA repair mechanisms in humans. Our preliminary data on cerumen type and cytologic dysplasia suggest that an additional genetic factor affecting breast secretion may indirectly influence exposure of breast epithelia to carcinogens. Further studies are indicated of possible genetic differences in the ability of breast epithelium to metabolize carcinogens as well as to respond to endocrine promoting agents.

ACKNOWLEDGMENTS

I would like to thank Doctors John Craig, Virginia Ernster, Larry Gruenke, Eileen King, Christopher Maack and Susan Sacks for their assistance. This research was supported in part by USPHS Grant PO1-CA 13556-09 from the National Cancer Institute, Bethesda, Maryland.

REFERENCES

Ames, B.N., J. McCann, and E. Yamasaki. 1975. Method for detecting carcinogens and mutagens with Salmonella/mammalian-microsome mutagenicity test. *Mutat. Res.* 31:347.

Bischoff, F. 1969. Carcinogenic effects of steroids. *Adv. Lipid Res.* 7:165.

Black, M.M., T.H. Barclay, S.J. Cutler, B.F. Hankey, and A.J. Asire. 1972. Association of atypical characteristics of benign breast lesions with subsequent risk of breast cancer. *Cancer* 29:338.

Brooks, P. 1980. Chemical carcinogenesis. *Br. Med. Bull.* 36:1.

Bruce, W.E., A.J. Varghese, R. Furrer, and P. Land. 1977. A mutagen in the feces of normal humans. *Cold Spring Harbor Conf. Cell Proliferation* 4:1641.

Feldmann, R.J. and H.I. Maibach. 1970. Absorption of some organic compounds through skin in man. *J. Invest. Dermatol.* 54:399.

Gray, M.F., T.D.V. Lawrie, and C.J.W. Brooks. 1971. Isolation and identification of cholesterol alpha-oxide and other minor sterols in human serum. *Lipids* 6:836.

Guerrero, R.R., D.E. Rounds, and T.C. Hall. 1979. Bioassay procedure for the detection of mutagenic metabolites in human urine with the use of sister chromatid exchange analysis. *J. Natl. Cancer Inst.* 62:805.

Hutchison, W.B., D.B. Thomas, W.B. Hamlin, G.J. Roth, A.W. Peterson, and W. Williams. 1980. Risk of breast cancer in women with benign breast disease. *J. Natl. Cancer Inst.* 65:13.

Imai, H., N.T. Werthessen, V. Subramaryam, P.W. LeQuesne, A.H. Soloway, and M. Kanisawa. 1980. Angiotoxicity of oxygenated sterols and possible precursors. *Science* 207:651.

Ing, R., N.L. Petrakis, and J.H. Ho. 1973. Evidence against association between wet cerumen and breast cancer. *Lancet* i:43.

Jose, J.G. 1979. Photomutagenesis by chlorinated phenothiazine tranquilizers. *Proc. Natl. Acad. Sci.* 76:469.

Kadis, B. 1978. Steroid epoxides in biologic systems: A review. *J. Steroid Biochem.* 9:75.

Kelsey, M.I. and R.J. Pienta. 1979. Transformation of hamster embryo cells by cholesterol-alpha-epoxide and lithocholic acid. *Cancer Lett.* 6:143.

King, E.B., D. Barrett, and N.L. Petrakis. 1975a. Cellular composition of the nipple aspirate specimen of breast fluid. II. Abnormal findings. *Am. J. Clin. Pathol.* 64:739.

King, E.B., D. Barrett, M.-C. King, and N.L. Petrakis. 1975b. Cellular composition of the nipple aspirate specimen of breast fluid. I. The benign cells. *Am. J. Clin. Pathol.* 64:729.

King, E.B., A.L. Zimmerman, D.L. Barrett, N.L. Petrakis, and M.-C. King. 1980. Cytopathology of abnormal mammary ductal epithelium. In *Prevention and detection of cancer, part II. Detection, vol. 2: Cancer detection in specific sites* (ed. H.E. Nieburgs), p. 1831. Marcel Dekker, New York.

Kodlin, D., E.E. Winger, N.L. Morgenstern, and U. Chen. 1977. Chronic mastopathy and breast cancer. A followup study. *Cancer* 39:2603.

Miller, W.R., R.A. Hawkins, R.S. Creel, and A.P.M. Forrest. 1977. Oestrogen in breast fluid. *Lancet* ii:1179.

Parsons, P.G. and P. Goss. 1978. Chromosome damage and DNA repair induced in human fibroblasts by UV and cholesterol oxide. *Austr. J. Exp. Biol. Med. Sci.* 56:287.

Petrakis, N.L. 1971. Cerumen genetics and human breast cancer. *Science* 173:347.

―――――. 1977a. Breast secretory activity in nonlactating women, postpartum breast involution and the epidemology of breast cancer. *Natl. Cancer Inst. Monogr.* 47:161.

―――――. 1977b. Genetic factors in the etiology of breast cancer. *Cancer* 39:2709.

Petrakis, N.L., L.D. Gruenke, and J.C. Craig. 1981. Cholesterol and cholesterol epoxides in nipple aspirates of breast fluids. *Cancer Res.* 41.

Petrakis, N.L., C.A. Maack, R.E. Lee, and M. Lyon. 1980. Mutagenic activity in nipple aspirates of human breast fluid. Letter. *Cancer Res.* **40**:188.

Petrakis, N.L., L.D. Gruenke, T.C. Beelen, J.C. Craig, and N. Castagnoli, Jr. 1978. Nicotine in breast fluid of nonlactating women. *Science* **199**:303.

Petrakis, N.L., L. Mason, R. Lee, B. Sugimoto, S. Pawson, and F. Catchpool. 1975. Association of race, age, menopausal status and cerumen type with breast fluid secretion in nonlactating women, as determined by nipple aspiration. *J. Natl. Cancer Inst.* **54**:829.

Petrakis, N.L., M.L. Mason, M. Doherty, M.E. Dupuy, G. Sadee, and C.S. Wilson. 1977a. Effects of altering diet fat on breast fluids in women. *Fed. Proc.* **36**:1163.

Petrakis, N.L., M. Doherty, R. Lee, L. Mason, S. Pawson, T.K. Hunt, and R. Schweitzer. 1977b. Immunoglobulin levels in breast fluids of women with breast cancer. *Clin. Immunol. Immunopathol.* **7**:386.

Sasano, N., H. Tateno, and G.N. Stemmermann. 1978. Volume and hyperplastic lesions of breasts of Japanese women in Hawaii and Japan. *Prev. Med.* **7**: 196.

Wynder, E.L. and P. Hill. 1977. Prolactin, estrogen, and lipids in breast fluid. *Lancet* **ii**:840.

COMMENTS

PIKE: Can I just go back to something that, in fact, Nick [Petrakis] said earlier on, because I think no one has yet responded to some of that. I have always been bothered by mutagens. Urine analysis for mutagens shows that because there is no more effective way to get mutagens to all parts of your body than by smoking cigarettes. Why is it then, if mutagens are important, that cigarette smokers get less breast cancer than noncigarette smokers?

On the model that I drew up yesterday, you would predict that smokers would get approximately 15% less breast cancer because they have an earlier age of menopause. But their urine is many times more mutagenic than the urine of nonsmokers, and if mutagens are important one would expect this to make up easily for the 15% deficit.

PETRAKIS: But you can't just say mutagens. You have to determine if and how they are metabolized. They must reach the target tissue to interact and they can't interact unless there is a metabolically active epithelium. You have got to have the right enzyme system that will metabolize the mutagens for breast epithelium to the active form. What we detect in breast fluid may only be mutagenically inert byproducts of carcinogens.

PIKE: But they have hundreds of mutagens.

PETRAKIS: If the cells take them up, you might have damage to DNA that might lead to activation of their repair mechanisms. There probably is DNA repair going on all the time, and some people probably do it better than others.

There is no simple answer. You have got to put together a lot of these factors.

KORENMAN: I would like to say one thing about what Malcolm [Pike] just said, and that is if there is a time when the breast is most susceptible and the women who are now age 50 didn't start smoking until after that time, then you might not expect much of a change.

PIKE: People almost always start smoking by age 25.

PETRAKIS: If I may make a comment here. M.-C. King et al. (1980) published a family study showing there is a linkage between a certain polymorphic genetic marker (glutamate-pyruvate transaminase [GPT]) on chromosome 10 and breast cancer susceptibility. You people keep ignoring the fact that underlying it all, there has to be a susceptible host. Now, who knows what the mechanism for susceptibility is? I mean, it could be genetically determined absence of repair mechanisms, or metabolic detoxifying system, of immune responses, or of other genetically influenced controlling factors. It could be almost anything. We don't really know. Therefore, you can't just say hormones are the key factor.

PIKE: One thing I am continually reminded of when studying Ames test mutation results is that there is considerable background mutation. Mutation does not require a mutagen. You don't have to have a carcinogen to have carcinogenesis. This is something we tend to ignore.

PETRAKIS: All right, but I want to come back to this. Cholesterol epoxide is a very potent transforming substance. It is equivalent to 3-methylcholanthrene (3-MC). We have unequivocally demonstrated that it is present in breast fluids. And now an important question is, what is its metabolism? For example, is there some difference in people and their ability to form cholesterol epoxides and destroy them? I think that is where you have got to go. The hormones might then interact through their influence on mechanisms that allow the epithelium to metabolize mutagens and transforming substances. But they won't directly cause cancer.

I presented our data on the mutagens in breast fluid because we first started looking for them using the Ames test because it was a simple test. I agree with Malcolm that many substances don't give a positive Ames test. Actually, cholesterol epoxide itself does not give a positive Ames test in any of the Ames testing systems. It has been tested by several groups, including us and there is no activity found. So there you are.

References

King, M.-C., R.C.P. Go, R.C. Elston, H.T. Lynch, and N.L. Petrakis. 1980. Allele increasing susceptibility to human breast cancer may be linked to glutamate-pyruvate transaminase locus. *Science* 208:406.

Breast Cancer: Diet and Hormone Metabolism

PETER HILL,* L. GARBACZEWSKI,* FUJIO KASUMI,† KEIJIRO KUNO,†
PERCY HELMAN,§ AND ERNST L. WYNDER*

*Naylor Dana Institute for Disease Prevention
American Health Foundation
Valhalla, New York 10595

†Cancer Institute Hospital
Tokyo, Japan

§Groote Schuur Hospital
Capetown, South Africa

Asian or African populations have a lower incidence of endocrine-related diseases than Western populations (Wynder and Hirayama 1977; Isaacson et al. 1978), although migration from a low- to high-risk area increases the incidence of these diseases (Haenszel and Kurihara 1968; Adelstein et al. 1979). Women living in rural vs urban areas have a lower incidence (Pederson 1978), but higher socioeconomic status and nulliparity increase the risk of this disease. Thus, the risk of breast cancer is associated with life-style, including diet, as well as reproductive and hormonal factors (MacMahon et al. 1973).

In 1969, Feinleib and Garrison (1969) suggested that "the risk from breast cancer is related to the frequency and quality of ovarian function which are, in turn, related to environmental factors." A tendency of breast cancer patients to have had fewer children (Salber et al. 1969; Hunt et al. 1980) and to have higher abortion rates in patients (Valaoras et al. 1969; Soini 1977) has been reported. In addition, Hems (1978) reported a correlation between breast cancer mortality and mean family size in 26 countries. An inverse association between risk and parity has been reported in Burmese (Thein-Hlaing and Thein-Maung-Myint 1978), Icelandic (Tulinius et al. 1978), Greek (Valaoras et al. 1969), and Finnish women (Soini 1977).

In spite of the fact that a high parity involves an early age of first pregnancy and number of children and that their interaction (Woods et al. 1980) or a late pregnancy may negate the effect of a high parity (Herity et al. 1975), an early pregnancy and number of live births depends on early establishment and maintenance of menstrual activity. In this regard, a higher proportion of anovulatory cycles are associated with nulliparity and higher socioeconomic status (Trichopoulos et al. 1980a,b) and increase in incidence with increasing number or risk factors (Bulbrook et al. 1978). Furthermore, luteal insufficiency is prevalent in women with benign breast disease (Mauvais-Jarvis et al. 1979), whereas a higher incidence of menstrual irregularity occurs in premenopausal women with breast cancer (Kodama et al. 1977: Grattarola 1978; Hunt et al. 1980).

Few comparative studies of plasma hormonal activity during the menstrual cycle have been published (Saxena et al. 1972; Haus et al. 1980; Hill et al. 1980b). Establishment at puberty and maintenance during reproductive life of menstrual activity requires a critical body weight and (or) percentage of body fat (Frisch and Revelle 1970). Excess weight, prolonged exercise (Dale et al. 1979), or stress (Drew 1961) result in menstrual dysfunction.

Failure to establish an adult hypothalamic-pituitary-ovarian axis (Grumbach et al. 1974) and (or) a balanced ovarian steroid metabolism (Vihko and Apter 1980) during early gynecological age may lead to anovulation and functional secondary amenorrhea. Such dysfunction is frequent in young girls (Widholm and Kantero 1971), with a higher frequency of irregular cycles in girls with a late onset of menarche (Wallace et al. 1978).

In adults, nutritional factors modify sleep patterns (Phillips et al. 1975; Lacey et al. 1978), which in turn are associated with release of pituitary hormones (Sassin et al. 1973) and modification of androgen (Feher and Halmy 1975) and estrogen (Fishman et al. 1975) metabolism.

Epidemiological comparison of the dietary habits of populations at different risk for breast cancer has suggested that dietary intake of sugar (Hems and Stuart 1975), animal protein, and especially fat (Carroll and Khor 1975) in Western vs Asian or African populations is associated with a higher risk of breast cancer (Wynder and Hirayama 1977; Miller 1980), an association that is evident even when anthropometric variables are controlled (Gray et al. 1979).

It was, therefore, of interest to determine if differences were evident in hormonal metabolism in pre- and postmenopausal women at different risk for breast disease and whether increased risk resulted from a diet modification of a hormone profile essential for normal menstrual function. The rationale for this approach was that environmental factors of a dietary nature in Western women adversely alter menstrual function or decrease parity or fertility, which are associated with increased risk of breast cancer.

Accordingly, we have investigated the effect of diet modification on hormonal metabolism in women at low risk (black South African and Japanese women) and in women at high risk (North American causasian women) for breast cancer.

METHODS AND MATERIALS

Healthy Volunteers

Healthy nonobese rural black and urban Japanese and caucasian women between 20 years and 30 years of age gave informed consent for the study. None of the women had or were using oral contraceptives. All menstruated regularly, had no illness during the last year, and were in general good health. Postmenopausal black South African women who were at least 2 years past their last mense, were not yet 60 years of age, and who were in general good health were selected.

Blood Sampling

In all cases, blood was withdrawn from an antecubital vein between 9 AM and 9:30 AM. In the premenopausal women, blood was drawn every 2 days during the menstrual cycle. In postmenopausal women, blood was drawn four times over 2 weeks. Overnight blood sampling was obtained by an indwelling catheter in the antecubital vein. Samples were withdrawn via a three-way valve and long catheter, which enables samples to be taken without awakening the subjects. Blood samples were taken as described previously (Hill and Wynder 1979). The pituitary response was determined using two i.v. injections of 100 μg luteinizing hormone-releasing factor (LRF) (Ayerst Laboratories) and 200 μg thyrotropin-releasing hormone (TRH) (Abbott Laboratories) given 2 hr apart. An initial blood sample was taken prior to the first injection, followed by serial blood samples over 4 hr. Plasma was separated and stored at $-20°C$, until analyzed. Samples taken in Tanskei, South Africa, and in Tokyo, Japan, were shipped airmail in freezing containers to the American Health Foundation in New York.

Diet Modification

White women were maintained on a Western diet, composed of customary foods (Hill et al. 1980b). Compliance was determined using a self-administered, 3-day diet record currently used in the Multi-Risk Factorial Intervention Trials sponsored by the National Institutes of Health, Bethesda, Maryland.

South African black women, whose diet consisted of a well-defined vegetarian diet comprised of few staple foods which supplied less than 20% fat calories and mainly plant protein (Table 1) (Lubbe 1973), were fed an isocaloric diet supplying meat, butter, milk, eggs, bread, and sugar for 8 weeks for premenopausal and 6 weeks for postmenopausal women, respectively. Urban premenopausal Japanese women who were ovo-lacto vegetarians, were fed a Western diet supplying meat, etc., as above, for 8 weeks. These diets supplied

Table 1
Population Characteristics

Population	Age of menarche (years)	Age of menopause (years)	Breast cancer per 100,000	Percent of total calories carbo-hydrate	fat	protein
North American white	12.6	49.7	21.8	48	40	12
South African white	12.8	51.4	22.7	47.5	38	15.5
South African black	14.9	50.7	6.0[a]	72	16.5	11.5
Japan	14.3	46.9	6.5	56.5	28	15.5

[a] Incidence rate.

40% calories from fat and approximately 65% of the protein from animal sources.

Giving away food or failure to collect the food cancelled participation in the study. The diet was well received and good compliance was obtained.

Hormone Assays

Samples from the same subject were assayed together, while samples from caucasian, Japanese, and black women were also assayed simultaneously. All samples were assayed in duplicate.

Luteinizing hormone (LH) and follicle stimulating hormone (FSH) in the plasma were determined by a double-antibody radioimmunoassay (RIA) method according to Midgley (1966, 1967), while prolactin was measured by an homologous RIA (Sinha et al. 1973) using human prolactin (V-L-S No. 3) and rabbit antiprolactin antibody, as described previously (Hill et al. 1980a).

Estradiol (E_2) was assayed in duplicate using ^{125}I-labeled E_2 and E_2 17β-carbomethylether BSA antisera (Radioassay Laboratory, California).

Androstenedione and dehydroepiandrosterone (DHEA) were measured by RIA after separation on Sephadex LH.20 (Hill et al. 1980a). Plasma testosterone was measured using a double-antibody technique, as described by Abraham et al. (1972).

Statistical analysis was performed using Student's t test for analysis of the hormone differences between different races of women. A comparison t test was carried out for paired samples for comparison of data before and after diet modification.

RESULTS

As shown in Figure 1, the plasma prolactin level throughout the menstrual cycle was lower in rural premenopausal black South African than in Japanese or caucasian women, the latter two having similar levels.

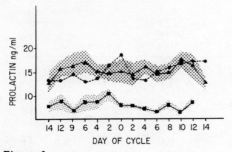

Figure 1
Plasma prolactin levels in caucasian women (▲) (n = 11), Japanese women (●) (n = 9), and South African black women (■) (n = 18). Results given as mean ± S.E.

When caucasian women were transferred to a vegetarian diet, plasma prolactin levels decreased, whereas prolactin levels increased in black South African women but not in Japanese women fed a Western diet (Fig. 2).

As shown in Figure 3, plasma testosterone is higher in caucasian vs Japanese or black South African women, whereas a vegetarian diet decreases testosterone in caucasian women and a Western diet increases testosterone in black South African and Japanese women (Fig. 4).

Following a previous study in caucasian women (Hill and Wynder 1979), five premenopausal Japanese nurses were fed a Western diet and overnight blood samples were taken while they were on their customary diet and on the Western diet. The overnight release was greater in Japanese women eating their customary diet than in caucasian women, confirming the finding of Haus et al. (1980). A nonsignificant decrease in prolactin occurred in Japanese women fed a Western diet (Fig. 5). To investigate further the relationship of diets on pituitary release of hormones, we determined the pituitary response to LRF/TRH in caucasian women maintained on their customary diet and when fed a vegetarian diet. As shown in Figures 6 and 7, the release of LH and FSH was reduced in the women fed their customary diet, but the release of FSH was increased (Fig. 8) in caucasian women fed a vegetarian diet.

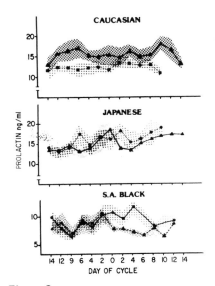

Figure 2

In caucasian women, plasma prolactin levels significantly decreased when transferred from customary (▲) to a vegetarian (■) diet ($P \leqslant 0.01$, $t = 7.45$), while in South African black women, prolactin levels increased in luteal phase when transferred from customary (▲) to a Western (●) diet ($P \leqslant 0.01$, $t = 3.86$). Comparison t test. Number of women as in Fig. 1. Results given as mean ± S.E.

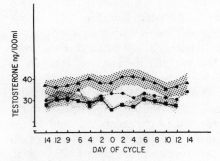

Figure 3

Plasma testosterone levels in caucasian (▲), Japanese (●), and South African black (■) women. Testosterone levels are significantly higher in caucasian than in South African black and Japanese women (one-way analysis of variance). Number of women as in Fig. 1. Results given as mean ± S.E.

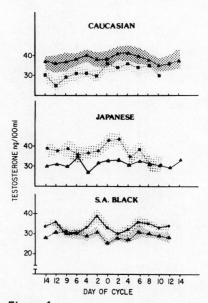

Figure 4

In caucasian women, plasma testosterone levels significantly decreased when transferred from a customary (▲) to a vegetarian (■) diet ($P \leqslant 0.01$, $t = 8.99$), while in South African black women ($P \leqslant 0.01$, $t = 5.87$) and in Japanese women ($P \leqslant 0.01$, $t = 5.05$), testosterone levels increased when transferred from a customary (▲) to a Western (●) diet. Comparison t test. Number of women per group as in Fig. 1. Results given as mean ± S.E.

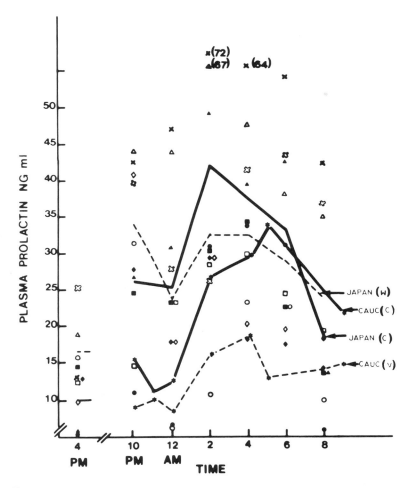

Figure 5

In caucasian women (n = 5), nocturnal release of prolactin was reduced when transferred to a vegetarian diet ($P \leqslant 0.01$, t = 3.74), but no significant change in prolactin occurred when Japanese women (n = 5) were transferred to a Western diet. Comparison t test.

DISCUSSION

Lower levels of plasma prolactin in premenopausal black South African than Japanese and caucasian women and the higher testosterone levels in caucasian vs black South African and Japanese women indicate differences in the hormonal profile during the menstrual cycle between the three races.

Diet-related increase in testosterone in black South African and Japanese women, and the increase in prolactin in black women fed a Western diet,

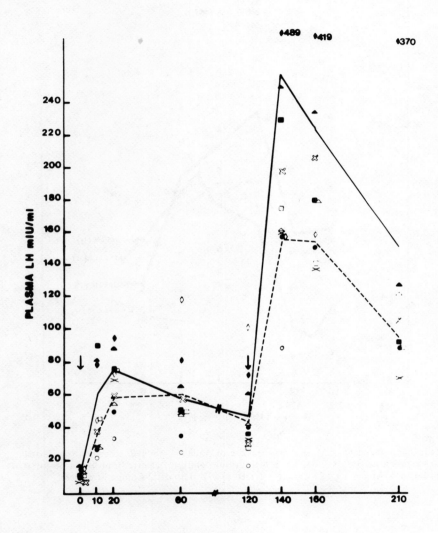

Figure 6

LH response to LRF injections given at 0 min and 120 min to premenopausal women
(n = 5) eating their customary diet (———) and then transferred to a vegetarian diet
(————) for 2 months. Significant decrease in response when fed a vegetarian diet
($P < 0.05$, t = 2.55). Comparison t test.

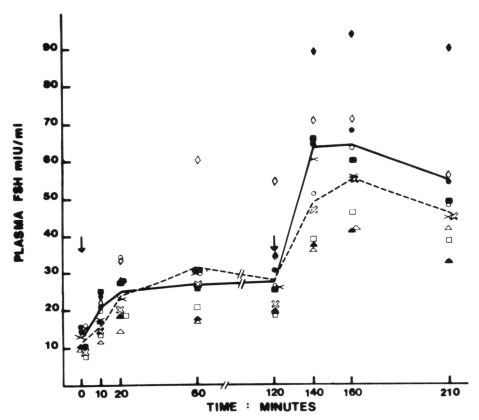

Figure 7
FSH response to LRF injections given at 0 min and 120 min to premenopausal women
($n = 5$) eating their customary diet (———) and then transferred to a vegetarian diet
(————) for 2 months. Significant decrease in response when fed a vegetarian diet
($P \leqslant 0.05, t = 2.66$). Comparison t test.

together with changes in E_2 and FSH in black women reported previously (Hill
et al. 1980b) indicate a change in menstrual activity. Opposite trends occur in
caucasian women fed a vegetarian diet, together with a shorter menstrual cycle
and a decreased menstrual flow.

Jones (1949) reported an association between short luteal phase and fertility. Subsequently, luteal deficiency characterized by decreased progesterone
and FSH levels (Strott et al. 1970) and changes in duration of the menstrual
cycle (Sherman and Korenman 1974) have been reported. Insufficient E_2 to trig-
ger LH release (Coutts et al. 1974), poor follicular growth related to depressed
FSH (Dodson et al. 1975), inadequate release of LH in response to estrogen

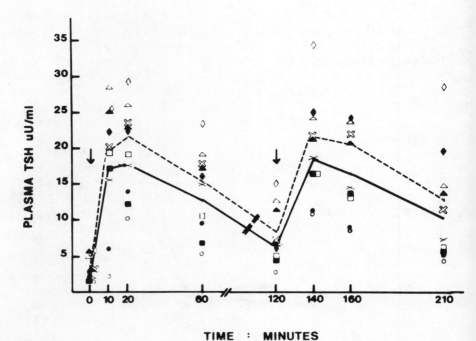

Figure 8
TSH response to TRH injections given at 0 min and 120 min to premenopausal women
(n = 5) eating their customary diet (———) and then transferred to a vegetarian diet
(————) for 2 months. Significant increase in response when fed a vegetarian diet ($P \leqslant 0.01$,
t = 5.83). Comparison t test.

feedback (VanLook et al. 1978), and (or) the possibility of inappropriate
gonadotropin release of LRF (Sheehan et al. 1979) are a few of the possible
changes associated with anovulation. In addition, many cases of infertility are
related to hyperprolactinemia, which can occur in a 28-day cycle (Lenton et al.
1977) and often in absence of galactorrhea (Franks et al. 1975). Loss of episodic
secretion of LH (Bohnet et al. 1975), reduced ovarian follicular activity without
any changes in plasma E_2 (McNatty 1979), and elevation of plasma DHEA
(Carter et al. 1977) are associated with hypoprolactinemia.

The importance of maintaining a physiological range of prolactin throughout the menstrual cycle has been postulated by Bohnet et al. (1977) and Lenton
et al. (1979) in regard to maintenance of the luteal phase and "conception level"
(e.g., 60 to 600 mU/liter or 3 to 25 ng/ml prolactin).

Thus, lower basal levels of prolactin in black South African women and
decreased levels in caucasian women fed a vegetarian diet may relate to the
number of conception cycles, whereas an increase in prolactin in black women
fed a Western diet may reverse this change.

Apart from such a basal range, the pituitary peak release pattern of prolactin in healthy women must be considered because Tarquini et al. (1978) have reported an abnormal evening prolactin level in women with a familial history of breast cancer, in nulliparous and obese women, and in women with breast cancer, and Malarkey et al. (1977a) reported a disordered nocturnal release in patients. Haus et al. (1980) recently reported a higher nocturnal release of prolactin in Japanese vs caucasian women, which we have confirmed. Our failure to find any significant change in the overnight release in Japanese women fed a Western diet may result from the fact that the study was carried out from April to June, Japanese women showing a seasonal variation in the magnitude of the overnight release (Haus et al. 1980). However, the decreased nocturnal release of prolactin in nonobese premenopausal caucasian women fed a vegetarian diet (Hill and Wynder 1979) and the delayed release (Copinschi et al. 1978) and impaired control of prolactin secretion (Kopelman et al. 1979) in obese women indicates that diet and excess weight modify prolactin metabolism.

As hyperprolactinemia is associated with changes in both hypothalamic-pituitary and ovarian activity, it is uncertain whether factors involving ovarian activity and (or) pituitary release of prolactin are of more significance. However, as breast cancer has been postulated to develop early in life, changes in release of prolactin and (or) differences in plasma prolactin levels, as reported in daughters of women with breast cancer by Henderson et al. (1975), should be evident at an early age.

Increased plasma testosterone levels in black South African and Japanese women fed a Western diet and a decrease in testosterone levels in caucasian women fed a vegetarian diet implies an alteration in testosterone metabolism and (or) peripheral conversion because 50% of plasma testosterone arises from androstenedione (Tait and Horton 1966) with the remainder secreted by the ovary and adrenals (Abraham 1974).

Early gynecological age is associated with a high frequency of anovulatory cycles where testosterone and LH levels are higher than in ovulatory cycles (Apter and Vihko 1977). Higher levels of testosterone and LH have been reported in late-maturing black South African than in early-maturing white girls (Hill et al. 1980a). Furthermore, elevated testosterone levels occur in infertile women (Steinberger et al. 1979), while increasing plasma testosterone levels are associated with decreasing length of luteal phase (Smith et al. 1979). Lowering plasma testosterone levels with prednisone administration reinitiates ovulatory cycles (Rodriguez-Rigau et al. 1979). This evidence suggests that plasma testosterone has a physiological level (35-59 ng/per 100 ml). Goebelsman et al. (1974) and Gibson et al. (1980) have suggested that excess ovarian androgen (testosterone) production, initiated by gonadotropin stimulation, inhibits granulosa cell proliferation. Thus, a relatively small change in ovarian production could lead to anovulatory cycles, but it is unknown whether dietary modification affects testosterone levels through a change in gonadotropin activity and (or) directly on ovarian steroid metabolism.

A survey of menopausal symptoms in unmarried women, women married with no children, or women with a late pregnancy or with a high socioeconomic status (Jaszmann et al. 1969) indicated an association between hormonal status and menopausal symptoms. During menopause, an imbalance in the hypo-thalamic-pituitary-ovarian axis develops, when LH and FSH increase and estrogen levels decrease (Sherman et al. 1976).

While episodic release of LRF (Seyler and Reichlin 1973) and LH and FSH (Medina et al. 1976), occurs after menopause, Meldrum et al. (1980) have reported a concomitant increase in LH with the presence of hot flushes, while Lightman and Jacobs (1979) reported Naloxone decreased the incidence of hot flushes.

In regard to environmental modification of hormonal status in post-menopausal women, Armstrong (1979) reported lower prolactin levels in vege-tarian women and this was also found in black South African women (Hill et al. 1980b). In our study, decreased LH and FSH response to LRF administration in premenopausal caucasian women fed a vegetarian diet suggests that diet modifies gonadotropin release and may also effect the episodic release of LH. Similar studies in postmenopausal caucasian and Japanese women may give leads to reduce the frequency and severity of menopausal symptoms.

Despite the fact that this study has selected dietary factors to be of prime importance, it should be noted that urbanization and socioeconomic status play an equally significant part in relation to environmental differences between populations. Although it can be argued that ongoing changes in the incidence of breast cancer (Brian et al. 1980) and dietary habits (Hirayama 1979) within populations are evident, at least in regard to caucasian and Japanese women, this is not true for rural black South African women who still maintain their traditional way of life.

While differences in pituitary response in circulating hormone levels and in duration of the menstrual cycle occur when a Western diet is interchanged for a vegetarian diet and vice versa, it remains to be determined how such modification takes place and whether dietary modification for the healthy Western women, and especially for the women with breast cancer, has thera-peutic value.

REFERENCES

Abraham, G. 1974. Ovarian and adrenal contribution to peripheral androgens during the menstrual cycle. *J. Clin. Endocrinol. Metab.* **39**:340.

Abraham, G.E., J.E. Buster, L.A. Lucas, P.C. Corrales, and R.C. Tailer. 1972. Chromatographic separation of steroid hormones for use in radioimmuno-assay. *Anal. Lett.* **5**:509.

Adelstein, A.M., J. Staszewski, and C.S. Muir. 1979. Cancer mortality in 1970-1972 among Polish born migrants to England and Wales. *Br. J. Cancer* **40**:464.

Apter, D. and R. Vihko. 1977. Serum pregnenolone, progesterone, hydroxyprogesterone, testosterone and 5α-dihydrosterone during female puberty. *J. Clin. Endocrinol. Metab.* **45**:1039.

Armstrong, B.K. 1979. Diet and hormones in the epidemiology of breast and endometrial cancers. *Nutrition and Cancer* **1**:90.

Bohnet, H.G., G.H. Dahlen, W. Wuttke, and H.P.G. Schneider. 1975. Hyperprolactinemic anovulatory syndrome. *J. Clin. Endocrinol. Metab.* **42**: 132.

Bohnet, H.G., D. Muhlenstedt, J.P.F. Hanker, and H.P.G. Schneider. 1977. Prolactin oversuppression. *Arch. Gynaekol.* **223**:173.

Brian, D.D., L.J. Melton, J.R. Goellner, R.L. Williams, and W.M. O'Fallon. 1980. Breast cancer incidence, prevalence, mortality and survivorship in Rochester, Minnesota. *Mayo Clin. Proc.* **53**:355.

Bulbrook, R.D., J.W. Moore, G.M.C. Clark, D.Y. Wang, D. Tong, and J. Hayward. 1978. Plasma oestradiol and progesterone levels in women with varying degrees of risk of breast cancer. *Eur. J. Cancer* **14**:1369.

Carroll, K.K. and H.T. Khor. 1975. Dietary fat in relation to tumorigenesis. *Prog. Biochem. Pharmacol.* **10**:308.

Carter, J.N., J.E. Tylon, G.L. Warne, A.S. McNeilly, C. Faiman, and H.G. Friesen. 1977. Adrenocorticoid function to hyperprolactinemic women. *J. Clin. Endocrinol. Metab.* **45**:973.

Copinschi, G., M.H. de Laet, J.P. Brion, R. LeClercq, M. l'Hermite, C. Robyn, E. Virasoro, E. Van Cauter. 1978. Simultaneous study of cortisol growth hormone and prolactin Nyctohemeral variations in normal and obese subjects. Influence of prolonged fasting in obesity. *Clin. Endocrinol.* **9**: 15.

Coutts, J.R.T., K. Dodson, and M.C. Macnaughtan. 1974. Hormone profiles in normally menstruating and infertile women. *Eur. J. Obsets. Gynecol. Reprod. Biol.* **4** (Suppl.):S169.

Dale, E., D.H. Gerlack, and A.L. Wilwhite, 1979. Menstrual dysfunction in distance runners. *Obstet. Gynecol.* **54**:47.

Dodson, K.S., M.C. Macnaughtan, and J.R.T. Coutts. 1975. Infertility in women with apparent ovulatory cycles. *Br. J. Obstet. Gynaecol.* **82**:615.

Drew, F.L. 1961. The epidemiology of secondary amenorrhea. *J. Chronic Dis.* **14**:396.

Feher, T. and L. Halmy. 1975. Dehydroepiandrostenone and dehydroepiandrosterone sulphate dynamics in obesity. *Can. J. Biochem.* **53**:215.

Feinleib, M. and R.J. Garrison. 1969. Interpretation of the vital statistics of breast cancer. *Cancer* **24**:1109.

Fishman, J., R.M. Boyar, and L. Hellman. 1975. Influence of body weight on estradiol metabolism in young women. *J. Clin. Endocrinol. Metab.* **41**:989.

Franks, S., M.A.F. Murray, A.M. Jequier, S.J. Steele, J.D.N. Nabarro, and H.S. Jacobs. 1975. Incidence and significance of hyperprolatinaemia in women with amenorrhea. *Clin. Endocrinol.* **4**:597.

Frisch, R.E. and R. Revelle. 1970. Height and weight at menarche and a hypothesis of critical body weight and adolescent events. *Science* **169**:397.

Gibson, M., R. Lackritz, I. Schiff,and T. Tulchinsky. 1980. Abnormal adrenal responses to adrenocorticotropic hormones in hyperandrogenic women. *Fertil. Steril.* **33**:43.

Goebelsman, U., J.J. Arce, I.H. Thorneycroft, and D.R. Mishell. 1974. Serum testosterone concentrations in women throughout the menstrual cycle and following HCG administration. *Am. J. Obstet. Gynecol.* 119:445.

Grattarola, R. 1978. Anovulation and increased androgenic activity in breast cancer risk in women with fibrocystic disease of the breast. *Cancer Res.* 38:3051.

Gray, G.E., M.C. Pike, and B.E. Henderson. 1979. Breast cancer incidence and mortality rates in different countries in relation to known risk factors and dietary practices. *Br. J. Cancer* 39:1.

Grumbach, M.M., J.C. Roth, S.L. Kaplan, and K.V. Kelch. 1974. Hypothalamic-pituitary regulation of puberty in man. In *Control of the onset of puberty* (ed. M.M. Grumbach et al.), p. 115. John Wiley & Sons, New York.

Haenszel, W. and M. Kurihara. 1968. Studies in Japanese migrants. I. Mortality from cancer and other diseases among Japanese in the United States. *J. Natl. Cancer Inst.* 40:43.

Haus, E., D.J. Lakatua, F. Halberg, E. Halberg, G. Cornelissen, L.L. Sackett, H.G. Berg, T. Kawasaki, M. Ueno, K. Uezono, M. Matsuoka, and T. Omae. 1980. Chronobiological studies of plasma prolactin in women in Kyusho, Japan and Minnesota, U.S.A. *J. Clin. Endocrinol. Metab.* 51:632.

Hems, G. 1978. The contributions of diet and childbearing to breast cancer rates. *Br. J. Cancer* 37:974.

Hems, G. and A. Stuart. 1975. Breast cancer rates in populations of single women. *Br. J. Cancer* 31:118.

Henderson, B.E., V. Gerkins, I. Rosario, J. Casagrande, and M.C. Pike. 1975. Elevated serum levels of estrogen and prolactin in daughters of patients with breast cancer. *N. Engl. J. Med.* 293:790.

Herity, B., M.J. O'Halloran, G.J. Bourke, and K. King-Davis. 1975. A study of breast cancer in Irish women. *Br. J. Prev. Soc. Med.* 29:176.

Hill, P. and E.L. Wynder. 1979. Effect of a vegetarian diet and dexamethasone on plasma prolactin, testosterone and dehydroepiandrosterone in men and women. *Cancer Lett.* 7:273.

Hill, P., L. Garbaczewski, E.L. Wynder, P. Helman, M. Hill, J. Spornangisa, and J. Huskisson. 1980a. Diet and menarche in different ethnic groups. *Eur. J. Cancer* 16:519.

Hill, P., L. Garbaczewski, P. Helman, J. Huskisson, J. Sporangisa, and E.L. Wynder. 1980b. Diet, lifestyle and menstrual activity. *Am. J. Clin. Nutr.* 33:1192.

Hirayama, T. 1979. Diet and cancer. *Nutrition and Cancer* 1:67.

Hunt, S.C., R.R. Williams, M.H. Skolnick, J.L. Lyon, and C.R. Smart. 1980. Breast cancer and reproductive history from genealogical data. *J. Natl. Cancer Inst.* 64:1047.

Isaacson, C., G. Selzer, V. Kaye, M. Greenberg, J.D. Woodruff, J. Davies, D. Niven, D. Vetten, and M. Andrew. 1978. Cancer in urban blacks in South Africa. *South African Cancer Bull.* 22:49.

Jazmann, L.J.B., N.D. Van Lith, and J.C.A. Zaat. 1969. The age of menopause in the Netherlands. *Int. J. Fertil.* 14:106.

Jones, G.S. 1949. Some newer aspects of management of infertility. *J. Am. Med. Assoc.* 141:1123.

Kodama, M., T. Kodama, S. Miura, and M. Yoshida. 1977. Hormonal status of breast cancer. Further analysis of ovarian-adrenal dysfunction. *J. Natl. Cancer Inst.* **59**:49.

Kopelman, P.G., T.R.E. Pilkington, N. White, and S.L. Jeffcoate. 1979. Impaired hypothalamic control of prolactin secretion in massive obesity. *Lancet* i:747.

Lacey, J.H., P. Stanley, M. Hartmann, J. Koval, and A.H. Crisp. 1978. The immediate effects of intravenous specific nutrients on EEG sleep. *Electroencephal. Clin. Neurophysiol.* **44**:275.

Lenton, E.A., O.S. Sobowale, and I.D. Cooke. 1977. Prolactin concentrations in ovulating, but infertile women. Treatment with bromocryptine. *Br. Med. J.* **2**:1179.

Lenton, E.A., L.M. Brook, O. Sobowale, and I.D. Cooke. 1979. Prolactin concentrations in normal menstrual cycles and conception cycles. *Clin. Endocrinol.* **10**:383.

Lightman, S.L. and H.S. Jacobs. 1979. Naloxone: Non-steroidal treatment for postmenopausal flushing. *Lancet* ii:1071.

Lipmann, M., G. Bolan, and K. Huff. 1976. The effects of estrogens and anti-estrogens on hormone responsive human breast cancer in long-term tissue culture. *Cancer Res.* **36**:4595.

Lubbe, A.M. 1973. Dietary survey in the Mount Ayliss District. *S. Afr. Med. J.* **47**:304.

MacMahon, B., P. Cole, and J. Brown. 1973. Etiology of human breast cancer: A review. *J. Natl. Cancer Inst.* **50**:21.

Malarkey, W.B., L.L. Schroeder, V.C. Stevens, A.G. James, and R.R. Lanese. 1977a. Disordered nocturnal prolactin regulation in women with breast cancer. *Cancer Res.* **37**:4650.

Mauvais-Jarvis, P., R. Sitruk-Ware, F. Kuttenn, and N. Sterkers. 1979. Luteal phase insufficiency: A common pathophysiologic factor in development of benign and malignant breast diseases. In *Commentaries on research in breast disease* (ed. R.D. Bulbrook et al.), vol. 1, p. 25. Alan R. Liss Inc., New York.

McNatty, K.P. 1979. Relationship between plasma prolactin and the endocrine microenvironment of the developing human antral follicle. *Fertil. Steril.* **32**:433.

Medina, M., H.E. Scaglia, G. Vazquez, S. Alatorre, and G. Perez-Palacios. 1976. Rapid oscillation of circulating gonadotrophins in postmenopausal women. *J. Clin. Endocrinol. Metab.* **43**:1015.

Meldrum, D.E., I.V. Tataryn, A.M. Frumar, V. Erlik, K.H. Lu, and H.L. Judd. 1980. Gonadotrophins, estrogens and adrenal steroids during the menopausal hot flash. *J. Clin. Endocrinol. Metab.* **50**:685.

Midgley, A.R. 1966. Radioimmunoassay for human LH. *Endocrinology* **79**:10.

———. 1967. Radioimmunoassay for human FSH. *J. Clin. Endocrinol. Metab.* **27**:295.

Miller, A.B. 1980. Nutrition and cancer. *Prev. Med.* **9**:189.

Miller, W.R. and A.P.M. Forrest. 1976. Oestradiol synthesis from C steroids by human breast cancer. *Br. J. Cancer* **33**:116.

Pederson, E. 1978. *Incidence of cancer in Norway 1972-1976.* Cancer Registry of Norway, Oslo.

Phillips, F., A.H. Crisp, B. McGuinness, E. Kalucy, C.N. Chen, J. Koval, R.S. Kalucy, and J.H. Lacey. 1975. Isocaloric diet changes and electroencephalographic sleep. *Lancet* ii:723.

Rodriguez-Rigau, L., K.D. Smith, R.K. Tcholakian, and E. Steinberger. 1979. Effect of prednisone and plasma testosterone levels on duration of phases of the menstrual cycle in hyperandrogenic women. *Fertil. Steril.* 32:408.

Salber, E.J., D. Trichopolous, and B. MacMahon. 1969. Lactation and reproductive histories of breast cancer patients in Boston 1965-1966. *J. Natl. Cancer Inst.* 43:1013.

Sassin, J.F., A.G. Frantz, S. Kapen, and E.D. Weitzman. 1973. The nocturnal rise of human prolactin is dependent on sleep. *J. Clin. Endocrinol. Metab.* 37:436.

Saxena, B.N., N. Dusitin, and V. Poshyachinda. 1972. Luteinizing hormone, oestradiol and progesterone levels in the serum of menstruating 'Thai' women. *J. Obstet. Gynaecol. Br. Commonw.* 84:113.

Seyler, I.E. and S. Reichlin. 1973. Luteinizing hormone releasing factor (LRF) in plasma of postmenopausal women. *J. Clin. Endocrinol. Metab.* 37:197.

Sheehan, K.L., R.F. Casper, and S.S.C. Yen. 1979. Effects of a superactive luteinizing releasing factor, agonist, on gonadotrophin and ovarian function during the menstrual cycle. *Am. J. Obstet. Gynecol.* 135:759.

Sherman, B.M. and S.G. Korenman. 1974. Inadequate corpus luteum function: A pathophysiological interpretation of human breast cancer epidemiology. *Cancer* 33:1306.

Sherman, B.M., J.H. West, and S.G. Korenman. 1976. The menopausal transition: Analysis of LH, FSH, estradiol and progesterone concentrations during menstrual cycles of older women. *J. Clin. Endocrinol. Metab.* 42:629.

Sinha, Y.N., F.W. Selby, V.J. Lewis, and W.P. Vanderlaan. 1973. A homologous radioimmunoassay for human prolactin. *J. Clin. Endocrinol. Metab.* 36:509.

Smith, K.D., L. Rodriguez-Rigau, R.K. Tcholakian, and E. Steinberger. 1979. The relationship between plasma testosterone levels and the length of phases of the menstrual cycle. *Fertil. Steril.* 32:403.

Soini, J. 1977. Risk factors of breast cancer in Finland. *Int. J. Epidemiol.* 6:365.

Steinberger, E., K.D. Smith, R.K. Tcholakian, and L. Rodriguez-Rigau. 1979. Testosterone levels in female partners of infertile couples. *Am. J. Obstet. Gynecol.* 133:133.

Strott, C.A., C.M. Cargille, G.T. Rose, and M.B. Lipsett. 1970. The short luteal phase. *J. Clin. Endocrinol. Metab.* 30:246.

Tait, J.F. and R. Horton. 1966. The in vivo estimation of blood production and interconversion rates of androstenedione and testosterone and the calculation of their secretion rates. In *Steroid dynamics* (ed. G. Pincus et al.), p. 393. Academic Press, New York.

Tarquini, A., L. DiMartino, A. Malloci, H.G. Kwa, A.A. Vander Gugten, R.D. Bulbrook, and D.Y. Ubang. 1978. Abnormalities in evening plasma prolactin levels in nulliparous women with benign or malignant disease. *Int. J. Cancer* 22:687.

Thein-Hlaing and Thein-Maung-Myint. 1978. Risk factors of breast cancer in Burma. *Int. J. Cancer* 21:432.

Trichopoulos, B., B. MacMahon, and J. Brown. 1980b. Socioeconomic status, urine estrogens and breast cancer risk. *J. Natl. Cancer Inst.* 64:753.

Tricholpoulos, D., P. Cole, J.B. Brown, M.B. Goldman, and B. MacMahon 1980a. Estrogen profiles of primiparous and nulliparous women in Athens, Greece. *J. Natl. Cancer Inst.* 65:43.

Tulinius, H., N.E. Day, T. Johannesson, O. Bearnason, and M. Gonzales. 1978. Reproductive factors and risk for breast cancer in Iceland. *Int. J. Cancer* 21:724.

Tyson, J.E. 1977. Neuroendocrine control of lactation infertility. *J. Biosoc. Sci.* (Suppl.) 4:23.

Valaoras, V.G., B. MacMahon, D. Trichopoulos, and A. Polychronopoulus. 1969. Lactation and reproductive histories of breast cancer patients in greater Athens, 1965–1967. *Int. J. Cancer* 4:350.

VanLook, P.F.A., W.M. Hunter, I.S. Frazer, and D.T. Baird. 1978. Impaired estrogen-induced luteinizing hormone release in young women with anovulatory dysfunctional uterine bleeding. *J. Clin. Endocrinol. Metab.* 46:816.

Vihko, R. and D. Apter. 1980. The role of androgens in adolescent cycles. *J. Steroid Biochem.* 12:389.

Wallace, P.B., B.M. Sherman, J.A. Bean, J.P. Leeper, and A.E. Treloar. 1978. Menstrual cycle pattern and breast risk factors. *Cancer Res.* 38:4021.

Widholm, O. and R.L. Kantero. 1971. A statistical analysis of the menstrual patterns of 8000 Finnish girls and their mothers. *Acta Obstet. Gynecol. Scand.* (Suppl.) 14:50.

Woods, K.L., S.R. Smith, and J.M. Morrison. 1980. Parity and breast cancer: Evidence of a dual affect. *Br. Med. J.* 2:419.

Wynder, E.L. and P. Hill. 1977. Prolactin, oestrogen, and lipids in breast fluid. *Lancet* ii:840.

Wynder, E.L. and T. Hirayama. 1977. Comparative epidemiology of cancers of the United States and Japan. *Prev. Med.* 6:567.

COMMENTS

TOPP: Is there any chance that we can pinpoint some chemical that is being fed to food-supplying animals in the feedlots or the hen houses to make them grow faster? It, rather than the diet, may actually be causing this effect on hormone levels.

HILL: I do not know the answer, except that in South Africa, farms generally use natural fertilizer. Egg production via battery hens is rare, and the cattle are grass fed. However, mutton was the South African meat source in this study. If estrogens are used on food animals, I do not know how much accumulates in this lean meat.

PIKE: Your question is premature in that other investigators (including Dr. Henderson and myself) have been unable to obtain these clear-cut results that Dr. Hill showed.

HILL: Perhaps the problem is related to our different diets. We have been interested in modifying protein composition. The vegetarian diet used in all our studies only reduced the fat from 40% to 33% fat calories per day (Hill and Wynder 1976). In each of our studies over the past 4 years, we have found a similar lowering of plasma prolactin in caucasian women fed a meatless, vegetarian diet. Concomitantly, we also find a shorter menstrual cycle and decreased menstrual flow. In black South African women, transfer from plant to animal protein, apart from changes in fat content, drastically modifies the amino acid content.

HENDERSON: We do get changes in the menstrual cycle, but no changes in the plasma prolactin level.

I might point out that the background for the hypothesis being tested in these experiments comes both from the animal experiments with fat and the observations that were published some years ago (Phillips 1975) that Seventh-day Adventists (SDAs) had a decreased mortality from breast cancer. The argument developed that their vegetarian diet, which is really a nonmeat diet and not a real vegetarian diet, protected them.

Just because we are here to talk about new information, I might point out that we now have some data on proportional incidence rates of breast cancer among SDAs in Los Angeles, and cannot confirm that they have a reduced rate of breast cancer. I think that is in keeping with Roland Phillips' latest information from the SDA Health Survey.

So it may be that that original hypothesis was based on incomplete information and that, in fact, there is no evidence in the human population that nonmeat eating lowers your risk of breast cancer.

SEGALOFF: I think there is another very crucial factor. I have often wondered if anybody has taken people on nonmeat diets of different kinds that have altered cholesterol-derived hormones and see whether or not they can make cholesterol at the same rate, say, from labeled acetate. In these populations, is their ability to make cholesterol as a steroid precursor different when you take away precursors in the form of meat in the diet?

HILL: We followed changes in lipoproteins, cholesterol, and triglycerides in this study. In black women, low-density lipoprotein (LDL) cholesterol increased. Normally, in South African black women, the daily cholesterol intake is low, less than 200 mg cholesterol per day, so that one assumes liver biosynthesis of cholesterol maintains the necessary study steroid precursors. Addition of meat therefore, would increase the supply of cholesterol. In malnourished women, it is possible that inadequate cholesterol biosynthesis could lead to a deficiency of steroid precursors. However, the women we studied were healthy and, as a group, have large families when eating their customary vegetarian diet.

SIRBASKU: But, in fact, though, the metabolic pathways are that acetyl coenzyme A (acetyl-CoA) is derived from glucose and the breakdown of fatty acids, and that protein contributes a very minor component to the acetyl numbers to begin forming cholesterol. So protein is not a major precursor of cholesterol, unless it becomes a total diet. If there is any carbohydrate or fat, it will be a preferential precursor going into cholesterol. These are the agents that are broken down to give acetyl-CoA, which is condensed hydroxy β-hydroxy-β-methyl glutaryl (HMG) CoA, and goes on from there.

HILL: As I stated, when one changes from a vegetarian to a Western diet or vice versa, one changes the protein, fat, and carbohydrate content simultaneously. In regard to protein, I was suggesting that this component modified hypothalamic-pituitary function and this in turn, affected steroid hormones, not that it acted as a precursor.

KORENMAN: Peter [Hill], there are two things I would like to introduce. One of them is that about a month of dietary change should play a very important role in sex-hormone-binding globulin (SHBG). I think Dr. Siiteri made the point about available steroid. So even if you did not get changes in the complete and total estrogen levels, certainly it would behoove you to examine the available steroid level. That is about the right time to find changes.

The other thing has to do with the possibility of a Hawthorn effect. When we first started studying menstrual cycles, we put the people in a clinical research center so that we could draw blood from them all the time, and they immediately became anovulatory. We stopped doing that, because there was too much change in their life pattern. (By the way, they worked their regular work during the day, and they just slept in the clinical research center, instead of sleeping at home.)

I think that what you have done with the Bantu, for example, is that you have brought in a lot of apparatus and a lot of people and have created a lot of change in their behavior patterns that might influence what their subsequent cycles are like. And I don't know whether you did a similar thing to the Japanese.

HILL: We have not measured SHBG, but I agree we should determine whether diet modifies the free vs bound steroid.

In answer to your second question, after the first visit, where the nutritionist, African fieldworker, and attendant physician visited the families, only the African fieldworker visited the villages. The women were, however, required to collect food every 2 days at a local village store and to have a blood sample taken at a clinic. Time of preparation of the diet vs preparation of their customary diet was comparable. Because we carried out a similar intervention in these normally physically active women on their customary diet and on the Western diet, we consider changes in hormonal patterns are caused predominantly by diet intervention. However, we have carried out a similar study in urban, black South African women, which, when analyzed, will provide an answer.

KORENMAN: I think that changing someone's dietary habit completely and sustaining that change in dietary habit for 2 months, is a major change in life-style, particularly in someone like that. For example, they didn't have to grub for the food; you gave it to them. I think that that is really quite a change.

COLE: You said that conception could not occur below a certain prolactin level.

HILL: I commented on the report of Lenton et al. (1979), who suggested conception occurred in women with prolactin levels less than 25 mg/ml serum. In regard to a minimum level of prolactin, Bohnet et al. (1977) reported an oversuppression of prolactin by bromoergocryptine produced a short luteal phase and suggested a minimum level of 3 ng/ml serum was necessary for normal luteal development.

COLE: I can see why conception wouldn't occur above a certain level, but I don't understand why a lower level would be necessary. Is this speculation?

HILL: Yes. The idea of a conception cycle where hormone levels are within certain limits is speculation, but it would explain several aspects of fertility.

ZUMOFF: I would just like to make a couple of comments about nocturnal prolactin levels from some data that we have. First, on the matter that you referred to in Malarkey's paper (Malarkey et al. 1977) about differences between nocturnal prolactin in postmenopausal breast cancer and normal women, we have shown preliminarily that in older women—and I leave that vague because I think that is the key to the problem—the nocturnal prolactin surge that you see in younger women doesn't occur. I am not sure at excatly what age that is. It is somewhere in the 55-60-year-old range. I can see that if that shows a splay with age—and I am sure it does—that you could accidentally find one group that didn't have a nocturnal surge and another one that did in the postmenopausal range. I would caution great care in age matching before making anything of that.

Second, our laboratory is engaged in a study of the influence of fat content, using isocaloric substitution of a 15% fat diet vs a 45% fat diet. In very preliminary data, the women on a 15% fat diet very definitely still have pronounced nocturnal surging of prolactin. They don't have a decrease of their nocturnal prolactins.

However, in a couple of people we did see the surge occurrring very early in the night period and ending within 1-2 hr. Conceivably, you could have missed it with the 4-hr interval that you used. So it is possible we may be talking about the same kind of data, but that your sampling isn't frequent enough to demonstrate the proper shape of the nocturnal curve.

References

Bohnet, H.G., D. Muhlenstedt, J.P.F. Hanker, and H.P.G. Schneider. 1977. Prolactin oversuppression. *Arch. Gynaekol.* 223:173.

Hill, P. and E.L. Wynder. 1976. Diet and prolactin release. *Lancet* ii:806.

Lenton, E.A., L.M. Brook, O. Sobowale, and I.D. Cooke. 1979. Prolactin concentrations in normal menstural cycles and conception cycles. *Clin. Endocrinol.* 10:383.

Malarkey, W.B., L.L. Schroeder, V.C. Stevens, A.G. James, and R.R. Lanese. 1977. Disordered nocturnal prolactin regulation in women with breast cancer. *Cancer Res.* 37:4650.

Phillips, R.L. 1975. Role of life-style and dietary habits in risk of cancer among Seventh-day Adventists. *Cancer Res.* (Suppl.) 35:3513.

SESSION 7:
Hormones and the Genesis and Progression of Murine Mammary Tumors

The Role of Ovarian Steroid Hormones in Mammary Carcinogenesis

THOMAS L. DAO
Department of Breast Surgery and Breast Cancer Research Unit
Roswell Park Memorial Institute
Buffalo, New York 14263

The mammary gland is an integral part of the female reproductive system and, as such, is subject to regulation by hormones from the pituitary, gonads, and adrenals for various phases of development. The influence of hormones on the etiology, pathogenesis, and control of mammary gland tumorigenesis in the murine species has been extensively investigated and reported (Bern and Nandi 1961; Dao 1964). The objective of this paper, therefore, is not to provide another lengthy review of this subject, but rather to undertake an in-depth examination of a few recently reported studies on the subject of hormone regulation of mammary carcinogenesis. It is hoped that such a discussion may contribute to our better understanding of the role of hormones in the pathogenesis of mammary cancer. It should be noted that extensive coverage of the literature is not the intent of this author.

When we consider the role of hormones in the carcinogenesis of the mammary gland, we must necessarily be concerned with two important questions: (1) Can a hormone or hormones be causative agents of mammary tumor development? (2) Do hormones act merely through their effect on cell proliferation and therefore on tumor growth? In other words, are they promotors of tumor growth? These questions are concerned with two aspects of the neoplastic process: The initiation phase of malignant transformation of the cells and the progression of the transformed cells to form palpable tumors, and the later phase of the maintenance and progression of tumor growth. It thus follows that steroid hormones may be able either to initiate neoplastic transformation as a carcinogen or promote tumor growth by the nature of their effects on cell proliferation, or both.

The gonadal hormones, specifically the estrogenic steroids, have the capacity to induce growth and neoplasia of various target tissues in murine species, including the pituitary, the testes, the uterus, the kidney, the lymphoid tissue, and the mammary gland. Whether estrogenic hormones can be considered carcinogens is a question that has yet to be answered by conclusive experimental data. Although mammary cancer can be induced by estrogenic hormones alone in a few strains of rats (Cutts and Noble 1964), no data have conclusively demonstrated that the cause of the mammary cancer was due solely to the administered estrogens. Unfortunately, there have been few, if any, in-depth studies to elucidate the mechanism by which estrogen induced mammary cancer in these strains of rats. The critical question to be answered is whether estrogens are capable of causing heritable changes in somatic cells during neoplastic transformation.

In the absence of "spontaneously" developing mammary cancers in the murine species as a suitable model for pathogenetic studies, we consider carcinogen-induced mammary cancers in the rat to be the best model for studies concerned with the regulation of growth by hormones for two reasons: (1) Mammary tumors can be readily induced by chemical carcinogens, and (2) the induced tumors are exquisitely hormone-responsive (Dao and Sunderland 1959; Huggins et al. 1959). This paper will describe the role of ovarian steroid hormones on the pathogenesis of mammary cancer in both in vivo and in vitro experiments. First, experiments are presented to demonstrate the critical importance of ovarian steroids in the initiation of carcinogenesis. Then the role of steroid hormones and the anterior pituitary hormone in regulating the growth of mammary cancer is described. Finally, in vitro experiments designed to examine and to identify the "key" hormone(s) in mammary carcinogenesis are discussed.

OVARIAN HORMONES IN THE INDUCTION
OF MAMMARY CANCER

The objective of the following experiments was to answer the question: Is an estrogenic hormone essential for the initiation of neoplastic transformation of mammary cells by a chemical carcinogen? The basic experimental design was based on the hypothesis that initiation of carcinogenesis may not occur if ovarian hormones are absent at the time the mammary cells are exposed to the carcinogen. To test this hypothesis, ovariectomy was performed at the time of carcinogen administration, and a source of these hormones was later restored by transplanting a pair of ovaries when tumors might normally be expected to appear. The failure of tumors to develop or a greatly decreased tumor incidence in the ovariectomized animals after the ovarian transplantation would strongly suggest the validity of the hypothesis that ovarian hormones are critical for the initiation of neoplastic transformation. The three experiments described below have all been published (Dao 1962).

Castration in Relation to the Induction of
Mammary Carcinogenesis in Female Rats

In this study, ovaries were removed 1, 3, 7, 15, and 20 days after a single dose of either 10 mg of 3-methylcholanthrene (3-MC) or 10 mg of 7,12-dimethylbenz-[a]anthracene (DMBA), or 20 mg of DMBA was given to 55-day-old female rats.

All animals subsequently received a pair of ovarian grafts 40-50 days after the administration of the carcinogen, to restore the source of ovarian hormones after the mammary cells had been exposed to the carcinogen in these castrated rats. The reason for using both 3-MC and DMBA was to investigate how ovarian hormones may influence the interaction of the target tissue with carcinogens of different potency. That the polycyclic aromatic hydrocarbons may be hormone-mimetic has been suggested by their unique molecular structural similarities (Yang et al. 1961) and the presence of certain common biochemical character-istics (Dao and Sinha 1975). A quantitative balance may exist between the carcinogenic hydrocarbons and the hormones that regulate the induction of mammary cancer in the rat.

The results summarized in Figures 1 and 2 clearly show that the removal of ovarian hormones from rats immediately after the administration of the carcinogen inhibited or profoundly reduced the incidence of mammary cancer.

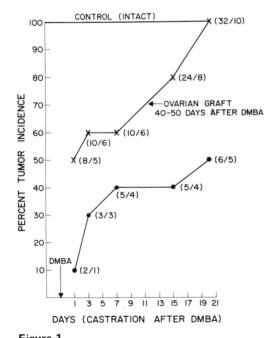

Figure 1
(●) Mammary tumor incidence in rats castrated on day 1, 3, 7, 15, and 21 after a single dose of 10 mg DMBA; (×) mammary tumor incidence in identical groups of castrated rats receiv-ing a pair of ovarian grafts 40-50 days after DMBA. Numbers in parentheses represent: Total number of tumors/number rats with tumors. Note the increase in tumor incidence in rats receiving ovarian grafts. Ovariectomy beyond 7 days after DMBA treatment failed to inhibit the tumor induction.

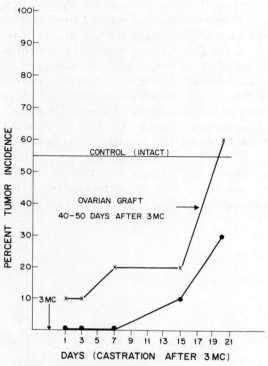

Figure 2

(●) Mammary tumor incidence in rats castrated on days 1, 3, 7, 15, and 21 after a single dose of 10 mg 3-MC; (✕) mammary tumor incidence in identical groups of castrated rats, except that they received a pair of ovarian grafts 40-50 days after 3-MC treatment. Note again the lack of effect of ovarian hormones to bring about an increase of tumor incidence if castration was done before 7 days after 3-MC treatment.

The data suggest that a suboptimal dose (10 mg) of either 3-MC or DMBA was unable to initiate carcinogenesis in the rat in the absence of ovarian hormones, because later treatment with ovarian hormones from a pair of functional ovarian grafts failed to produce any significant increase in the mammary tumor incidence. However, the excision of ovaries beyond 7 days after the oral dose of the carcinogen did not prevent or reduce significantly the incidence of mammary cancer in these rats. Castration 15 or 20 days after carcinogen treatment had no effect on tumor incidence.

Figure 3 summarizes the results in rats given an optimal dose of a potent carcinogen (DMBA). It appears that a 20-mg dose of DMBA is able to elicit few mammary cancers, even when ovarian hormones were absent at the time the carcinogen was administered. This finding, however, does not mean that DMBA may induce mammary cancer without the presence of ovarian hormones. The

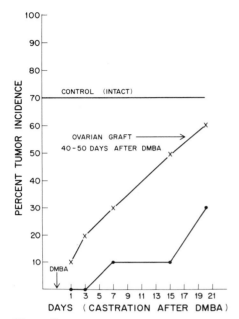

Figure 3
Similar experiments as shown in Fig. 1, except that a 20-mg dose of DMBA was given.

data simply suggest that a potent carcinogen may induce changes leading to neoplasia in mammary gland cells in which metabolic activities are declining as a result of the deprivation of ovarian hormones.

Even as potent a carcinogen as DMBA, however, does not induce any cancers in rats castrated for a long period of time, as shown in the following experiments. These experiments were done to examine the effect of administering the carcinogen at different intervals to castrated female rats. The experiment consisted of three groups of rats fed a single 20-mg dose of DMBA at 7, 15, and 30 days after castration. Each of these three groups had five subgroups receiving ovarian grafts on different days, as shown in Table 1.

The results demonstrate that when a 20-mg dose of DMBA was given to the rats 7 days after castration, 43% of the rats so treated developed mammary cancer, if ovaries were transplanted on the same day as DMBA treatment. Delayed grafting of the ovaries did not significantly influence the tumor incidence. The tumor incidence in the 15-day-old castrates was similar, and, as before, there was no effect on the development of mammary tumors if the interval between ovarian grafting and DMBA treatment was prolonged. In contrast, mammary tumors failed to develop in the 30-day-old castrates, either in the castrated control group or in those receiving a pair of functioning ovaries.

Table 1
Effects of Ovarian Grafts on Incidence of Breast Cancer in Castrated Female Rats Receiving a Single Dose of 20 mg DMBA

Groups	DMBA 7 days after castration			DMBA 15 days after castration			DMBA 30 days after castration
	number rats with tumors[a]	total number tumors	appearance of palpable tumors (days)	number rats with tumors[a]	total number tumors	appearance of palpable tumors (days)	number rats with tumors[a]
Control (castrated)	1/20 (5%)	1	95	0/20			0/20
Ovarian graft 0 days after DMBA	3/7 (43%)	9	43, 47, 50	3/7 (43%)	4	43, 45, 59	0/7
Ovarian graft 7 days after DMBA	2/6 (33%)[b]	4	43, 43	3/7 (43%)	3	34, 40, 72	0/7
Ovarian graft 15 days after DMBA	3/7 (43%)	7	43, 43, 49	2/7 (29%)	2	75, 85	0/7
Ovarian graft 30 days after DMBA	2/7 (29%)	2	92, 101	2/7 (29%)	2	84, 85	0/7

Reprinted, with permission, from Dao (1962).
[a]Number rats with tumors/number rats.
[b]One rat died 1 wk after feeding of DMBA.

These findings led to two conclusions: (1) In rats deprived of ovarian hormones, the incidence of mammary tumors in DMBA-treated rats decreased as the interval between castration and carcinogen treatment lengthened, and (2) the interval between DMBA treatment and subsequent ovarian transplantation had little or no effect on the mammary tumor incidence.

Castration and Induction of Mammary Cancer in Male Rats

Four groups of rats were used in this experiment. In group 1 are rats castrated on day 50 and given a single dose of 3-MC 1 day later. This group served as a control. In group 2, castration and transplantation were carried out simultaneously. These rats were given a single dose of 3-MC 25 days later. Rats in group 3 were castrated and given a single dose of 3-MC a day later. A pair of ovaries was transplanted into each of these 3-MC-treated, orchiectomized rats 25 days later. In group 4, a single 3-mg dose of 3-MC was given to mature male rats. Castration was perfomed 25 days later, and a pair of ovaries was grafted into each of these rats.

The results summarized in Table 2 disclose that castrated male rats bearing a pair of functional ovarian grafts and receiving a single dose of 3-MC have a tumor incidence of 53%. If, however, the carcinogen was given to the castrated rats first and ovaries were transplanted 30 days later, mammary tumor incidence was only 13%. In noncastrated male rats, administering the carcinogen prior to ovarian transplantation was similarly ineffective in inducing any mammary

Table 2
Induction of Mammary Cancer in Male Rats by 3-MC

Group[a]	Number rats	Number rats with palpable tumors	Total number tumors
Castrated males	10	1 (10%)	1
Castrated males + ovarian graft → 3-MC[b]	19	10 (53%)	11
Castrated males + 3-MC → ovarian grafts[c]	23	3 (13%)	3
Intact males + 3-MC → castration + ovarian grafts[d]	27	1 (3%)	1

Reprinted, with permission, from Dao (1962).
[a]3-MC, 30 mg, was given as a single dose in all groups.
[b]Castration and ovarian graft done simultaneously in 35-day-old males, 3-MC 25 days later.
[c]3-MC fed to 35-day-old male rats just being castrated; ovaries were transplanted to these rats 25 days later.
[d]3-MC fed to intact 35-day-old male rats; 25 days later castration and ovarian graft done simultaneously.

tumors. These experiments again demonstrated that the time that ovarian hormones are introduced is critical. The fact that grafting ovaries into castrated rats receiving the carcinogen prior to the transplantation failed to induce any mammary tumors is conclusive evidence that initiation of carcinogenesis cannot take place in the absence of ovarian hormones.

Induction of Mammary Tumors by Local Application of the Carcinogen

The objective of this experiment was to elucidate how an estrogen and a chemical carcinogen interact in initiating neoplastic transformation of mammary cells. We particularly wished to determine whether estrogen exerted its effect directly on the mammary epithelium.

The technique we developed was the induction of mammary tumors by direct application of a minute quantity of the carcinogen (Sinha and Dao 1972). In this experiment, a specific amount of DMBA, diethylstilbestrol (DES), or a combination of the two, was "dusted" over the surgically exposed right inguinal mammary gland. Since the amounts of DMBA and DES used for local application were very small, cholesterol powder was used as a vehicle. A suitable amount of DES or DMBA was weighed out and uniformly mixed with an appropriate amount of cholesterol powder, so that 2 mg of the final mixture contained the desired dose of DES or DMBA. In the control group, the rats received 2 mg cholesterol.

The results showed conclusively that an estrogen in combination with DMBA induced a significantly greater incidence of mammary cancer than did DMBA given alone. The optimal dose of DMBA for tumor induction appeared to be 1 mg. When 0.1 mg DMBA was applied locally to the mammary gland, the tumor incidence was only 14%. The addition of 50 μg DES at this dose level of DMBA again resulted in an increase in tumor incidence to 42% (Table 3).

Interestingly, the local application of DES in these rats did not have an effect on the endocrine system. Neither the organ weights nor the histologic appearance of the ovaries, uteri, and anterior pituitaries showed any differences between groups receiving DMBA alone or in combination with DES (Sinha and Dao 1972). Perhaps the most interesting and important observation of this study is the demonstration that an estrogen acts synergistically with a chemical carcinogen to induce mammary cancer in the rat.

Conclusions

The data from the above three experiments led to the following conclusions:

1. These experiments strongly suggest that neoplastic transformation of mammary gland cells cannot take place if ovarian hormones are absent.
2. The data suggest that there may be a quantitative balance between the carcinogenic hydrocarbons and the hormones governing the induction of mammary cancer in rats.

Table 3
Effect of Estrogen on Mammary Tumorigenesis by DMBA

Treatment	Number rats	Rats with tumors	%	Average latency period (days)	Average tumor size (cm)
1 mg DMBA	12	11	91.6	65	1.2
1 mg DMBA + 100 μg DES	12	12	100.0	54	2.5
0.5 mg DMBA	14	6	42.8	83	1.1
0.5 mg DMBA + 100 μg DES	12	8	66.6[a]	65	2.0
0.5 mg DMBA + 50 μg DES	5	3	60.0[b]	65	1.1
0.1 mg DMBA	7	1	14.0	112	0.7
0.1 mg DMBA + 100 μg DES	7	3	42.0[c]	92	1.4

Reprinted, with permission, from Sinha and Dao (1972).
All P values were calculated by the Student's t-test.
[a] $P < 0.01$ (from 0.5 mg DMBA).
[b] $P < 0.01$ (from 0.5 mg DMBA).
[c] $P < 0.1$ (from 0.1 mg DMBA).

3. Estrogen may act in synergism with a carcinogen, and in some way the hormone appears to enhance the interaction between the carcinogen and the target tissue in the initiation of carcinogenesis.

RELATIONSHIP BETWEEN PROLACTIN AND ESTROGEN IN MAMMARY TUMOR GROWTH

Mitogenic hormones are apparently effective in accelerating tumor growth. There is now abundant evidence that prolactin and estrogen are the hormones regulating the growth of mammary tumors. Several studies seem to suggest that prolactin can promote mammary tumor growth in the absence of ovarian hormones (Nagasawa and Yanai 1970; Meites 1972; Welsch 1972). Studies from our laboratory as described above and published earlier (Sinha and Dao 1972) suggest that estrogen influences tumor growth, apparently without increasing the release or secretion of prolactin from the pituitary in rats receiving a direct application of estrogen to the mammary gland.

The following experiments demonstrate the interaction between ovarian hormones and prolactin in the regulation of mammary tumor growth (Sinha et al. 1973). In these experiments, mammary tumors were induced in female Sprague-Dawley rats by a single intravenous injection of an emulsion containing 5 mg DMBA. When the tumors were palpable and measured 1.0 cm in diameter, electrolytic lesions were placed in the median eminence (ME) of the hypothalamus of a group of rats by using a stoelting stereotoxic instrument. Placement of electrolytic lesions in the tuber cinereum enhanced only prolactin release and secretion by the pituitary by inhibiting the pituitary inhibitory factor (PIF), whereas the secretion of all other pituitary hormones was inhibited. In another group of rats, ovariectomy was performed 3 weeks after ME lesion to determine whether mammary tumors regress over ovariectomy. In the third experiment, a group of ovariectomized, ME-lesioned rats with regressing mammary tumors received a pair of ovarian grafts to determine whether regrowth of the tumors occurs after ovarian transplantation.

The effects of the ME lesion, ovariectomy, and ovarian grafts on serum prolactin (determined by radioimmunoassay) were examined. Figure 4 shows that the plasma prolactin level in rats rose rapidly above that of the control after placement of ME lesions. Ovariectomy in intact female rats induced a

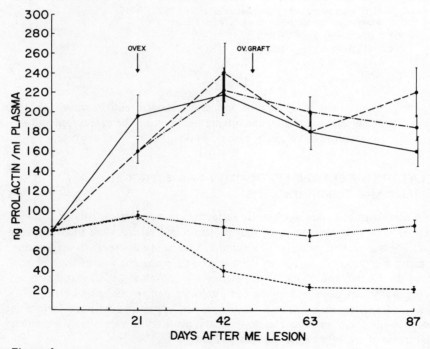

Figure 4

Effect of ME lesions, ovariectomy, and ovarian graft on plasma prolactin levels in rats. Each point on the graph represents the mean of prolactin values from 5 rats at different time intervals. (– · · · –) Control (intact); (– – – –) ovariectomy (ovex); (– · –) rats with ME lesions; (———) ovariectomized rats with ME lesions; (– –) ovariectomized rats with ME lesions and ovarian (Ov) grafts.

marked decrease in plasma prolactin levels, but it failed to alter the plasma prolactin levels in those rats having electrolytic lesions in the ME. Grafting a pair of ovaries in ovariectomized rats with ME lesions likewise had no effect on plasma prolactin levels. These results conclusively demonstrate that prolactin secretion and release are not affected by the presence or absence of ovarian hormones, once ME lesions are placed in these rats.

Figure 5 summarizes the results of the interaction of prolactin and ovarian hormones on mammary tumor growth. The data show that the placement of ME lesions greatly enhanced tumor growth, paralleling the rise of plasma prolactin. Ovariectomy brought about the regression of tumors in rats in the control group as well as in those with ME lesions, even though the plasma prolactin level remained high. Transplantation of a pair of ovaries in rats in the ME-lesioned, ovariectomized group caused the regressing tumors to resume a rapid growth rate.

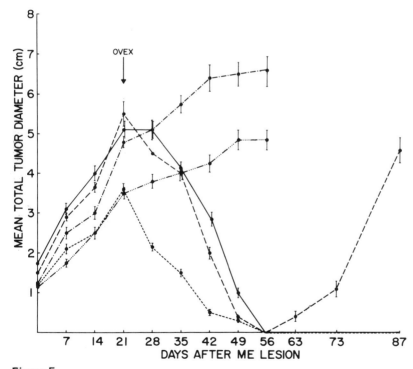

Figure 5
Effect of ME lesions, ovariectomy (ovex), and ovarian grafts in mammary tumor growth. The experimental groups and the animals are the same ones used for prolactin assays in Fig. 4. The curves are the measurements of tumor growth rats as expressed in mean total tumor diameter. The symbols are the same as in Fig. 4.

The above experiments clearly demonstrate that prolactin alone fails to sustain tumor growth in the absence of ovarian hormones. The study, however, does not clearly delineate whether the effect is due primarily to estrogen, to progesterone, or to both. Examination of the ovarian grafts removed at the end of the experiments revealed that all surviving grafts contained follicular cysts with well-developed thecal cells, but there was no active corpus luteum. The uterine weights decreased significantly after ovariectomy in both the control rats and the rats with ME lesions, but grafting a pair of ovaries in the ovariectomized, ME-lesioned rats led to a significant rise in uterine weights to values comparable to those in rats with ME lesions only (Sinha et al. 1973).

In a recent study, we repeated these experiments except that instead of transplanting a pair of ovaries to the ovariectomized, ME-lesioned rats, replacement therapy with either 1 μg estrone, 1 mg progesterone, or a combination of estrone (E_1) and progesterone was given daily to similar experimental groups, as shown in Figure 5. The objective of these experiments was to determine which ovarian hormone is of primary importance in stimulating mammary growth. The results are summarized in Figure 6. The data clearly show that whereas E_1 alone was capable of restoring the tumor growth in overiectomized, ME-lesioned rats, progesterone alone failed to induce tumor growth. Progesterone, however, appeared to have a synergistic effect when it was given together with an estrogen.

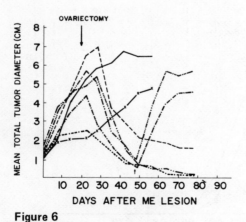

Figure 6
Effect of ME lesions, ovariectomy, and ME lesion + ovariectomy and ovarian hormones on mammary tumor growth. (· − − ·), ME lesion + ovariectomy; (− · · −) ovariectomy; (−−−) ME-ovariectomy + progesterone; (· − ·) ME lesion-ovariectomy + E_1; (− · · · −) ME lesion-ovariectomy + E_1 + progesterone; (————) ME lesion only; and (×) control. Note that the administration of E_1 alone on ME-lesioned, ovariectomized rats can restore the tumor growth rate.

Conclusion

Results from these in vivo experiments convincingly demonstrate the interaction between prolactin and estrogen in regulating the growth of mammary cancer, although the mechanism(s) by which estrogen enhances the action of prolactin have yet to be elucidated. Data clearly show that increased release of pituitary prolactin as a result of placement of electrolytic lesions in the ME of the hypothalamus greatly accelerates tumor growth, yet ovariectomy in these rats induced rapid tumor regression in spite of high plasma prolactin levels. Grafting a pair of ovaries or injection of E_1 alone in these ovariectomized, ME-lesioned rats caused resumption of tumor growth. These observations led to the conclusion that the prolactin stimulus to mammary tumor growth is dependent on the presence of estrogens. The most plausible explanation is that estrogen-responsive tissues, including carcinogen-induced mammary cancer, contain receptor protein binding units that bind estrogen specifically to initiate increased macromolecular synthesis and increased cell proliferative activity thereafter. Prolactin is not mitogenic (Oka and Topper 1972), but it may act indirectly as a mitogen by rendering the cells susceptible to mitogens such as estrogens.

IN VITRO STUDIES OF MAMMARY CARCINOGENESIS

Elucidation of the mode of action of hormones in the pathogenesis of mammary cancer requires a suitable in vitro system in which the role of individual principles can be evaluated.

In our laboratory, we have successfully cultured mammary tissues in a chemically defined medium for 6 and 12 days, the length of time that we believe is suitable for studies of carcinogenesis (Koyama et al. 1972). In that study, we found that insulin was essential for maintenance of the mammary explants in culture. Among the hormones investigated, progesterone was found to be most effective in stimulating the growth of the mammary explants, as measured by labeling and mitotic indexes. The combinations of insulin, estrogen, progesterone, and prolactin induced a maximal rise of labeling and mitotic indexes in the mammary explants in culture for 6-12 days. The increased DNA synthesis as a result of hormonal stimulation, however, did not alter the duration of DNA synthesis. The data suggest that the parallel increase in labeling and mitotic indexes was due to this increased number of cells entering DNA synthesis, rather than to a shortening of the S phase of the cycle (Koyama et al. 1972).

We then investigated the effect of DMBA on mammary glands grown in organ culture and subsequent tumorigenesis in them after transplantation into isologous hosts.

In the in vitro carcinogenesis study, a combination of four hormones, 5 μg/ml insulin, 0.001 μg/ml estradiol-17β, 1.0 μg/ml prolactin, and 1.0 mg/ml progesterone, was added to the base medium (Eagle's medium containing penicillin and 10% inactivated fetal bovine serum at 37°C for 9-12 days and fungizone,

0.5 μg/ml). This combination of hormones was chosen because it gave optimal maintenance and growth of the mammary gland in culture. DMBA (1.0 μg/ml medium, dissolved in absolute ethanol) was added to the medium, and the media containing hormones were changed (with or without DMBA) every third day of the culture. At the end of 9 days in culture, four pieces of mammary explants were transplanted into the interscapular fat pad of isologous hosts (Dao and Sinha 1972).

The results of four experiments are summarized in Table 4. In 16 surviving explants, 10 tumors developed. Of these 10, 8 were papillary adenocarcinomas and 2 were fibromas. All tumors were discernible grossly at autopsy (90 days after transplantation). Although abnormal changes, including squamous metaplasias and anaplasias, were seen frequently, in no instance did we observe the presence of hyperplastic alveolar nodules. Control explants (cultured in media containing hormones but not DMBA) transplanted to isologous hosts did not develop tumors.

Conclusion

The study demonstrated the in vitro transformation of mammary epithelial cells in culture by a chemical carcinogen. That the neoplastic transformation occurred in the mammary cells in vitro prior to transplantation into the isologous hosts was convincingly demonstrated by the presence of anaplastic changes in the mammary tissues after 9 days in culture. It was also unlikely that the explants, after a single treatment with DMBA and continued culture for 6 more days in a medium containing no carcinogen, still retained DMBA at transplantation.

We have since carried out experiments to determine whether there is a key hormone that is essential for the initiation of carcinogenesis. Our preliminary experiments show that the minimal hormonal combination that is necessary

Table 4
Induction of Mammary Tumors in Organ Culture

Dose of DMBA[a]	Number rats with surviving surviving transplants/total number rats	Number rats with tumors in surviving transplants
1 μg/ml × 3	3/5	2
1 μg/ml × 2	4/5	3[b]
1 μg/ml × 1	5/5	2
4 μg/ml × 1	4/5	3[b]

Reprinted, with permission, from Dao and Sinha (1972).

[a]Amount of DMBA/ml medium, which also contained combinations of 5 μg/ml insulin, 1 μg/ml prolactin, 0.001 μg/ml estradiol-17β, and 1 μg/ml progesterone. Total volume of medium/culture dish was 4 ml.

[b]One in each group was a fibroma.

for initiation of carcinogenesis is insulin, estrogen, and progesterone. The absence of prolactin does not inhibit initiation of carcinogenesis. It appears that one prerequisite to initiate neoplastic transformation by a chemical carcinogen is that the target cell must be in an active proliferative state.

REFERENCES

Bern, H. and S. Nandi. 1961. Recent studies of the hormonal influence in mouse mammary tumorigenesis. *Prog. Exp. Tumor Res.* 2:90.

Cutts, J.H. and R.L. Noble. 1964. Estrogen-induced mammary tumors in the rat. I. Induction and behavior of tumors. *Cancer Res.* 24:1116.

Dao, T.L. 1962. The role of ovarian hormones in initiating the induction of mammary cancer in rats by polynuclear hydrocarbons. *Cancer Res.* 22: 973.

————. 1964. Carcinogenesis of mammary gland in rat. *Prog. Exp. Tumor Res.* 5:157.

Dao, T.L. and J. Sunderland. 1959. Mammary carcinogenesis by 3-methylcholanthrene. I. Hormonal aspects in tumor induction and growth. *J. Natl. Cancer Inst.* 23:567.

Dao, T.L. and D. Sinha. 1972. Mammary adenocarcinoma induced in organ culture. *J. Natl. Cancer Inst.* 49:591.

————. 1975. Effect of carcinogen on pituitary prolactin release and synthesis. *Proc. Am. Assoc. Cancer Res.* 16:28 (#112).

Huggins, C., G. Briziarelli, and H. Sutton, Jr. 1959. Rapid induction of mammary carcinoma in the rat and the influence of hormones on the tumors. *J. Exp. Med.* 109:25.

Koyama, H., D. Sinha, and T.L. Dao. 1972. Effects of hormones and 7,12-dimethylbenz(a)anthracene on rat mammary tissue grown in organ culture. *J. Natl. Cancer Inst.* 48:1671.

Meites, J. 1972. The relation of estrogen and prolactin to mammary tumorigenesis in the rat. In *Estrogen target tissues and neoplasia* (ed. T.L. Dao), p. 275. University of Chicago Press, Chicago.

Nagasawa, H. and R. Yanai. 1970. Effect of prolactin or growth hormone on growth of carcinogen-induced mammary tumors of adreno-ovariectomized rats. *Int. J. Cancer* 6:488.

Oka, T. and Y.J. Topper. 1972. Is prolactin mitogenic for mammary epithelium? *Proc. Natl. Acad. Sci.* 69:1093.

Sinha, D. and T.L. Dao. 1972. Estrogen and induction of mammary cancer. In *Estrogen target tissues and neoplasia* (ed. T.L. Dao), p. 307. University of Chicago Press, Chicago.

Sinha, D., D. Cooper, and T.L. Dao. 1973. The nature of estrogen and prolactin effect on mammary tumorigenesis. *Cancer Res.* 33:411.

Welsch, C.W. 1972. Effects of brain lesions on mammary tumorigenesis. In *Estrogen target tissues and neoplasia* (ed. T.L. Dao), p. 317. University of Chicago Press, Chicago.

Yang, N.C., A.J. Castro, M. Lewis, and T.W. Wong. 1961. Polycyclic aromatic hydrocarbons, steroids and carcinogenesis. *Science* 134:386.

COMMENTS

HENDERSON: In Dr. Dao's presentation on ovarian steroids, he made reference to the fact that progesterone, if anything, seems to enhance the effect of estrogen. Is it thus valid to conclude that for breast tissue progesterone does not have an antiestrogen effect?

DAO: Brian [Henderson], I think in the mammary tumor systems that we have been studying for many years that progesterone doesn't play an essential role in terms of the induction of mammary tumors. However, progesterone and estrogen do have some synergistic effect in promoting tumor growth. In an in vitro study, we found progesterone to be one of the most effective mitogenic agents that induces an increase in the synthesis of DNA. We have a paper that was published on that study (Koyama et al. 1972).

But there is no convincing evidence in humans that progesterone inhibits the action of estrogens on tumor growth.

WELSCH: I would like to comment on this, Brian. We have an array of experimental animal models to study the question you are asking, i.e., does progesterone enhance the mammary tumorigenic effect of estrogen? It depends upon which experimental model you use. If you use the GR mouse model, for example, it is unequivocal that estrogen plus progesterone is better than either hormone alone in stimulating growth of this particular neoplasm. There are other models in which estrogen alone is more effective; the addition of progesterone produces no effect whatsoever. There are other models in which progesterone alone is better than estrogen alone.

HENDERSON: But are there models where progesterone plus estrogen is less effective than estrogen alone?

WELSCH: Yes. The classical example of that is the work done by Huggins et al. (1962). They observed that rats bearing either DMBA- or 3-MC-induced mammary tumors, when treated with estrogen plus progesterone, showed an inhibition of mammary tumor growth.

DAO: It was a large dose.

WELSCH: Yes; it was 20 μg estrogen and 4 mg progesterone.

MOON: Large doses of estrogen and physiological doses of progesterone inhibit DMBA-induced mammary tumorigenesis. If one gives a large dose of estrogen, tumorigenesis is inhibited. Thus, one may increase the latency of tumor appearance with estrogen alone, but the tumor incidence is not

of tumor appearance with estrogen alone, but the tumor incidence is not reduced. However, if you administer progesterone with estrogen, a reduction in incidence is seen. On the other hand, if one gives progesterone alone, depending upon when it is applied, tumor enhancement occurs. So I think you have to consider what model is used, what time the hormone manipulations are applied, and what is being measured.

COLE: But, if you have to consider the model, which means, as far as I understand it, the strain of the animal that you are using, what relevance could any of this have to people? If every different strain gives you a different observation, how are we going to pick which one we should generalize to people?

SEGALOFF: The model includes the stimulus as well as the strain.

COLE: What are the principles emerging from it?

DAO: Brian's question is whether progesterone can have an antagonist effect on estrogen. I say there is no model to demonstrate this effect, and I am right. There is no model to demonstrate it. But I think that Phil's [Cole] question will take too long a time to resolve here. I think the model has great significance to human studies.

SIRBASKU: There is an important model—a kidney tumor that is published, beginning in about 1933 and running through 1959. The best monograph is by Hadley Kirkman (Kirkman 1959) at Stanford. He showed that if you administer estrogen to Syrian hamsters, they all get clear-cell carcinomas of the kidney tubule. You can completely block carcinogenesis by the simultaneous administration of progesterone. Furthermore, once the tumors have developed and you transplant them to estrogen-treated animals, you can inhibit the growth of the tumor with progesterone at an equal dose to estrogen. That is the model. But that one completely suppresses carcinogenesis. It is the only one that I know of that has that dramatic effect.

HENDERSON: My question is: Is there experimental evidence to support Korenman's hypothesis that progesterone is an antiestrogen on breast tissue mitogenesis?

WELSCH: I would like to respond to that. In experimental murine mammary tumorigenesis, one can administer estrogens to a wide variety of strains of mice and markedly enhance mammary tumorigenesis. Progesterone, on the other hand, is different. Fewer strains of mice respond to the administration of progesterone. Oral contraceptives, which usually contain progesterone and an estrogen, are less effective in enhancing mouse mammary tumorigenesis than is estrogen alone. This suggests that the addition of progesterone to the hormonal milieu is inhibitory to this tumorigenic process.

ZUMOFF: It is not progesterone in any of those pills.

WELSCH: Well, progestational compounds.

ZUMOFF: Don't slide over that distinction. These are abnormal compounds and each has its own spectrum of activity.

MOON: The same thing occurs in the rat with norgesterol as with progesterone.

WELSCH: But estrogen appears to be far more stimulatory than are oral contraceptives in enhancing murine mammary tumorigenesis.

SEGALOFF: As long as you are talking about models, though, remember that the dog is exactly backwards.

WELSCH: Correct! The dog mammary tumor model responds dramatically to progesterone, not to estrogen.

References

Huggins, C., R.C. Moon, and S. Morii. 1962. Extinction of experimental mammary cancer. I. Estradiol 17-β and progesterone. *Proc. Natl. Acad. Sci.* 48:379.
Kirkman, H. 1959. Estrogen-induced tumor of the kidney in the Syrian hamster. *Natl. Cancer Inst. Monogr.* 1:1.
Koyama, H., D. Sinha, and T.L. Dao. 1972. Effect of hormones and 7,12-dimethylbenzanthracene on rat mammary tissue grown in organ culture. *J. Natl. Cancer Inst.* 48:1671.

Prolactin and Growth Hormone in the Development, Progression, and Growth of Murine Mammary Tumors

CLIFFORD W. WELSCH
Department of Anatomy
Michigan State University
East Lansing, Michigan 48824

An extensive amount of information is available that correlates the level of ovarian steroids, i.e., estrogen or progesterone with the genesis, progression, and growth of murine mammary tumors. In comparison, considerably less data are available relating the role of prolactin and growth hormone (GH), two anterior pituitary peptides, to this neoplastic process. Thus, the purpose of this paper is to examine the role of these peptides in the development and growth of spontaneous rodent mammary tumors; the growth of transplantable rodent mammary tumors; and the development and growth of carcinogen-induced rat mammary tumors.

SPONTANEOUS RODENT MAMMARY TUMORS

It is unequivocal that anterior pituitary hormones are critical, perhaps essential, for the genesis of spontaneous murine mammary tumors, for hypophysectomized rodents do not develop tumors of the mammary gland (Moon et al. 1951). Since early ovariectomy or ovariectomy-adrenalectomy also sharply reduces or totally prevents mammary tumorigenesis in rodents (Durbin et al. 1966; Richardson 1967), it seems logical to assume that a lack of gonadotropin secretion is responsible for the absence of mammary tumors in hypophysectomized rodents. Interest in the mammary tumorigenic potential of anterior pituitary peptides other than the gonadotropins was generated in 1931 by Evans and Simpson, who studied the action of prolonged administration of GH to intact male and female Long-Evans rats. Mammary tumors appeared in 10/16 female rats treated over a 16-month period. No mammary tumors were observed in similarly treated male rats. In 1950, Moon et al. reported that fibroadenomas of the mammary gland occurred more frequently, were larger, and were often multiple in intact female Long-Evans rats treated six times weekly with an improved purified preparation of GH. However, long, continued administration of GH to hypophysectomized adult Long-Evans rats, though producing continuous body growth, did not produce the numerous mammary tumors that developed in intact rats that were similarly treated (Moon et al. 1951).

In the 1950s, interest was focused more on prolactin, rather than GH, as potentially the key anterior pituitary peptide in the genesis of spontaneous murine mammary tumors. This shift in interest was derived primarily from the studies of Loeb and Kirtz (1939) and Mühlbock, Boot, and colleagues (1959), who demonstrated that the grafting of multiple pituitary isografts to a variety of strains of female mice markedly increased the incidence of mammary tumors in that species. Subsequently, we reported that grafting of pituitaries to female Sprague-Dawley rats also sharply increased the incidence of spontaneous mammary tumors (Welsch et al. 1970a) (Table 1). In 1972, Yanai and Nagasawa demonstrated that the transplantation of multiple pituitaries to mature multiparous C3H/He mice deficient in (or lacking) ovarian steroids (adrenalectomized-ovariectomized) also resulted in increased incidence of mammary tumors when compared to mice that were only adrenalectomized-ovariectomized. From the pioneering studies of Desclin (1950) and Everett (1954), it is now well established that the transplanted rodent pituitary, free from direct hypothalamic influence, secretes increased amounts of prolactin and reduced secretion of all other anterior pituitary hormones. Additional support for the concept that prolactin is an important pituitary hormone in rodent spontaneous mammary gland tumorigenesis comes from the report of Boot et al. (1962), who showed that daily administrations of prolactin to hybrid female mice ($O_{20} \times$ DBA) ($O_{20} \times$ IF) increased the incidence of mammary tumors; from the study of Lacassagne and Duplan (1959), who showed that the administration of reserpine, a potent stimulator of prolactin secretion, to female C3H mice increased mammary tumor incidence, and from the reports of Bruni and Montemurro (1971) and our laboratory (Welsch et al. 1970b) (Table 2) showing that lesions in the hypothalamus that increase prolactin secretion (female C3D2 F_1 mice and female Sprague-Dawley rats, respectively) result in increased incidence of mammary tumors.

Table 1
Effects of Multiple Pituitary Homografts on Development of Mammary Tumors in Female Sprague-Dawley Rats

Treatment[a]	Total number rats	Number and % rats with tumors[b]
Controls, nulliparous	12	1/12 (8%)
Pituitary grafts, nulliparous	12	9/12 (75%)
Controls, multiparous	16	3/16 (19%)
Pituitary grafts, multiparous	13	8/13 (61%)

Data from Welsch et al. (1970a).

[a]Each noncontrol nulliparous and multiparous rat was grafted beneath the kidney capsule and subcutaneously with 7 pituitaries at 2 and 8 months of age, respectively, prior to the onset of palpable mammary tumors. All rats were sacrificed 9 months after grafting.

[b]$P < 0.001$.

Table 2
Effects of Induced Hypothalamic Lesions (ME) on Development of Mammary Tumors in Female Sprague-Dawley Rats

Treatment[a]	Total number rats	Serum prolactin levels (ng/ml)[b]	Number and % rats with tumors[b]	Total number tumors[b]
Controls, sham lesion	21	50.9 ± 9.6	4 (19%)	4
Hypothalamic lesions	23	179.8 ± 23.9	12 (52%)	20

Data from Welsch et al. (1970b).
[a] All rats were sacrificed 25 wk after placement of hypothalamic lesions or sham lesions.
[b] $P < 0.001$.

With the advent of drugs that suppress the secretion of prolactin, e.g., the ergot alkaloids and the ergoline derivatives (Brooks and Welsch 1974), further support for a critical role for this peptide in spontaneous murine mammary tumorigenesis has been provided. For example, 2-bromo-α-ergocryptine (CB-154) or bromotriphenylethylene induced inhibition of prolactin secretion in pituitary isograft-bearing female C3H/He mice and female C3Hf mice, respectively, results in a sharp reduction in incidence of mammary tumors (Yanai and Nagasawa 1972; Drasdowsky et al. 1980). Furthermore, the reduction of prolactin secretion below basal levels in female C3H/HeJ mice by chronic administration of CB-154 or the ergoline derivative 6-methyl-8-β-ergoline acetonitrile, either sharply suppressed the incidence of spontaneously developing mammary tumors (Welsch et al. 1974) or virtually totally blocked this neoplastic process (Welsch and Gribler 1973) (Table 3). It appears, therefore, that

Table 3
Effect of Chronic Suppression of Prolactin Secretion by Daily Administration of 2-Bromo-α-ergocryptine (CB-154) on the Development of Mammary Tumors in Female C3H/HeJ Mice

Treatment[a]	Total number of mice	Number and % mice with tumors[b]
Controls, nulliparous	90	24/90 (24%)
CB-154-treated, nulliparous	90	1/90 (1%)
Controls, multiparous	70	36/70 (51%)
CB-154-treated, multiparous	70	9/70 (13%)

Data from Welsch and Gribler (1973).
[a] Daily administration of CB-154 was begun at 2 months of age for nulliparous mice and 7 months of age for multiparous mice. Nulliparous mice were sacrificed at 24 months of age, multiparous mice were sacrificed at 19 months of age.
[b] $P < 0.001$.

not only may prolactin be an important hormonal stimulant of mammary tumorigenesis but it may also be an essential hormone for neoplastic transformation of the mouse mammary gland. The genesis of spontaneous rodent mammary tumors is profoundly enhanced by increased secretory levels of prolactin; the growth of established spontaneous mammary tumors in the rat (but not generally in the mouse) also appears to be controlled by this hormone, as chronic ergot alkaloid treatment of female Sprague-Dawley rats bearing these tumors causes significant tumor regression (Quadri and Meites 1971). In the aforementioned studies, essentially all of the rat mammary tumors were histopathologically benign fibroadenomas, whereas, in contrast, virtually all the mouse mammary tumors were adenocarcinomas.

TRANSPLANTABLE RODENT MAMMARY TUMORS

In the 1930s, a number of studies began to emerge demonstrating that a variety of rodent mammary tumors could be successfully transplanted to recipients of the same strain. Furthermore, these neoplasms usually retained their responsiveness to the secretory activity of the endocrine system. In 1936, Heiman and Krehbiel reported that the administration of estrogen to castrated male and female white rats bearing a transplantable mammary fibroadenoma resulted in little or no alteration of growth of the transplant. However, upon administration of a crude GH preparation with the ovarian steroid, a sharp increase in growth of the transplanted mammary tumor was observed. Subsequently, it was reported by Millar and Noble (1954) that crude beef and sheep pituitary preparations stimulated growth of a transplantable mammary fibroadenoma in intact female Sprague-Dawley rats; a GH preparation, however, did not alter the growth or morphology of the transplanted neoplasm.

Mammary fibroadenomas can be transplanted successfully to hypophysectomized rats, although these neoplasms, at least initially, grow poorly when grafted to such animals. It was reported by Huggins et al. (1956a) that growth of these transplanted neoplasms in the hypophysectomized Sprague-Dawley rat was not stimulated by estrone (E_1), progesterone, prolactin, or GH administered separately. The administration of E_1 and progesterone, in combination, moderately stimulated growth, whereas supplementing these steroids with GH restores the growth rate of the tumors to that occurring in intact female rats. Prolactin was not effective as a replacement for GH in the steroid-peptide hormonal combination. In a similar study in the same laboratory, hypophysectomized Sprague-Dawley rats bearing a transplantable mammary fibroadenoma were treated with E_1 and progesterone. Moderate tumor growth was observed in these animals. Growth of the tumors was accelerated, however, by the additional administration of prolactin or GH (Huggins et al. 1956b). None of the pituitary peptides, administered separately, stimulated the growth of the tumor. The steroid hormones exerted a greater influence on growth of the tumor than the peptide hormones; synergism between these two classes of hormones, however, was most apparent.

In the early 1960s, reports by Kim, Clifton, and Furth (Kim and Furth 1960a,b,c; Kim et al. 1960) provided evidence that hormones secreted by a grafted rat pituitary tumor would markedly stimulate growth of a variety of transplantable rat mammary tumors. The transplantable pituitary tumors (MtT) used in these studies secrete large amounts of prolactin, GH, and variable amounts of adrenocorticotropin (ACTH); these neoplasms were maintained in female Wistar-Furth rats. The transplantable mammary tumors used in these studies were originally induced by irradiation or polycyclic hydrocarbon treatment of Wistar-Furth rats (adenocarcinomas) or were derived from spontaneously developing mammary tumors in this strain of rat (fibroadenomas). It is clear from these studies that the secretory products of MtT pituitary tumor are efficacious growth stimulators of these transplantable mammary tumors not only in intact female rats but also in male rats, ovariectomized rats, or hypophysectomized rats (Kim et al. 1960). These studies were in effect the first to direct attention actively toward pituitary hormones (in particular prolactin and GH), as opposed to ovarian steroids, as the key hormones in this oncogenic process.

In the mid 1960s, studies by MacLeod and colleagues (MacLeod et al. 1964) drew attention to the synergistic effect of anterior pituitary and steroid hormones for growth of transplantable rat mammary tumors. Using a transplantable mammary tumor (MTW9), a carcinoma obtained from Furth and colleagues, and a transplantable rat pituitary tumor (MtTW5) or pituitary homografts as sources of pituitary hormones, they observed a lack of growth of MTW9 in ovariectomized pituitary-tumor-bearing Wistar-Furth rats unless these rats were injected with estrogen and progesterone. Homografts of pituitary glands transplanted beneath the kidney capsule in intact and hypophysectomized Wistar-Furth rats (without MtTW5) also stimulated the growth of MTW9. However, ovariectomy of rats bearing pituitary homografts inhibited mammary tumor growth and the administration of estrogen and progesterone to ovariectomized pituitary-homograft-bearing rats promoted MTW9 growth. MtTW5 secretes large amounts of prolactin and GH, whereas pituitary homografts secrete only large amounts of prolactin, thus implicating prolactin rather than GH as the key pituitary peptide in these growth processes.

That prolactin is the key pituitary peptide for growth stimulation of transplantable rat mammary tumors is also supported by the studies of Bogden et al. (1974) and Harada (1976). Treatment of female Fischer-344 rats bearing the transplantable mammary carcinoma 13762-MT with perphenazine sharply increased growth of the transplanted mammary tumor and concurrently markedly increased serum prolactin levels. The 13762-MT transplantable mammary tumor was originally induced in Fischer rats by the administration of polycyclic hydrocarbons. Treatment of hypophysectomized female Sprague-Dawley rats bearing a polycyclic-hydrocarbon-induced transplantable mammary carcinoma (MRMT-1) with prolactin or transplantation of pituitary homografts to these animals resulted in a reactivation of mammary tumor growth and metastasis.

The authors concluded that 13762-MT and MRMT-1 are prolactin-dependent mammary carcinomas.

Although the aforementioned studies provide evidence that prolactin and perhaps GH are important hormones for stimulating growth of a variety of transplantable rat mammary tumors, it should be pointed out that not all transplanted rat mammary tumors are stimulated by increased secretion of these peptides. Indeed, there are two transplantable rat mammary tumors (R3230AC and 35-MT) whose growth appears to be inhibited by increasing prolactin secretion. Elevation of blood prolactin levels by grafting of pituitary tumors (MtTF4) (Hilf et al. 1967) or by injection of perphenazine and its derivatives (Hilf et al. 1971; Bogden et al. 1974) in these mammary-tumor-bearing rats inhibited growth of these transplanted neoplasms. The R3230AC is a transplantable carcinoma originally induced by polycyclic hydrocarbons and was maintained in female Fischer rats. The 35-MT is a carcinomatous subline of the Huggins transplantable fibroadenoma and was maintained in female Sprague-Dawley rats. MtTF4 is a transplantable pituitary tumor that unlike MtTW5 secretes large amounts of ACTH in addition to prolactin and GH. The mechanism by which perphenazine treatments and pituitary tumor grafting causes inhibition of mammary tumor growth in these studies is not clear. It is conceivable that the hormonal milieu, caused by these treatments, induced secretory activity of the tumor cells, a physiological phenomenon that could oppose tumor cell proliferation. Indeed, the transplantable 13762-MT carcinoma, whose growth was stimulated by perphenazine treatment (Bogden et al. 1974) (enhanced secretion of only prolactin), showed growth inhibition by coimplantation of MtTF4 (secretes large amounts of prolactin, GH, and ACTH) (Segaloff 1966). Histological examination of the 13762-MT tumor cells in MtTF-4 bearing hosts indicated secretory activity.

Transplantable mouse mammary tumors have received little attention from endocrinologists, as most advanced (palpable) mouse mammary tumors are not responsive to pituitary and ovarian hormones. One exception to this generalization is the GR mouse mammary tumor. These neoplasms are induced by the chronic administration of estrogen and progesterone or repeated pregnancies. The primary neoplasms appear to be estrogen, progesterone, and prolactin responsive (Briand et al. 1977; Welsch et al. 1979a) and can be transplanted to syngeneic hosts. The growth of the transplanted tumor is suppressed after ovariectomy and is stimulated in intact or ovariectomized hosts by the administration of estrogen and progesterone, or by the administration of prolactin (Briand et al. 1977). This is an interesting neoplasm in that it appears that prolactin can stimulate growth of these tumors in ovariectomized mice (Briand et al. 1977) and that estrogen-progesterone may be a growth stimulant in hypophysectomized mice (Sluyser and Van Nie 1974).

The hormonal responsiveness of preneoplastic mouse mammary-nodule transplant lines (Balb/c hosts) has been reported by Medina (1977). Although growth of a number of these lines was inhibited by ovariectomy or an estrogen antagonist (nafoxidine), chronic prolactin suppression by CB-154 administration did not effect the growth rate of these preneoplasias. In contrast, Singh et al. (1972) reported that the chronic administration of ergocornine to Balb/c mice bearing a preneoplastic mammary nodule line resulted in suppression of nodule growth. Ergocornine, like CB-154, is an effective inhibitor of prolactin secretion but, unlike CB-154, causes a general insalubrious condition in rodents when administered for prolonged periods of time (Cassell et al. 1971).

CARCINOGEN-INDUCED RAT MAMMARY TUMORS

Carcinogen-induced mammary tumors in the rat (almost invariably adeno-carcinomas) have been extensively studied in recent years and their dependency on pituitary hormones has been clearly established. In general, most treatments that increase blood levels of prolactin in female rats bearing carcinogen-induced mammary tumors cause an increase in growth of these tumors. For example, adrenalectomy, pregnancy, pseudopregnancy, pituitary homografts, pituitary tumors, and hypothalamic lesions all cause an increase in blood prolactin levels and also stimulate carcinogen-induced mammary tumor growth (Dao and Sunderland 1959; Kim and Furth 1960b,c; Welsch et al. 1969; Chen et al. 1976). Certain neuroendocrine-influencing drugs that sharply increase prolactin secretion in rodents, e.g., reserpine, perphenazine, and haloperidol, also marked-ly increased growth of these neoplasms (Pearson et al. 1969; Welsch and Meites 1970; Quadri et al. 1973a). Drugs that decrease prolactin secretion, e.g., certain ergot alkaloids, cyclic imide derivatives, lysergic acid, ergoline derivatives, L-dopa, and pargyline, also caused a regression of carcinogen-induced mammary carcinomas (Fig. 1) (Mückter et al. 1970; Welsch et al. 1973; Quadri et al. 1973b; Sweeney et al. 1975).

Whether or not GH can stimulate growth of carcinogen-induced rat mammary carcinomas is not totally clear at this time. For example, median eminence (ME) hypothalamic lesions in female Sprague-Dawley rats suppress the secretion of GH and increase prolactin secretion; such lesions markedly stimulate growth of these neoplasms (Welsch et al. 1969). The administration of GH to carcino-gen-induced mammary-tumor-bearing female Sprague-Dawley rats has been reported to have no effect (Pearson et al. 1969; Nagasawa and Yanai 1970) or a slight but significant stimulatory effect (albeit less than prolactin) on growth of these tumors (Li and Yang 1974).

Although growth of carcinogen-induced rat mammary carcinomas is un-doubtedly regulated by prolactin, it appears that ovarian steroids are also impor-tant in these growth processes. Ovariectomy of Sprague-Dawley rats bearing this neoplasm resulted in a prompt regression of these tumors. Concurrent enhancement of prolactin secretion by placement of ME hypothalamic lesions in these animals prevented this regression; tumor growth actually was stimulated by this experimental procedure (Welsch et al. 1969). This enhanced mammary tumor growth, however, did not persist for long periods unless ovaries were reimplanted into these animals (Sinha et al. 1973). Daily injections of prolactin

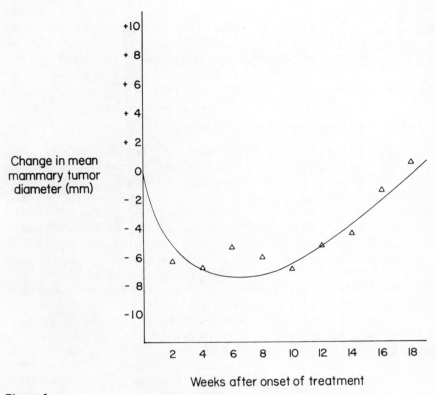

Figure 1
Effect of CB-154 treatment on growth of DMBA-induced mammary tumors in 20 female Sprague-Dawley rats.

into ovariectomized-adrenalectomized Sprague-Dawley rats bearing these tumors resulted in an initial increased growth of these neoplasms (Pearson et al. 1969; Nagasawa and Yanai 1970). These results suggest that prolactin can stimulate growth of carcinogen-induced rat mammary tumors in animals lacking ovarian steroids, but for persistent growth of these tumors, despite high blood prolactin, ovarian hormones may be essential.

In the induction of mammary carcinomas in rats by chemical carcinogens, pituitary and ovarian hormones are also very important. We have shown that ovariectomy of Sprague-Dawley rats 30 days prior to carcinogen treatment prevented the occurrence of the induced tumors despite high blood levels of prolactin (Welsch et al. 1968). If ovariectomy of Sprague-Dawley rats was performed only 7 days prior to carcinogen treatment, concurrent treatment with prolactin and GH increased mammary tumor incidence above that observed in ovariectomized controls (Talwalker et al. 1964). We have demonstrated that suppression of prolactin secretion prior to, during, or shortly after carcinogen treatment also sharply reduced mammary tumor incidence in female Sprague-Dawley and Lewis rats (Figs. 2 and 3) (Welsch et al. 1979b; Welsch et al. 1980). It appears, therefore, that ovarian hormones and prolactin are critical in the chemical transformation of the epithelium of the rat mammary gland. GH may

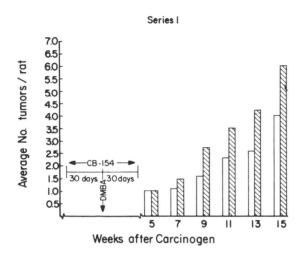

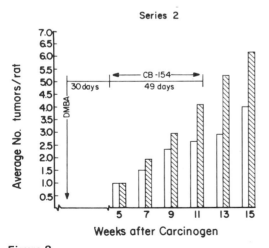

Figure 2
Effect of CB-154 treatment on DMBA-induced mammary tumorigenesis in female Sprague-Dawley rats (30 rats/group). Number of mammary tumors, controls (▨) vs CB-154 (□) treatment ($P < 0.05$).

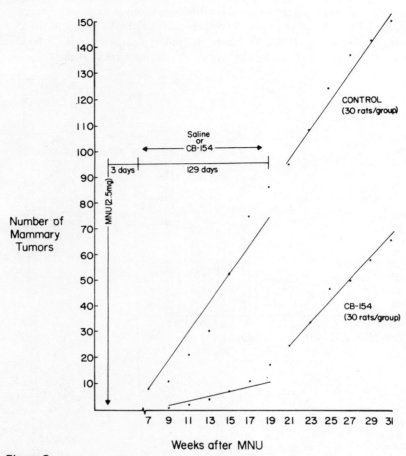

Figure 3
Effect of CB-154 treatment on N-methyl-N-nitrosourea (MNU)- induced mammary tumorigenesis in female Sprague-Dawley rats (30 rats/group). Number of mammary tumors, controls vs CB-154 treatment ($P < 0.005$). (Data from Welsch et al. 1980.)

also be important in this process, however, as Young (1961) has demonstrated the successful chemical induction of mammary carcinomas in hypophysectomized female Sprague-Dawley rats that were chronically treated with estrogen, progesterone, and large doses of GH. Carcinogen-treated hypophysectomized female rats that are not treated with hormones do not develop mammary carcinomas (Moon et al. 1952; Noble and Walters 1954; Huggins and Briziarelli 1959).

It is paradoxical that both a low and a high rate of prolactin secretion prior to and during carcinogen treatment results in a reduction of incidence of mammary carcinomas. When prolactin secretion in female Sprague-Dawley rats was increased by ME hypothalamic lesions, pituitary homografts, or reserpine prior to carcinogen treatment, mammary tumor incidence was sharply reduced (Welsch et al. 1968; Welsch et al. 1969; Welsch and Meites 1970). Furthermore, lactation at the time of carcinogen treatment and lactation in mammary-tumor-bearing rats resulted in a decreased incidence and diminution of growth, respectively, of these mammary carcinomas (Dao et al. 1960). The inhibitory effect of prolactin in this neoplastic process may be a function of prolactin-induced cellular differentiation (as opposed to proliferation), a phenomenon that could suppress chemical carcinogenesis (initiation) and tumor growth (promotion).

The effect of hormones on growth of carcinogen-induced rat mammary carcinomas in vitro has been studied by a number of laboratories. In 1972, we first demonstrated that the addition of prolactin to media containing organ cultures of rat mammary carcinomas resulted in a striking increase in DNA synthesis of these explants (Welsch and Rivera 1972). This effect of prolactin subsequently was confirmed and extended by a number of laboratories (Lewis and Hallowes 1974; Pasteels et al. 1976; Aspegren and Trope 1977). Prolactin also appears to increase protein synthesis of organ cultures of carcinogen-induced rat mammary carcinomas, an effect that is enhanced by the concurrent addition of estrogen to the culture media (Lee et al. 1975). The effects of the addition of GH to organ cultures of carcinogen-induced rat mammary carcinomas have also been reported (Iturri and Welsch 1976) (Table 4). Generally, a mild DNA synthetic stimulatory effect of this peptide has been observed, although this effect appears quantitatively to be considerably less than that obtained with prolactin. In contrast to organ cultures, cell cultures of carcinogen-induced rat mammary carcinomas have been examined seldom and have yielded conflicting results. In 1976, Chan et al. reported that prolactin alone or estrogen alone did not enhance growth of monolayers of carcinogen-induced rat mammary carcinomas. Prolactin, however, could reverse the growth-inhibitory action of high levels of estradiol. On the other hand, Hallowes et al. (1977) and Rudland et al. (1977) reported that prolactin alone was capable of promoting

Table 4
Effect of Ovine Prolactin and Ovine GH on DNA Synthesis of 5-Day Organ Cultures of DMBA-induced Rat Mammary Tumors

Treatment	[^{3}H]Thymidine/μg DNA[a] (cpm)
Control	108 ± 42
GH, 5 μg/ml	188 ± 46
Prolactin, 5 μg/ml	265 ± 54[b]

Data from Iturri and Welsch (1976).
[a] Mean ± S.E. of 4 mammary tumors.
[b] $P < 0.05$.

DNA synthesis of cell cultures of carcinogen-induced rat mammary carcinomas. In general, the effect of these hormones on growth processes (DNA synthesis) in vitro appears to reflect what is observed in vivo and provides substantial evidence that the primary action of these pituitary peptides is at the site of the mammary tissue. It is conceivable, however, that these peptides (prolactin and GH) may also act, at least in part, by enhancing the production and secretion of tissue growth factors as has been postulated for estrogenic hormones (Sirbasku and Benson 1979).

SUMMARY

1. Prolactin is an important hormone in both the initiating and promoting phases of murine mammary tumorigenesis.
2. Under certain endocrinic conditions, prolactin can be a potent growth stimulant to a number of murine mammary tumors; under other endocrinic conditions this pituitary peptide may inhibit mammary tumor growth processes.
3. Under certain conditions, prolactin can stimulate growth of murine mammary tumors in animals that are deficient (perhaps lacking?) ovarian steroids (ovariectomized-adrenalectomized), although a growth synergism between these two classes of hormones is most often encountered.
4. In rodents, prolactin exerts its effect, at least in part, by acting directly on the mammae and (or) indirectly via its luteotropic effect on the ovary.
5. GH appears to be less important than prolactin in murine mammary tumorigenesis; its role in this oncogenic process remains to be determined.

ACKNOWLEDGMENTS

Sincere appreciation is extended to the U.S. National Cancer Institute and the American Cancer Society for the continuous support of the research activities of the author's laboratory.

REFERENCES

Aspegren, K. and C. Trope. 1977. In vitro effects of prolactin and hydrocortisone on 7,12-DMBA-induced mammary tumour and virus-induced sarcoma in the rat. *Acta Pathol. Microbiol. Scand.* 85:57.

Bogden, A.E., D.J. Taylor, E.Y.H. Kuo, M.M. Mason, and A. Speropoulos. 1974. The effect of perphenazine-induced serum prolactin response on estrogen-primed mammary tumor-host systems, 13762 and R-35 mammary adenocarcinomas. *Cancer Res.* 34:3018.

Boot, L.M., O. Mühlbock, and G. Ropcke. 1962. Prolactin and the induction of mammary tumors in mice. *Gen. Comp. Endocrinol.* 2:601.

Briand, P., S.M. Thorpe, and J.L. Daehnfeldt. 1977. Effect of prolactin and bromocriptine on growth of transplanted hormone-dependent mouse mammary tumours. *Br. J. Cancer* 35:816.

Brooks, C.L. and C.W. Welsch, 1974. Reduction of serum prolactin in rats by 2 ergot alkaloids and 2 ergoline derivatives: A comparison. *Proc. Soc. Exp. Biol. Med.* 146:863.

Bruni, J.E. and D.G. Montemurro. 1971. Effect of hypothalamic lesions on the genesis of spontaneous mammary gland tumors in the mouse. *Cancer Res.* 31:854.

Cassell, E.E., J. Meites, and C.W. Welsch. 1971. Effects of ergocornine and ergocryptine on growth of 7,12-dimethylbenzanthracene-induced mammary tumors in rats. *Cancer Res.* 31:1051.

Chan, P.C., J.Tsuang, J. Head, and L.A. Cohen. 1976. Effects of estradiol and prolactin on growth of rat mammary adenocarcinoma cells in monolayer cultures. *Proc. Soc. Exp. Biol. Med.* 151:362.

Chen, H.J., C.J. Bradley, and J. Meites. 1976. Stimulation of carcinogen-induced mammary tumor growth in rats by adrenalectomy. *Cancer Res.* 36:1414.

Dao, T.L. and H. Sunderland. 1959. Mammary carcinogenesis by 3-methylcholanthrene. I. Hormonal aspects in tumor induction and growth. *J. Natl. Cancer Inst.* 23:567.

Dao, T.L., F.G. Bock, and M.J. Greiner. 1960. Mammary carcinogenesis by 3-methylcholanthrene. II. Inhibitory effect of pregnancy and lactation on tumor induction. *J. Natl. Cancer Inst.* 25:991.

Desclin, L.A. 1950. Propos du mécanisme d'action des oestrogènes sur le lobe antérieur de l'hypophyse chez le rat. *Ann. Endocrinol.* 11:656.

Drosdowsky, M., M. Edery, M. Guggiari, A. Montes-Rendon, G. Rudali, and C. Vives. 1980. Inhibition of prolactin-induced mammary cancer in C3Hf(XVII) mice with the trans isomer of bromotriphenylethylene. *Cancer Res.* 40:1674.

Durbin, P.W., M.H. Williams, N. Jeung, and J.S. Arnold. 1966. Development of spontaneous mammary tumors over the life-span of the female Charles River (Sprague-Dawley) rat: The influence of ovariectomy, thyroidectomy, and adrenalectomy-ovariectomy. *Cancer Res.* 26:400.

Evans, H.M. and M.E. Simpson. 1931. Hormones of the anterior hypophysis. *Am. J. Physiol.* 98:511.

Everett, J.W. 1954. Luteotrophic function of autografts of the rat hypophysis. *Endocrinology* 54:685.

Hallowes, R.C., P.S. Rudland, R.A. Hawkins. D.J. Lewis, D. Bennett, and H. Durbin. 1977. Comparison off the effects of hormones on DNA synthesis in cell cultures of nonneoplastic and neoplastic mammary epithelium from rats. *Cancer Res.* 37:2492.

Harada, Y. 1976. Pituitary role in the growth of metastasizing MRMT-1 mammary carcinoma in rats. *Cancer Res.* 36:18.

Heiman, J. and O.F. Krehbiel. 1936. The influence of hormones on breast hyperplasia and tumor growths in white rats. *Am. J. Cancer* 27:450.

Hilf, R., C. Bell, and I. Michel. 1967. Influence of the mammotropic tumor MtTF4 on the growth and biochemistry of the R3230AC mammary carcinoma and mammary glands. *Cancer Res.* 27:482.

Hilf, R., C. Bell, H. Goldenberg, and I. Michel. 1971. Effect of fluphenazine HCl on R3230AC mammary carcinoma and mammary glands of the rat. *Cancer Res.* 31:1111.

Huggins, C., and G. Briziarelli. 1959. Prevention of mammary cancer by endocrinologic methods. *Science* 129:1285.

Huggins, C., Y. Torralba, and A. Charr. 1956a. Endocrine influences on growth of a benign transplantable mammary tumor. *Science* 123:674.

Huggins, C., Y. Torralba, and K. Mainzer. 1956b. Hormonal influences on mammary tumors of the rat. I. Acceleration of growth of transplanted fibroadenoma in ovariectomized and hypophysectomized rats. *J. Exp. Med.* 104:525.

Iturri, G. C. and C.W. Welsch. 1976. Effects of prolactin and growth hormone on DNA synthesis of rat mammary carcinomas in vitro. *Experientia* 32:1045.

Kim, U. and J. Furth. 1960a. Relation of mammary tumors to mammotropes. I. Induction of mammary tumors in rats. *Proc. Soc. Exp. Biol. Med.* 103: 640.

————. 1960b. Relation of mammary tumors to mammotropes. II. Hormone responsiveness of 3-methylcholanthrene induced mammary carcinomas. *Proc. Soc. Exp. Biol. Med.* 103:643.

————. 1960c. Relation of mammary tumors to mammotropes. IV. Development of highly hormone dependent mammary tumors. *Proc. Soc. Exp. Biol. Med.* 105:490.

Kim, U., J. Furth, and K.H. Clifton. 1960. Relation of mammary tumors to mammotropes. III. Hormone responsiveness of transplanted mammary tumors. *Proc. Soc. Exp. Biol. Med.* 103:646.

Lacassagne, A. and J.F. Duplan. 1959. Le mécanisme de la cancérisation de la mamelle chez la souris consideré d' après les résultats d'experiences au moyen de la réserpine. *Comptes. Rendues. Acad. Sci.* 249:810.

Lee, C., R. Oyasu, and C. Chen. 1975. In vitro interaction of estrogen and prolactin on hormone-dependent rat mammary tumors. *Proc. Soc. Exp. Biol. Med.* 148:224.

Lewis, D. and R.C. Hallowes. 1974. Correlation between the effects of hormones on the synthesis of DNA in explants from induced rat mammary tumours and the growth of the tumours. *J. Endocrinol.* 62:225.

Li, C.H. and W. Yang. 1974. The effect of bovine growth hormone on growth of mammary tumors in hypophysectomized rats. *Life Sci.* 15:761.

Loeb, L. and M.M. Kirtz. 1939. The effects of transplants of anterior lobes of the hypothesis on the growth of the mammary gland and the development of mammary gland carcinoma in various strains of mice. *Am. J. Cancer* 36:56.

MacLeod, R.M., M.S. Allen, and V.P. Hollander. 1964. Hormonal requirements for the growth of mammary adenocarcinoma (MTW9) in rats. *Endocrinology* 75:249.

Medina, D. 1977. Tumor formation in preneoplastic mammary nodule lines in mice treated with nafoxidine, testosterone, and 2-bromo-α-ergocryptine. *J. Natl. Cancer Inst.* 58:1107.

Millar, M.J. and R.L. Noble. 1954. Effects of exogenous hormones on growth characteristics and morphology of transplanted mammary fibroadenoma of the rat. *Br. J. Cancer* 8:495.

Moon, H.D., M.E. Simpson, and H.M. Evans. 1952. Inhibition of methylcholanthrene carcinogenesis by hypophysectomy. *Science* 116:331.

Moon, H.D., M.E. Simpson, C.H. Li, and H.M. Evans. 1950. Neoplasms in rats treated with pituitary growth hormone. III. Reproductive organs. *Cancer Res.* 10:549.

_____. 1951. Neoplasms in rats treated with pituitary growth hormone. V. Absence of neoplasms in hypophysectomized rats. *Cancer Res.* 11: 535.

Mückter, H., E. Frankus, and E. Moré. 1970. Experimental investigations with 1-(morpholinomethyl)-4-phthalimido-piperidindione-2,6 and drostanolone propionate in dimethylbenzanthracene-induced tumors of Sprague-Dawley rats. *Cancer Res.* 30:430.

Mühlbock, O. and L.M. Boot. 1959. Induction of mammary cancer in mice without the mammary tumor agent by isografts of hypophysis. *Cancer Res.* 19:402.

Nagasawa, H. and R. Yanai. 1970. Effects of prolactin or growth hormone on growth of carcinogen-induced mammary tumors of adreno-ovariectomized rats. *Int. J. Cancer* 6:488.

Noble, R.L. and J.H. Walters. 1954. The effect of hypophysectomy on 9,10-dimethyl-1-2-benzanthracine-induced carcinogenesis. *Proc. Am. Assoc. Cancer Res.* 1:35.

Pasteels, J.L., J.C. Heuson, J. Heuson-Stiennon, and N. Legros. 1976. Effects of insulin, prolactin, progesterone, and estradiol on DNA synthesis in organ culture of 7,12-dimethylbenzanthracene-induced rat mammary tumors. *Cancer Res.* 36:2162.

Pearson, O.H., O. Llerena, L. Llerena, A. Molina, and T. Butler. 1969. Prolactin dependent rat mammary cancer: A model for man? *Transactions Assoc. Am. Physicians* 82:255.

Quadri, S.K. and J. Meites. 1971. Regression of spontaneous mammary tumors in rats by ergot drugs. *Proc. Soc. Exp. Biol. Med.* 138:999.

Quadri, S.K., J.L. Clark, and J. Meites. 1973a. Effects of LSD, pargyline and haloperidol on mammary tumor growth in rats. *Proc. Soc. Exp. Biol. Med.* 142:22.

Quadri, S.K., G.S. Kledzik, and J. Meites. 1973b. Effects of L-dopa and methyldopa on growth of mammary cancers in rats. *Proc. Soc. Exp. Biol. Med.* 142:759.

Richardson, F.L. 1967. Effect of ovariectomy at different ages on development of mammary tumors in (C3H X R111) F$_1$ mice. *J. Natl. Cancer Inst.* 39: 347.

Rudland, P.S., R.C. Hallowes, H. Durbin, and D. Lewis. 1977. Mitogenic activity of pituitary hormones on cell cultures of normal and carcinogen-induced tumor epithelium from rat mammary glands. *J. Cell Biol.* 73: 561.

Segaloff, A. 1966. Hormones and breast cancer. *Recent Prog. Hormone Res.* 22: 351.

Singh, D.V., J. Meites, L. Halmi, K.H. Kortright, and M.J. Brennan. 1972. Effect of ergocornine on transplanted mammary tumor growth and pituitary prolactin level in Balb/c mice. *J. Natl. Cancer Inst.* 48:1727.

Sinha, D., D. Cooper, and T.L. Dao. 1973. The nature of estrogen and prolactin effect on mammary tumorigenesis. *Cancer Res.* 33:411.

Sirbasku, D.A. and R.H. Benson. 1979. Estrogen-inducible growth factors that may act as mediators (estromedins) of estrogen-promoted tumor cell growth. *Cold Spring Harbor Conf. Cell Proliferation* 6:477.

Sluyser, M. and R. Van Nie. 1974. Estrogen receptor content and hormone responsive growth of mouse mammary tumors. *Cancer Res.* 34:3253.

Sweeney, M.J., G.A. Poore, E.C. Kornfeld, N.J. Bach, N.V. Owen, and J.A. Clemens. 1975. Activity of 6-methyl-8-substituted ergolines against the 7,12-dimethylbenzanthracene-induced mammary carcinoma. *Cancer Res.* 35:106.

Talwalker, P.K., J. Meites, and H. Mizuno. 1964. Mammary tumor induction by estrogen or anterior pituitary hormones in ovariectomized rats given 7,12-dimethyl-1,2, benzanthracine. *Proc. Soc. Exp. Biol. Med.* 116:531.

Welsch, C.W. and J. Meites. 1970. Effects of reserpine on development of 7,12-dimethylbenzanthracene-induced mammary tumors in female rats. *Experientia* 26:1133.

Welsch, C.W. and E.M. Rivera. 1972. Differential effects of estrogen and prolactin on DNA synthesis in organ cultures of DMBA-induced rat mammary carcinomas. *Proc. Soc. Exp. Biol. Med.* 139:623.

Welsch, C.W. and C. Gribler. 1973. Prophylaxis of spontaneously developing mammary carcinoma in C3H/HeJ female mice by suppression of prolactin. *Cancer Res.* 33:2939.

Welsch, C.W., J.A. Clemens, and J. Meites. 1968. Effects of multiple pituitary homografts or progesterone on 7,12-dimethylbenzanthracene-induced mammary tumors in rats. *J. Natl. Cancer Inst.* 41:465.

_____. 1969. Effects of hypothalamic and amygdaloid lesions on development and growth of carcinogen-induced mammary tumors in the female rat. *Cancer Res.* 29:1541.

Welsch, C.W., T.W. Jenkins, and J. Meites. 1970a. Increased incidence of mammary tumors in the female rat grafted with multiple pituitaries. *Cancer Res.* 30:1024.

Welsch, C.W., H. Nagasawa, and J. Meites. 1970b. Increased incidence of spontaneous mammary tumors in female rats with induced hypothalamic lesions. *Cancer Res.* 30:2310.

Welsch, C.W., G. Iturri, and J. Meites. 1973. Comparative effects of hypophysectomy, ergocornine and ergocornine-reserpine treatments on rat mammary carcinoma. *Int. J. Cancer* 12:206.

Welsch, C.W., C. Gribler, and J.A. Clemens. 1974. 6-methyl-8-β-ergoline-acetonitrile (MEA)-induced suppression of mammary tumorigenesis in C3H/HeJ female mice. *Eur. J. Cancer* 10:595.

Welsch, C.W., M. Goodrich-Smith, C.K. Brown, and M. Wilson. 1979a. Inhibition of mammary tumorigenesis in GR mice with 2-bromo-α-ergocryptine. *Int. J. Cancer* 24:920.

Welsch, C.W., C.K. Brown, M. Goodrich-Smith, J. Chiusana, and R.C. Moon. 1980. Synergistic effect of chronic prolactin suppression and retinoid treatment in the prophylaxis of N-methyl-N-nitrosourea-induced mammary tumorigenesis in female Sprague-Dawley rats. *Cancer Res.* 40:3095.

Welsch, C.W., C.K. Brown, M. Goodrich-Smith, J. Van, B. Denenberg, T.M. Anderson, and C.L. Brooks. 1979a. Inhibition of mammary tumorigenesis in carcinogen-treated Lewis rats by suppression of prolactin secretion. *J. Natl. Cancer Inst.* 63:1211.

Yanai, R. and H. Nagasawa. 1972. Inhibition of mammary tumorigenesis by ergot alkaloids and promotion of mammary tumorigenesis by pituitary isografts in adreno-ovariectomized mice. *J. Natl. Cancer Inst.* 48:715.

Young, S. 1961. Induction of mammary carcinoma in hypophysectomized rats treated with 3-methylcholanthrene, oestradiol-17β, progesterone and growth hormone. *Nature* 190:356.

The Actions of Insulin as a Hormonal Factor in Breast Cancer

RUSSELL HILF
Department of Biochemistry and University of Rochester Cancer Center
University of Rochester
School of Medicine and Dentistry
Rochester, New York 14642

In a multihormonal disease such as breast cancer, it is not surprising that tentative assignments of relative importance of hormones have arisen. Hormones categorized as having primary roles are the estrogens and prolactin, and perhaps progestagens. Owing to either lack of data or inconclusive evidence, a secondary status can be assigned to the following hormones: glucocorticoids, androgens (as precursors for estrogens), thyroid, and insulin. Hormones that can be considered as not yet categorized but potentially influential are growth hormone (GH), oxytocin, relaxin, and a variety of growth factors, such as epidermal growth factor (EGF). Although this extensive list includes those hormones defined by Lyons et al. (1958) as essential for growth and development of the normal rodent mammary gland, viz., estrogens, progesterone, glucocorticoids, prolactin, and GH, there remains a need to identify the exact roles of these and the other hormones in the neoplastic mammary cell. This paper offers evidence to implicate insulin as one of the hormones involved in growth of breast cancer in animals, describes some of the actions of insulin that relate to neoplastic growth, and reviews the modest amount of clinical data.

EXPERIMENTAL ANIMAL TUMORS

Definitions are required prior to discussion of the role of insulin in tumor growth. It is reasonable to conclude that decreased growth or regression of neoplastic mass as a consequence of reduction or removal of a hormone from the milieu is an adequate criterion for hormone dependence. Hormone independence would be demonstrated by continued tumor growth in the presence of altered hormonal environment. A second set of terms pertains to responsiveness and can be defined as altered tumor growth as a result of treatment, i.e., therapeutic or pharmacologic administration of hormones. These terms are not mutually exclusive, since within a given neoplastic mass, a spectrum of these properties can occur because of the presence of different cell populations or changes in properties of cells as they adapt to the altered environment. The following

317

discussion is limited to insulin-dependent neoplasms, and to insulin-independent but responsive tumors.

Insulin-dependent Tumors

There are several reports indicating that growth of transplantable tumors was retarded in diabetic animals, as exemplified by studies of Walker 256 carcinoma (Goranson and Tilser 1955), a spontaneously arising transplantable mammary tumor in C3H mice (Puckett and Shingleton 1972), Ehrlich ascites and solid tumors (Pavelic et al. 1979), a thymoma in mice (Pavelic and Slijepcevic 1978), and a methylcholanthrene-induced fibrosarcoma (Pavelic 1980). Curiously, transplantation of this fibrosarcoma into diabetic mice resulted in faster growth after each susbequent transfer, an effect that was attributed to production by the tumor of insulin, as measured by radioimmunoassay procedures. The question of severity of the diabetic state and the nutritional status of the host, however, needs to be considered; both Ingle (1958) and Puckett and Shingleton (1972) pointed out that inhibition of tumor growth was greatest in the most severely diabetic animals.

In an interesting series of papers, Heuson and his colleagues demonstrated that insulin caused proliferation of 7,12-dimethylbenz[a]anthracene (DMBA)-induced tumors studied by an explant culture technique in vitro (Heuson et al. 1967), that this effect was not mediated through increased glucose consumption (Heuson and Legros 1968), and that actual tumor regression occurred in DMBA tumors when rats were made diabetic (Heuson and Legros 1970). Extending these studies, they (Heuson et al. 1972) reported that administration of estrogens failed to prevent tumor regression resulting from alloxan-induced diabetes. Furthermore, in hypophysectomized hosts, insulin administration, along with prolactin, reactivated tumor growth; prolactin alone in this situation was inactive as a stimulator of neoplastic growth. It was concluded that insulin played a role in stimulating growth of DMBA-induced tumors and, along with estrogens and prolactin, should be considered as an important hormonal factor in mammary cancer.

Studies in our laboratory regarding the role of insulin in mammary tumors were prompted by our investigations directed at hormonal regulation of carbohydrate metabolism, particularly for the estrogens, and in a broader sense, at defining biochemical parameters that would distinguish between hormone-dependent and -independent lesions. We (Cohen and Hilf 1974) chose streptozotocin as the diabetes-inducing agent, defining diabetes as blood glucose >250 mg/100 ml, urinary glucose >0.5 gm/ml, and serum insulin $<10^{-10}$ M. Our overall experience with DMBA tumor growth behavior after induction of diabetes has been 86/161 (53.4%) lesions regress ($>20\%$ decrease in size), 47/161 (29.2%) lesions continue to grow ($>20\%$ increase in size), and 28/161 (17.4%) lesions remain static ($<20\%$ change in size). Although these results show fewer regressions than Heuson and Legros (1970), some difference is likely due to the severity of diabetes and weight loss seen in Heuson's study using alloxan as the diabetogenic agent. Compared to lesions growing in diabetic rats, tumors classified as regressing have demonstrated lower activities of pyruvate kinase, phosphofructokinase (PFK), and glucose 6-phosphate dehydrogenase, reduced utilization of labeled glucose in vitro, lowered transport of glucose, elevated levels of cAMP but not cGMP, increased binding of insulin, and decreased estrogen receptor (ER) content (Cohen and Hilf 1974; Matusik and Hilf 1976; Gibson and Hilf 1976; Shafie and Hilf 1978). The altered glucose utilization, and the activities of the glycolytic enzymes measured, were restored after treatment with insulin, concomitant with stimulation of tumor growth (Cohen and Hilf 1974). Thus, for the criterion befitting hormonal dependence in vivo, these data strongly support consideration of insulin as another hormonal factor in DMBA-induced mammary tumors.

To examine the effects of insulin under more controlled conditions, Pasteels et al. (1976) studied DMBA-induced mammary tumors in the organ explant system earlier devised for study of the normal gland (Topper and Oka 1974). Of these tumors, 17 of 20 were considered as insulin-dependent for DNA synthesis, as measured by thymidine incorporation into DNA; in the presence of insulin, variable additional responses to prolactin, progesterone, and estrogen were observed. While prolactin and progesterone were stimulating in 9/12 lesions, estrogens were inhibitory in the presence of prolactin. Welsch et al. (1976) reported similar results for both mouse and rat (DMBA-induced) mammary tumors, in which insulin dramatically increased thymidine incorporation into DNA in the mouse tumors and significantly enhanced precursor incorporation in the rat tumors. Interestingly, prolactin had an additive effect on the insulin response in rat, but not mouse, adenocarcinomas. The mitogenic effects of insulin have also been demonstrated for certain human breast cancer cells in long-term tissue culture. Osborne et al. (1976) reported that MCF-7 cells were quite sensitive to insulin; increases in cell number of 50% and 100% were seen after addition of 0.1 nM and 10 mM insulin, respectively. Similar results were obtained for the ZR75-1 cell line, but the MVA-MB-231 and EVSA-T lines (Osborne et al. 1978) did not demonstrate such results. Curiously, all four cell lines demonstrate the presence of insulin receptors. Extending these observations by examination of labeled precursor incorporation into macromolecules yielded data (Osborne and Lippman 1978) suggestive of the following sequence of events: Rapid, early effects of insulin to stimulate protein and fatty acid synthesis (within 1 hr), stimulation of uridine incorporation into RNA by 3 hr, and later effects on thymidine incorporation into DNA (10-15 hr). A similar sequence of events was reported by Rillema and Linebaugh (1977). Insulin dependence of MCF-7 cells in vivo was incontrovertibly demonstrated by Shafie (1980). In diabetic nude mice, MCF-7 cells did not form tumors; tumors were obtained with 100% frequency in diabetic mice treated with insulin. The growth stimulation by insulin was similar in MCF-7 cells from the continuous culture line and in cultured cells derived by enzymatic dissociation of MCF-7 tumors from nude mice.

It would appear that insulin can act as a growth-stimulating hormone for mammary carcinomas, a conclusion based on data obtained from experimental model systems originating from rat, mouse, and human.

Insulin-responsive Tumors

As defined earlier, neoplasms that demonstrate altered growth or metabolism as a result of insulin status are considered responsive tumors. Responsive tumors differ from those lesions defined as dependent, because the former grow quite adequately in the absence of insulin, i.e., diabetes. Administration of insulin could produce inhibition of tumor growth, as was reported for Walker 256 carcinosarcomas (Salter et al. 1958), and there was a report by Wieser et al. (1967) indicating that the Zajdela hepatoma grew faster in diabetic animals.

Our interest in insulin arose from studies on glucose metabolism in the transplantable R3230AC mammary adenocarcinoma, a tumor of Fischer rats that we had characterized as estrogen-responsive (Hilf et al. 1965, 1967). The unusual feature of this neoplasm was its ability to respond to estrogen treatment with lactation-like features: Enhanced secretory activity, presence of a milk-like fluid that contained casein, lactose, and short-chain fatty acids, and an enzyme activity profile that resembled the mammary gland during pregnancy (Hilf 1967). Others have reported the presence of α-lactalbumin in the tumor (Schultz and Ebner 1977), confirming the existence of the enzymatic requirements for production of lactose. As insulin was shown to be a necessary hormone for lactation, we examined the effects of insulin removal and treatment on growth of the R3230AC tumor. In the diabetic rat, this neoplasm grew somewhat faster than that seen in the intact animal; a dose-response inhibition of tumor growth was obtained as a result of insulin treatment (Cohen and Hilf 1975). Estrogen treatment inhibited tumor growth in diabetic rats, but an additive effect was obtained when insulin was administered with estrogens. We considered these effects to be independent actions of the two hormones, but, as will be pointed out below, this may not be the case.

The ability of insulin to inhibit tumor growth was not unique to the R3230AC tumor system. During studies of DMBA-induced tumors in diabetic rats, we performed experiments to examine the effects of insulin replacement on tumor growth and biochemical parameters. As expected, tumors regressing in diabetic rats resumed growth after insulin treatment. Interestingly, tumors growing in diabetic rats, which were classified as insulin-independent, frequently were caused to regress by insulin treatment: 9/19 lesions regressed, 1/19 became static, and 9/19 continued to grow (Gibson and Hilf 1980). Taken together with the data on the R3230AC tumors, administration of insulin can retard mammary tumor growth, tumors that would be classified as insulin-independent but insulin-responsive. This duality of action, i.e., removal or administration of the hormone, resembles to some extent the well-known paradoxical effects of estrogens (Hilf 1979).

MECHANISMS OF ACTION OF INSULIN

In attempting to elucidate the processes that would offer insight as to how insulin may regulate growth of mammary tumors, consideration was given to those cellular events thought to be affected by insulin, as shown in studies of normal tissues.

Insulin Receptors and Their Regulation

It is most likely that if a cell or tissue responds to a hormonal perturbation, specific receptors for the hormone are present in the target cell, because the interaction of the hormone with its receptor represents the initial step in a programmed sequence of events. Specific receptors for insulin have been characterized in the R3230AC (Harmon and Hilf 1976a), DMBA-induced (Shafie and Hilf 1978), and several continuous culture human mammary tumor cell lines (Osborne et al. 1978), as well as in Zajdela ascites hepatomas (Capeau et al. 1978) and transformed fibroblasts (Thomopoulos et al. 1976). Properties of insulin receptors in neoplastic cells were found to be similar to those of normal cells based on saturability, estimated K_D, specificity for ligand, and curvilinearity of the Scatchard binding plot. Although considerable discussion has arisen regarding the interpretation of the curvilinear Scatchard plot, i.e., multiple classes of receptors vs one class of sites demonstrating negative cooperative interactions, it would appear that no significant alterations in the properties of insulin receptors have been identified in neoplastic tissues. The number of receptors per neoplastic cell may show some differences from their normal counterparts, but difficulties in quantitating the number of sites due to the curvilinear Scatchard plots suggests that caution is needed in reaching any conclusions.

Insulin receptors appear to be under negative control, i.e., down-regulation: Binding of insulin is inversely related to circulating levels of the hormone (Kahn et al. 1973). This was demonstrated for both the R3230AC and DMBA-induced mammary tumors (Harmon and Hilf 1976b; Shafie et al. 1977; Shafie and Hilf 1978), because enhanced insulin binding occurred in tumors from diabetic rats and reduced binding was obtained in lesions from diabetic rats treated with insulin. A most interesting finding was a negative regulation of insulin receptors by estrogens (Shafie et al. 1977). Insulin binding was increased in R3230AC tumors from ovariectomized rats and reduced after treatment with estrogens. In DMBA-induced tumors, lesions that continued to grow after ovariectomy showed increased insulin binding, although neoplasms regressing after ovariectomy demonstrated a decrease in insulin binding (Shafie and Hilf 1978). Taken together, these data indicate that insulin receptors in mammary tumors are subject to hormonal regulation, and this may offer an exploitable parameter for hormonal therapy. The recent report by Bertoli et al. (1980) regarding changes in insulin binding to monocytes at different phases of the menstrual cycle implies a regulatory role for sex hormones even at physiological levels.

Insulin and Glucose Transport

One of the most extensively studied responses to hormones is the insulin-induced stimulation of glucose transport; this subject has been reviewed frequently (Morgan and Whitfield 1974; Czech, 1977; Clausen 1977). Considerable recent attention has turned toward elucidation of the mechanisms for insulin action and studies have invoked roles for sulfhydryl status, Ca^{++} and Mg^{++}, membrane protein phosphorylation, and membrane fluidity as offering insight into the response to the hormone (see review by Hilf et al. 1981). Hatanaka (1974), in reviewing the literature on glucose transport in tumor cells, concluded that a feature common to transformed cells is the existence of an increased initial rate of sugar transport compared with their normal cells of origin. Thus, in keeping with the proposal of Holley (1972), in which cell growth could be related to nutrient uptake, the enhanced uptake of glucose by neoplastic cells may be one critical factor in regulation of growth of cancer cells. It seemed logical, then, to ascertain whether insulin perturbed glucose transport in mammary tumors and to seek out correlations with neoplastic growth behavior.

Heuson and Legros (1968) examined the role of glucose and insulin on thymidine incorporation into explants of DMBA-induced tumors and concluded that the insulin-stimulated increase in thymidine incorporation was not mediated through the simple expediency of enhanced glucose uptake and utilization, which was measured as disappearance of glucose from the medium over a 24-hour period. However, their data also indicated that at low glucose levels thymidine incorporation into DNA was low but was raised by addition of insulin, indicating that glucose was rate-limiting. They concluded that growth stimulation and glucose uptake were apparently dissociated in this tumor system. However, we observed that glucose utilization by slices of DMBA-induced tumors regressing in diabetic hosts was reduced compared with that from tumors growing in intact hosts; production of $^{14}CO_2$ from uniformly labeled glucose or glucose labeled at C-1 was diminished during a 3-hr incubation (Cohen and Hilf 1974). A desirable measurement of insulin action on glucose utilization can be obtained by the study of glucose transport, i.e., carrier-mediated entry of glucose. We (Harmon and Hilf 1976c) performed such a study on three lesions from the same diabetic animal, one that was regressing, one that was static, and one that was growing. In the absence of insulin in vitro, glucose transport was lowest in the regressing lesion and highest in the growing lesion, suggesting a relationship between glucose transport and growth behavior. Exposure of cells to 10^{-10} M insulin for 15 min in vitro produced a 55% increase in glucose transport in the cells from the regressing lesion (insulin-dependent), had no effect on cells from the static lesion, and caused a 50% decrease in transport in cells from the growing lesion (insulin-independent). These data demonstrate that insulin can produce an alteration in glucose transport in DMBA-induced tumors. Of particular interest was the unusual finding of a decrease in glucose transport after insulin treatment in vitro, which, in light of our more recent findings of insulin-induced regressions of so-called insulin-independent tumors (see above), offers a possible explanation for the biological behavior of such lesions.

A more detailed study of glucose transport was performed with dissociated R3230AC tumor cells (Harmon and Hilf 1976d). The facilitated uptake of glucose occurred by a carrier system that demonstrated saturability, substrate specificity, inhibition by phloretin and temperature sensitivity. The K_m for glucose transport was 3-4 mM. Effects of 10^{-9} M insulin in vitro on glucose transport in cells from diabetic rats showed a time-related decrease in initial velocity (v_i), resulting in an increased calculated K_m. This result occurred when glucose was present in the medium at 2 mM and 5 mM. The effect of insulin to decrease v_i was dose-related, with the major effects seen at 10^{-10} M to 10^{-8} M. The temporal relationship of this response in transport to insulin binding was consistent with the hormonal interaction preceding the response on transport. The apparent decrease in glucose transport seen in vitro in response to insulin may in part explain the ability of insulin to reduce tumor growth in vivo.

An interesting well-known observation is the ability of phloretin to inhibit facilitated glucose transport. Phloretin, a hydroxyphenyl trihydroxypropiophenone, is weakly estrogenic; diethylstilbestrol (DES) was reported to inhibit glucose transport (LeFevre 1959). We examined the steroidal estrogens and found that estradiol-17β, estrone (E_1), and estriol (E_2) demonstrated activity to inhibit glucose transport (Gay and Hilf 1980). These data pose an interesting consideration for actions of estrogens at the membrane level, and, as agents that interfere with substrate entry, may offer a partial explanation for inhibition of tumor cell growth by estrogens.

Insulin and Amino Acid Transport

Insulin regulates entry of neutral amino acids into cells. Data have been obtained in numerous tissues indicating that there is specificity to this response; amino acid entry by the A system is enhanced by insulin, whereas entry by the L system is unaffected (Guidotti et al. 1978). We have conducted experiments with the R3230AC carcinoma, in which we demonstrated that alteration of the insulin milieu of the tumor-bearing animal produced changes in transport by the A system but not by the L system (Hissin and Hilf 1978a,b). For example, faster growing tumors from diabetic rats demonstrated increased entry of proline but not leucine; treatment with insulin reduced tumor growth and decreased entry of amino acids via the A, but not the L, system (Hissin and Hilf 1978c). Even though these effects might appear to be contrary to those usually seen with insulin, we have also shown that insulin in vitro can stimulate transport of amino acids via the A system in tumor cells from diabetic rats (Hissin and Hilf 1978c). These data suggest that the action of insulin in vivo may be influenced by the presence of other hormonal factors, which would be absent under the conditions used in vitro.

To explore this, we undertook studies of estrogens and their effects on transport, since estrogens alter growth of this tumor (Hilf et al. 1967). Analogous to our findings with insulin, enhanced tumor growth resulting from ovariectomy, or reduced tumor growth occurring in response to estrogen treatment, was accompanied by changes in proline (A system) transport (Table 1). These changes correlated with changes in the growth behavior of the R3230AC carcinoma. Specificity for the A system was greater than that seen with the L system (Hissin and Hilf 1979). A similar specificity was seen in vitro; E_2 inhibited proline transport with little or no effect on phenylalanine (L system) entry. An interesting observation was the ability of estradiol-17β to antagonize the insulin-induced increase in proline transport under in vitro conditions. It is tempting to propose that the additive inhibitory effects of insulin and E_2 on R3230AC tumor growth in vivo may result from their actions to inhibit substrate transport.

Our most recent efforts to characterize the effects of estrogens on transport have yielded kinetic data indicating that estradiol-17β has properties of a classical noncompetitive inhibitor of proline transport (see Fig. 1). These data, when analyzed as a Dixon plot or by the the graphical method of Cornish-Bowden (1974) gave an estimated K_i of ~ 2 μM. Comparable values were obtained for DES, whereas lower relative potency as inhibitors was obtained for E_1, estriol (E_3), and estradiol-17α. No effects on L-system transport were observed in the same cells. Thus, our efforts to elucidate mechanisms whereby insulin altered tumor growth have yielded information on a heretofore unrecognized action of pharmacological doses of estrogens as they relate to the effects of insulin on transport of substrates. Interestingly, significant inhibition of growth of a human pituitary cell line (Wyche and Noteboom 1979) and the human breast cancer cell line MCF-7 (Weichselbaum et al. 1980) was observed in the presence of E_2 at concentrations around 2 μM, suggesting that at these concentrations of the hormone, inhibition of substrate transport could play a role.

Table 1
Relationship of Hormonal Effects In Vivo on Growth, Receptors, and Amino Acid Transport in R3230AC Mammary Adenocarcinomas

Host and treatment	Tumor growth response	Hormone binding		Amino acid transport	
		insulin	estradiol	A system	L system
Diabetic; none	increase	increase	decrease	increase	static
Diabetic; insulin	decrease	decrease	increase	decrease	static
Ovariectomy; none	increase	increase	increase	increase	static
Ovariectomy; estrogen	decrease	decrease	decrease	decrease	decrease
Diabetic; estrogen	decrease	decrease	decrease	decrease	decrease

Changes recorded are relative to untreated hosts.

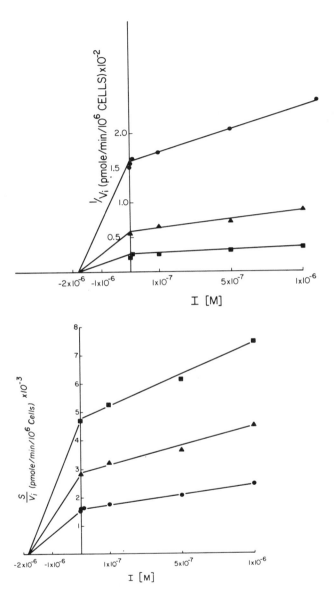

Figure 1
Inhibition of proline transport by estradiol-17β (10^{-10} M to 10^{-6} M). Dissociated cells were incubated initially for 90 min in the presence of varying concentrations of E_2. Transport (initial velocity) was determined by linear regression analysis of triplicate samples at 20, 40, and 60 sec, using proline at 0.1 mM ($\bullet$), 0.5 mM ($\blacktriangle$). and 2.0 mM ($\blacksquare$) as substrate. Each point represents the average of 3 or more separate experiments. *Top:* Plot according to method of Dixon. Correlation coefficients for lines exceeded 0.97. *Bottom:* Plot according to method of Cornish-Bowden. Correlation coefficients for lines exceeded 0.98.

Insulin as a Regulator of ERs

The ability of insulin to regulate certain intracellular proteins is well known, as classically exemplified by its regulatory action on glucokinase in the liver. Since there are several instances of one hormone regulating receptors for another hormone, e.g., estrogen regulation of progesterone receptors and prolactin regulation of ERs, we initiated studies to examine the effects of insulin on ER. Initially, we reported that DMBA-induced tumors regressing in diabetic rats demonstrated significantly lower estrogen-binding capacity (Gibson and Hilf 1976), whereas insulin-independent lesions had ER levels comparable to those found in growing tumors from intact rats. These studies have been extended to examine the effects of insulin administration on ER levels (Gibson and Hilf 1980). As indicated above (Insulin-responsive Tumors), treatment with insulin produced regrowth of most tumors regressing in diabetic hosts; the resulting lesions had ER levels equal to those found in tumors from intact hosts. Even insulin-independent lesions, i.e., those grown in diabetic rats, had a modest reduction of ER levels (see Table 2). However, whenever insulin treatment resulted in an alteration in the tumor growth pattern, either stimulation or inhibition, the level of ER was elevated. This was observed even in the case of those neoplasms that were static at the outset of treatment or responded by becoming static; ER levels were increased compared with static lesions that remained static after insulin treatment. The changes in estrogen binding capacity reflected a change in the number of ER rather than an alteration in the affinity for the hormonal ligand. We concluded that insulin played a role in regulation of ER independent of growth.

Table 2

Effects of Diabetes and Insulin Treatment on Growth and ER Levels in DMBA-induced Tumors

Animal	Treatment	Tumor behavior pre-R_x	post-R_x	ER levels (fmoles/mg protein)[a]	Average K_D ($\times 10^{-9}$ M)
Intact	none	growth		39.4 ± 3.8	1.5
Diabetic	none	growth		24.2 ± 2.9	1.2
Diabetic	none	regrowth		8.5 ± 0.7	1.2
Diabetic	insulin	regrowth	growth	52.8 ± 9.9	1.9
Diabetic	insulin	growth	regrowth	39.9 ± 6.0	0.4
Diabetic	insulin	growth	growth	27.5 ± 10.5	1.8
Diabetic	none	static		8.0 ± 0.4	1.2
Diabetic	insulin	static	growth	58^b	1.0

[a] ER data presented as mean ± S.E. with 4–8 samples/group.
[b] Value from one lesion.

Support for such a regulatory role for insulin has also come from preliminary experiments with R3230AC carcinoma cells in short-term culture; higher ER levels were observed when insulin was added to the culture medium compared with ER in cells grown in the absence of insulin supplementation (Shafie et al. 1977). Gentry et al. (1977) have reported a reduction in nuclear uptake of $[^3H]E_2$ in the hypothalamus and pituitary from diabetic rats. The inability of estrogen to activate tumor growth in the diabetic rat (Heuson et al. 1972) may have been due to decreased ER and its subsequent role in hormone response.

ROLE OF INSULIN IN HUMAN BREAST CANCER

Recently, we (Harmon and Hilf 1979) surveyed the existing literature dealing with epidemiological studies of the relationship between diabetes and breast cancer. Although no clear cut picture has emerged, reports were found suggesting that the incidence of diabetes was lower in breast cancer patients vs all other cancer patients (Glicksman et al. 1956). In contrast, Repert (1952) found a higher percentage of diabetes in his breast cancer patients vs the general population, and Muck et al. (1975, 1976), using matched-pairs analysis, found a considerably higher incidence of diabetes in breast cancer patients vs patients with benign breast disease. Another approach taken was to examine cancer risk among diabetics, and there is a suggestion that the diabetic may have an increased risk for certain cancers, including breast cancer (Lancaster 1954; Lancaster and Maddox 1958). Recently, D.C. Deubner (pers. comm.) has also noted that diabetes appears to be associated with breast cancer. There is a need to include the criteria for classifying diabetes, since juvenile and mature onset diabetes have significant differences in course and therapy. In the absence of such information, a conclusion regarding diabetes and breast cancer cannot be made.

Use of insulin as a therapeutic agent for cancer has been mentioned in several anecdotal reports in the older literature (Silberstein et al. 1927) and more recently (Koroljow 1962; Neufeld 1962). A most interesting paper was authored by Rhomberg (1975), who studied 130 women with advanced breast cancer treated with hormones and cytostatic drugs. In this group of patients, 30 women were classified as diabetics. He suggested that the course of the disease was more protracted in the diabetics. Most intriguing was his finding that the diabetic patients may have been more responsive to hormone therapy, since 18 out of 24 diabetic patients demonstrated objective response to hormone therapy compared to one-third of the remaining patients. Abnormalities in glucose tolerance have been observed in women with breast cancer, with diabetic-type glucose tolerance curves and delayed insulin responses (Pearson et al. 1968; Carter et al. 1975). The implication that this metabolic imbalance may alter the course of the disease, as well as the response to hormonal therapy, is surely worthy of further investigations.

CONCLUSIONS ON ACTIONS OF INSULIN IN BREAST CANCER

From the foregoing data, certain tentative conclusions can be offered regarding the roles of insulin in mammary tumor growth. These can be divided into direct and indirect, or facilitative, roles, based on studies with various experimental neoplastic models.

Direct effects include the following:

1. Insulin stimulates growth of tumors. As an anabolic hormone, insulin can stimulate growth of certain rodent and human tumors, probably via its effects on enhancement of substrate entry and stimulation of protein synthesis. Removal of insulin by induction of diabetes can result in regression of tumor mass. These results are similar to those reported for estrogens and prolactin in experimental models.

2. Insulin can inhibit tumor growth. A somewhat surprising action, this has now been observed in two different rodent systems, R3230AC and certain DMBA-induced mammary carcinomas. These lesions can be considered as hormone-independent but -responsive. Data indicate that one possible mechanism can be attributed to inhibition of substrate transport in these systems, a result compatible with reduced cell growth. Inhibition of proliferation of the Cloudman S91 melanoma cells in vitro by insulin has recently been reported (Kahn et al. 1980), although uptake of A1B was stimulated by insulin in the inhibited cells. Thus, inhibition of neoplastic cell growth can be caused by insulin, but the mechanisms in vivo and in vitro need to be established.

Indirect (facilitative) effects include the following:

1. Insulin regulates ERs. Data have been obtained suggesting that insulin may play a regulatory role for ERs, analogous to other systems of hormonal regulation of receptors. Because many breast cancers are estrogen-dependent or -responsive, growth or inhibition of growth of neoplasms may arise through the indirect effects of insulin on ER.

2. Antagonism of insulin effects by estrogens. Studies have demonstrated that estrogens can down-regulate insulin receptors in rodent mammary tumors. In human monocytes (Bertoli et al. 1980), reduced insulin binding occurred during the secretory phase of the menstrual cycle. Reduction in insulin binding may produce reductions in response to insulin. Similarly, antagonism of insulin-induced increases in substrate transport may be another action of estrogens. All these results implicate an insulin-estrogen axis that requires elucidation for mammary tumor growth (Hilf et al. 1978).

SUMMARY AND SPECULATIONS

If it is valid to assume that effects of hormones on rodent mammary tumors may have a counterpart in the human, then it would appear that insulin should be added to the list of hormones considered to play a role in breast cancer. From the data obtained, insulin may stimulate or inhibit mammary tumor growth, depending on the animal model examined. Such a spectrum of effects is reminiscent of, although not entirely analogous to, the paradoxical effects of estrogens, in which removal or addition may produce the desired inhibition of neoplastic growth. For insulin, effects on substrate transport offer a measurable parameter to relate to cell growth and such a relationship was seen to occur with the rodent models being studied. The possible regulatory effects of insulin on ER are potentially exploitable for therapeutic application; if insulin can stimulate ER levels, might not an enhanced response to estrogen treatment result? The effects of estrogens at pharmacological doses need to be elucidated and their apparent ability to down-regulate insulin receptors and inhibit transport of glucose and certain amino acids offers a possible mechanism to explain reduction in tumor growth. The fact that the effects of estrogens demonstrate specificity for the same carrier systems that respond to insulin is further support for an insulin-estrogen interrelationship in mammary tumor growth.

ACKNOWLEDGMENTS

The studies presented here and those cited from the author's laboratory were supported by U.S. Public Health Service grant CA-16660. The continued interest and support of the University of Rochester Cancer Center (CA-11198) and its Animal Tumor Research Facility is gratefully noted. The research summarized here resulted from the dedicated efforts of former and current students N.D. Cohen, J. Feldman, R.J. Gay, J.T. Harmon, P.J. Hissin, R.J. Matusik, and L.K. Sorge; post-doctoral fellow S.M. Shafie; and my very able laboratory technicians, S.L. Gibson and D. Helton. I wish to thank A. Stevenson for her good spirits during the typing of this manuscript, especially given the considerable pressure of time.

REFERENCES

Bertoli, A., R. De Pirro, A. Fusco, A.V. Greco, R. Magnatta, and R. Lauro. 1980. Differences in insulin receptors between men and menstruating women and influences of sex hormones on insulin binding during the menstrual cycle. *J. Clin. Endocrinol. Metab.* 50:246.

Capeau, J., J. Picard, and M. Caron. 1978. Insulin receptors in Zajdela rat ascites hepatoma cells and their sensitivity to certain enzymes and lectins. *Cancer Res.* 38:3930.

Carter, A.C., B.W. Lefkon, M. Farlin, and E.B. Feldman. 1975. Metabolic parameters in women with metastatic breast cancer. *J. Clin. Endocrinol. Metab.* 40:260.

Clausen, T. 1977. Calcium, glucose transport and insulin action. In *Biochemistry of membrane transport* (ed. G. Semenza and E. Carafoli), p. 481. Springer-Verlag, New York.

Cohen, N.D. and R. Hilf. 1974. Influence of insulin on growth and metabolism of 7,12-dimethylbenz(a)anthracene-induced mammary tumors. *Cancer Res.* 34:3245.

————. 1975. Influence of insulin on estrogen-induced responses in the R3230AC mammary carcinoma. *Cancer Res.* 35:560.

Cornish-Bowden, A. 1974. A simple graphical method for determining the inhibition constants of mixed, uncompetitive and non-competitive inhibitors. *Biochem. J.* 137:143.

Czech, M. 1977. Molecular basis for insulin action. *Annu. Rev. Biochem.* 46: 359.

Gay, R.J. and R. Hilf. 1980. Paradoxical effects of 17β-estradiol on glucose transport in primary cell cultures of a rat mammary tumor. *Biochem. Biophys. Res. Comm.* 92:1180.

Gentry, R.T., G.N. Wade, and J.D. Blauskin. 1977. Binding of [^{3}H]estradiol by brain cell nuclei and female rat sexual behavior: Inhibition by experimental diabetes. *Brain Res.* 135:146.

Gibson, S.L. and R. Hilf. 1976. Influence of hormonal alteration of host on estrogen binding capacity in 7,12-dimethylbenz(a)anthracene-induced mammary tumors. *Cancer Res.* 36:3736.

————. 1980. Regulation of estrogen-binding capacity by insulin in 7,12-dimethylbenz(a)anthracene-induced mammary tumors in rats. *Cancer Res.* 40:2343.

Glicksman, A.S., W.P.L. Meyers, and R.W. Rawson. 1956. Diabetes mellitus and carbohydrate metabolism in patients with cancer. *Med. Clin. N.A.* 40:887.

Goranson, E.S. and G.J. Tilser. 1955. Studies on the relationship of alloxan-diabetes and tumor growth. *Cancer Res.* 15:626.

Guidotti, G.G., A.F. Borghetti, and G.C Gazzola. 1978. The regulation of amino acid transport in animal cells. *Biochim. Biophys. Acta* 515:329.

Harmon, J.T. and R. Hilf. 1976a. Identification and characterization of the insulin receptors in the R3230AC mammary adenocarcinoma of the rat. *Cancer Res.* 36:3993.

————. 1976b. Insulin binding and glucose transport in the R3230AC mammary adenocarcinoma. *J. Supramol. Struct.* 4:233.

————. 1976c. Effect of insulin on glucose transport in DMBA-induced mammary tumors. *Eur. J. Cancer* 12:933.

————. 1976d. Effect of insulin to decrease glucose transport in dissociated cells from the R3230AC mammary adenocarcinoma of diabetic rats. *Biochim. Biophys. Acta* 508:401.

————. 1979. Insulin and mammary cancer. In *Influences of hormones on tumor development* (ed. J.A. Kellen and R. Hilf), vol. II, p. 111. CRC Press, Boca Raton, Florida.

Hatanaka, M. 1974. Transport of sugars in tumor cell membranes. *Biochim. Biophys. Acta* 355:77.

Heuson, J.C. and N. Legros. 1968. Study of the growth-promoting effect of insulin in relation to carbohydrate metabolism in organ culture of rat mammary carcinoma. *Eur. J. Cancer* 4:1.

————. 1970. Effect of insulin and of alloxan diabetes on growth of the rat mammary carcinoma in vivo. *Eur. J. Cancer* 6:349.

Heuson, J.C., A. Coune, and R. Heimann. 1967. Cell proliferation induced by insulin in organ culture of the rat mammary carcinoma. *Exp. Cell Res.* 45:351.

Heuson, J.C., N. Legros, and R. Heimann. 1972. Influence of insulin administration on growth of the 7,12-dimethylbenz(a)anthracene-induced mammary carcinoma in intact, oophorectomized and hypophysectomized rats. *Cancer Res.* **32**:233.

Hilf, R. 1967. Milk-like fluid in a mammary adenocarcinoma: Biochemical characterization. *Science* **155**:826.

—————. 1979. Dose-time relationships in the effect of estrogens on mammary cancer. In *Reviews on endocrine-related cancer* (ed. B.A. Stoll), p. 11. Imperial Chemical Industries, Ltd., Cheshire, England.

Hilf, R., I. Michel, and C. Bell. 1965. Biochemical and morphological properties of a new lactating mammary tumor line in the rat. *Cancer Res.* **25**:286.

—————. 1967. Biochemical and morphological responses of normal and neoplastic mammary tissue to hormonal treatment. *Recent Prog. Horm. Res.* **23**:229.

Hilf, R., P.J. Hissin, and S.M. Shafie. 1978. Regulatory interrelationships for insulin and estrogen action in mammary tumors. *Cancer Res.* **38**:4076.

Hilf, R., L.K. Sorge, and R.J. Gay. 1981. Insulin binding and glucose transport. *Int. Rev. Cytol.* **72**:147.

Hissin, P.J. and R. Hilf. 1978a. Characteristics of proline transport into R3230AC mammary tumor cells. *Biochim. Biophys. Acta* **508**:401.

—————. 1978b. α-Aminoisobutyrate transport into cells from R3230AC mammary adenocarcinoma. Evidence for sodium ion-dependent and -independent carrier mediated entry and effects of diabetes. *Biochem. J.* **176**:205.

—————. 1978c. Effects of insulin in vivo and in vitro on amino acid transport into cells from the R3230AC mammary adenocarcinoma and their relationship to tumor growth. *Cancer Res.* **38**:3646.

—————. 1979. Effects of estrogen to alter amino acid transport in R3230AC mammary carcinomas and its relationship to insulin action. *Cancer Res.* **39**:3381.

Holley, R.W. 1972. A unifying hypothesis concerning the nature of malignant growth. *Proc. Natl. Acad. Sci.* **69**:2840.

Ingle, D.J. 1958. Urinary glucose and tumor growth in partially depancreatized force-fed rats. *Endocrinology* **62**:78.

Kahn, C.R., D.M. Neville, Jr., and J. Roth. 1973. Insulin-receptor interaction in the obese-hyperglycemic mouse. A model of insulin resistance. *J. Biol. Chem.* **248**:244.

Kahn, R., M. Murray, and J. Pavelic. 1980. Inhibition of proliferation of Cloudman S91 melanoma cells by insulin and characterization of some insulin-resistant variants. *J. Cell Physiol.* **103**:109.

Koroljow, S. 1962. Two cases of malignant tumors with metastases apparently treated successfully with hypoglycemic coma. *Psychiatr. Q.* **36**:262.

Lancaster, H.O. 1954. The mortality in Australia from cancer of the pancreas. *Med. J. Aust.* **1**:596.

Lancaster, H.O. and J.K. Maddox. 1958. Diabetic mortality in Australia. *Australas. Ann. Med.* **7**:145.

LeFevre, P.G. 1959. Molecular structural factors in competitive inhibition of sugar transport. *Science* **130**:104.

Lyons, W.R., C.H. Li, and R.E. Johnson. 1958. The hormonal control of mammary growth and lactation. *Recent Prog. Horm. Res.* 14:219.

Matusik, R.J. and R. Hilf. 1976. Relationship of adenosine 3',5'-cyclic monophosphate and guanosine 3', 5'-cyclic monophosphate to growth of dimethylbenz(a)anthracene-induced mammary tumors in rats. *J. Natl. Cancer Inst.* 56:659.

Morgan, H.E. and C.E. Whitfield. 1974. Regulation of sugar transport in eukaryotic cells. *Curr. Top. Membr. Transp.* 4:225.

Muck, B.R., S. Trotnow, and G. Hommel. 1975. Cancer of the breast, diabetes, and pathologic glucose tolerance. *Arch. Gynaekol.* 220:73.

Muck, B.R., S. Trotnow, H. Egger, and G. Hommel. 1976. Altered carbohydrate metabolism in breast cancer and benign breast affections. *Arch. Gynaekol.* 221:83.

Neufeld, O. 1962. Insulin therapy in terminal cancer: A preliminary report. *J. Am. Geriatr. Soc.* 10:274.

Osborne, C.K. and M.E. Lippman. 1978. Human breast cancer in tissue culture. The effects of hormones. In *Breast cancer* (ed. W.K. McGuire), vol. 2, p.103. Plenum Publishing Corp., New York.

Osborne, C.K., G. Bolan, M.E. Monaco, and M.E. Lippman. 1976. Hormone responsive human breast cancer in long-term tissue culture: Effect of insulin. *Proc. Natl. Acad. Sci.* 73:4536.

Osborne, C.K., M.E. Monaco, M.E. Lippman, and C.R. Kahn. 1978. Correlations among insulin binding, degradation and biologic activity in human breast cancer cells on long-term tissue culture. *Cancer Res.* 38:94.

Pasteels, J.L., J.C. Heuson, J. Heuson-Stiennon, and N. Legros. 1976. Effects of insulin, prolactin, progesterone, and estradiol on DNA synthesis in organ culture of 7,12-dimethylbenz(a)anthracene-induced rat mammary tumors. *Cancer Res.* 36:2162.

Pavelic, K. 1980. Growth of a methylcholanthrene-induced fibrosarcoma in mice with diabetes mellitus. *Eur. J. Cancer* 16:279.

Pavelic, K. and M. Slijepcevic. 1978. Growth of a thymoma in diabetic mice treated with insulin. *Eur. J. Cancer* 14:675.

Pavelic, K., M. Slijepcevic, J. Pavelic, J. Ivic, S. Andy-Jurkovic, Z.P. Pavelic, and M. Boranic. 1979. Growth and treatment of Ehrlich tumor in mice with alloxan-induced diabetes. *Cancer Res.* 39:1807.

Pearson, O.H., O. Llerana, N. Samaan, and D. Gonzalez. 1968. In *Prognostic factors in breast cancer* (ed. A.P.M. Forrest and P.B. Kunkler), p. 421. Williams & Wilkins, Baltimore, Maryland.

Puckett, C.L. and W.W. Shingleton. 1972. The effect of induced diabetes on experimental tumor growth in mice. *Cancer Res.* 32:789.

Repert, R.W. 1952. Breast carcinoma study: Relation to thyroid disease and diabetes. *J. Mich. State Med. Soc.* 51:1315.

Rhomberg, W. 1975. Metastasierendes Mammakarzinom und Diabetes mellitus-seine prognostich günstige Krankheitskombination. *Dtsch. Med. Wochenschr.* 100:2422.

Rillema, J.A. and B.E. Linebaugh. 1977. Characteristics of the insulin stimulation of DNA, RNA and protein metabolism in cultured human mammary carcinoma cells. *Biochim. Biophys. Acta* 475:74.

Salter, J.M., R. Meyer, and C.H. Best. 1958. Effect of insulin and glucagon on tumour growth. *Br. Med. J.* 2:5.

Schultz, G.S. and K.E. Ebner. 1977. Measurement of α-lactalbumin in serum and mammary tumors of rats by radioimmunoassay. *Cancer Res.* 37:4482.

Shafie, S.M. 1980. Estrogen and the growth of breast cancer: New evidence suggests indirect action. *Science* 209:701.

Shafie, S.M. and R. Hilf. 1978. Relationship between insulin and estrogen binding to growth response in 7,12-dimethylbenz(a)anthracene-induced rat mammary tumors. *Cancer Res.* 38:759.

Shafie, S.M., S.L. Gibson, and R. Hilf. 1977. Effect of insulin and estrogen on hormone binding in the R3230AC mammary adenocarcinoma. *Cancer Res.* 37:4641.

Silberstein, F., J. Freud, and T. Revesz. 1927. Versuche, inoperable Carcinome mit Insulin zu behandeln. *Z. Gesamte Exp. Med.* 55:78.

Thomopoulos, P., J. Roth, E. Lovelace, and I. Pastan. 1976. Insulin receptors in normal and transformed fibroblasts: Relationship to growth and transformation. *Cell* 8:417.

Topper, Y.J. and T. Oka. 1974. Some aspects of mammary gland development in the mature mouse. In *Lactation: A comprehensive treatise* (ed. B.L. Larson and V.R Smith), vol. I, p. 327. Academic Press, New York.

Weichselbaum, R.R., J.B. Little, J. Nove, S. Hellman, and A.J. Piro. 1980. Lack of selective killing by steroids in normal and malignant cells. *J. Cell. Physiol.* 103:429.

Welsch, C.W., G.C. de Iturri, and M.J. Brennan. 1976. DNA synthesis of human, mouse and rat mammary carcinomas in vitro. *Cancer* 38:1272.

Wieser, O., M. Pool, and U. Mohr. 1967. Wachstum von Transplantations Tumoren auf Ratten mit Alloxan-diabetes. *Z. Naturwiss. Med. Grundlagenforsch.* 54:23.

Wyche, J.H. and W.D. Noteboom. 1979. Growth regulation of cultured human pituitary cells by steroidal and nonsteroidal compounds in defined medium. *Endocrinology* 104:1765.

COMMENTS

SIITERI: Regarding Dr. Hilf's studies showing effects of estrogen interacting with insulin and also acting on amino acid transport, I would like to ask whether he has looked at the steroid specificity of this effect. Dr. Hilf, do you get the same effect with progesterone, testosterone, or unrelated steroids?

HILF: Yes, we have looked at some other steroids that are representative of other classes. We looked at testosterone and progesterone, as other sex steroids, and at dexamethasone, as a glucocorticoid. All were able to inhibit proline transport, but only dexamethasone was as potent as estradiol-17β based on the estimated inhibition constant (K_i) calculated from the Dixon plot. There were some subtle differences, however, in that dexamethasone also inhibited leucine transport. Testosterone and progesterone also had slight effects on leucine transport. I would also repeat that the effects of estradiol-17β were dose-related, such that significant effects were seen at 10^{-8} M.

SIITERI: I asked that question because we did a study on the effects of steroids on thymidine and glucose uptake by lymphocytes. Using a variety of steroids, you can inhibit uptake of many substances in the concentration range from 1 μM to 10 μM.

HILF: Yes. I think if you get up high enough, you can do that. The highest we looked at was 1 μM.

SIITERI: We have wondered about estrogens producing tumor regressions by a direct effect on the tumor cell, which is what you were proposing. I would suggest that there may be several alternatives. One of them that I favor is that, in fact, you provided a stimulus to the immune system. It has been known for 30 or 40 years that estrogen is a prime stimulator of antibody formation. More recently, it has been shown that the cell-mediated system also can be stimulated by E_2.

So when we see a remission to large doses of estrogen, it may be an indirect effect where the immune system is stimulated to knock off some tumor cells.

HILF: Certainly that is possible. This particular tumor, the R3230AC carcinoma, arose spontaneously in the Fischer rat and has been transplanted in the Fischer rat for the past 15 years. On this basis, the tumor is reasonably compatible with the host.

Again, the question of effects of estrogens relative to the doses employed is certainly an important consideration. We see significant inhibition at 10^{-8} M for estradiol-17β. We also see this with dexamethasone, but not with progesterone and testosterone. What has excited me is that the effect to inhibit entry of substrates is consonant with reduction in growth.

SHELLABARGER: Dr. Hilf, when you make your animals diabetic, some tumors grow, some regress, and some are static. If you don't make your animals diabetic, some tumors grow, some regress, and some are static.

HILF: You are referring to DMBA-induced tumors. Yes, it is true that with this animal model, you will see all types of behavior in the endocrine-intact host. The major difference is in the proportion of tumors that demonstrate progressive growth. Our overall experience is that about 75%-80% of the lesions grow in the intact animal and the remainder either become static or regress. There are several factors here, including the dose of carcinogen used, the way it is administered, the time of the year, etc.

SHELLABARGER: You also must consider the health of the animals.

HILF: Yes, although that is difficult to assess. However, there is little doubt that the proportion of growing, static, and regressing tumors in diabetic rats is significantly different than that seen in the intact animals.

SHELLABARGER: Can you look under a microscope and predict which one is going to regress?

HILF: No.

KORENMAN: Russ [Hilf], are you familiar with the work out of Fred Kerns' group concerning the effect of estrogens on bile flow transport across the hepatic cell membrane? In more or less the same doses that you are using in this case, estrogens have a very interesting effect on the cell membrane of hepatic cells in which they increase the cholesterol ester concentration, increase membrane stiffness, and impair the transport of bile into the bile canaliculus. This effect, by the way, is not a transcriptional effect, in that it is reversible instantaneously by the use of a triton derivative, the specific one that they use in these lipid studies. These results suggest that this is at least a low-dose pharmacologic effect, although it could be achievable in an animal or a person by giving a high enough dose, and that it is a direct effect of the incorporation of estrogen into the cell membrane.

HILF: I am familiar with these data. I also feel that the effects are probably not a transcriptional effect, because we have some very preliminary data on vesicles prepared from membranes of these tumors. We are pursuing this finding, as such a system would allow us to study the membrane effects in the absence of other cellular components.

KORENMAN: Have you tried triton-1368?

HILF: No, we have not tried that.

ROSEN: Russell, do you have any direct evidence that insulin can stimulate the ER content without changing the population of cells. Most of the studies you are doing are in time periods, and you know, receptor levels can be changed in 24 hours. They are cell-cycle-dependent as well. All your studies to me would suggest that you are just changing cell populations and growing static and regressing tumors.

HILF: Do you mean cell size?

ROSEN: No, cell populations. These are heterogeneous populations of cells, some of which have a lot of receptors, some of which have very few receptors. There is no evidence that I know of, but it seems to me that insulin can directly stimulate the synthesis of ER without changing the populations of cells.

HILF: Certainly this is a legitimate concern. Of course, we do not have a technique to assess the alteration in relative proportions of cell populations. For example, if there were cells with high ER and others with low ER, it is possible that removal of insulin causes the high-ER cells to decrease, leaving a lesion with a predominance of low-ER cells and, hence, low ER values. Administration of insulin reverses this process. We then have to consider that insulin treatment, which causes regression of some tumors, would reduce the low ER cell population, because the resulting tumors have higher ER. Although I can't rule this out, we have data from the R3230AC tumor that also implies a role for insulin in regulation of ER, and this tumor system is a more homogeneous system.

NANDI: That is not true. That is impossible.

HILF: What is not true, that the R3230AC tumor is homogeneous?

NANDI: Unless you have a clonally derived line.

HILF: I don't have a clonally derived line.

NANDI: Even the clonally derived lines can change in time.

HILF: I agree. I was referring to the effects seen with cultured R3230AC cells in vitro, in which insulin added to the medium appeared to increase the ER levels.

ROSEN: How long do the changes take? What are the kinetics of the response in vitro?

HILF: In the R3230AC cells, these changes were examined at the end of 4-6 days in culture.

ROSEN: Such changes, if they are really affecting receptor synthesis or turn-over, should be occurring in very rapid kinetics. All of the studies that Jim Clark and other people have done regarding estrogen regulation of its own receptor in the uterus suggest that these kinetics are very rapid. You had very small changes in your cells.

HILF: At this time, the in vitro changes are modest and less than those seen in vivo.

ROSEN: As a result, then, you can't make the statement at the present time that insulin regulates the ERs.

HILF: I didn't say it did regulate them. I said that the data are suggestive of a role of insulin for regulation of ERs.

Pituitary and Steroid Hormones in Radiation-induced Mammary Tumors

CLAIRE J. SHELLABARGER
Medical Department
Brookhaven National Laboratory
Upton, New York 11973

RADIATION-INDUCED CARCINOGENESIS

The radiation-induced *rat* mammary tumor system is, perhaps, the best animal-model system for radiation-induced breast cancer in the human female. This argument (Segaloff 1978; Shellabarger 1978) is based on the following demonstrations:

1. Radiation exposure of the human female increases the risk of breast cancer development. This association between radiation and breast cancer has been accepted by the National Cancer Institute (NCI) ad hoc committee (Upton et al. 1977), the BEIR III Committee (NAS 1980), the United Nations (UNSCEAR 1977), and the National Council on Radiation Protection and Measurements (NCRP) (NCRP 64 1980; NCRP 66 1980). Similarly, radiation exposure of female rats increases mammary carcinogenesis (Shellabarger et al. 1957).

2. Radiation-induced mammary carcinogenesis occurs by a scopal mechanism in both the human female and the female rat. (The word *scopal* means *an effect ascribable to radiation exposure and observed in a region of the body within the irradiation field.*) The evidence for a scopal mechanism of action in the human female comes from the report of Mettler and colleagues (Mettler et al. 1969), who noted an increased risk of breast cancer in women whose breasts were irradiated as a treatment for acute postpartum mastitis, and from the report of MacKenzie (1965), who found breast cancer largely confined to the irradiated breast in unilaterally fluoroscoped patients. Similarly, most of the breast tumors appear in the irradiated mammary tissue in rats receiving partial-body irradiation (Bond et al. 1960b). There is no evidence for a scopal mechanism in the other three species (mice, dogs, and guinea pigs) known to exhibit radiation-induced mammary carcinogenesis. In fact, it is possible to interpret some irradiated mouse data (Furth and Furth 1936) as being consistent with an abscopal mechanism.

In relating some of the radiation studies in rats to the human breast cancer situation in irradiated human females and to chemically-induced mammary carcinogenesis, one must bear in mind that the estrus cycle of rodents is largely a shift in the levels of estrogen, whereas the human menstrual cycle is a shift in levels of both estrogen and progesterone. Thus, any attempt to extrapolate results obtained in rats to the human is complicated not only by the usual unknown factors, but also by this only partially understood difference in endocrinology. Also, the animal data are better used for qualitative extrapolations than for quantitative extrapolations. I agree with Clifton (1978) on this point: "It is almost surely true that absolute dose extrapolation cannot be made from experimental animals to man. However, it seems very likely that the nature of the dose-response curve and probably the effects of fractionation will be found to be similar across species lines."

The important question concerning radiation-induced breast cancer of the human female is a two-part question, with probably interrelated answers. What is the shape of the dose-effect curve, and is there a smaller effect when the dose is spread out in time? That is, does the effect per rad decrease with dose and time between successive doses? Many review groups of the human breast cancer data (UNSCEAR 1977; NCRP 64 1980; NRCP 66 1980) believe it would be prudent to accept a linear dose-effect with no dose-rate sparing effect. The BEIR III report (NAS 1980) is an exception. This committee believes that "the linear model probably leads to overestimates of the risk of most cancers" and that "the quadratic model may be used to define the lower limits of risk," and it recognizes, somewhat paradoxically, "that dose rate may affect the risk of cancer induction, but believes that the information available in man is insufficient to adjust for it." The BEIR III committee did not unanimously agree, as there were two minority opinions.

The rat data concerned with dose-effect are, in my opinion, not very helpful. In the first instance, some of the data have been reported in terms of mammary neoplasia, where mammary neoplasia includes mostly mammary fibroadenomas and only a few mammary adenocarcinomas. Some of the data have been reported only over relatively short periods of time, which means the process of radiation-induced acceleration was studied rather than an increase in tumor incidence. Some of the studies were done on hormonally stimulated animals, which complicates interpretation (Bond et al. 1960a, Shellabarger et al. 1969; Clifton and Crowley 1978). Within these limitations, these authors believe their data are consistent with a linear dose-effect relationship. It must be pointed out that the dose range studied probably included doses large enough to produce cell-killing, and, in my opinion, the statistical analysis was often not rigorous enough to exclude other shapes of the dose-effect curve.

I know of only a single report in which mammary adenocarcinoma incidence in rats not treated with hormones was studied after X-rays over the entire life-span (Shellabarger et al. 1980a). This study included 167 control rats, and 95, 48, and 48 rats exposed to 28, 56, and 85 rad, respectively. The authors concluded that "the number of radiation-induced adenocarcinomas is too small to permit definite statements on the dose-effect relationships."

If the rat studies have not been productive in regard to the understanding of dose-effect relationships, and if it is unlikely, because of the large sample size required (Dethlefsen et al. 1978), that studies of irradiated human females will be helpful, where do we go from here? As has been pointed out by my colleague Dr. V.P. Bond (1979), there are good theoretical reasons for believing that dose and dose-rate are interrelated (for a detailed presentation of the following argument, see pages 5-21 of NCRP 64 1980). Briefly, it is assumed that initiation occurs by the way of a lesion, presumably in DNA. Each lesion is made up of two combined sublesions, each of which can undergo repair. The maximum buildup of sublesions, maximum interaction, and lack of repair will occur at high dose rates and at high doses. With either a lowering of dose rate or a lowering of dose, the buildup of sublesions will be less, interaction will be less, and the time for possible repair will increase. Thus, the effect of lowering dose or dose rate will be the same. Rather than studying dose-effect relationships at smaller and smaller doses, with vanishingly smaller and smaller responses, it may be more efficient to select a single dose that produces a measurable effect and study this dose at lower dose rates to see if the effect is lost or reaches a limiting value. For several animal tumor systems (NCRP 64 1980), the carcinogenic effect does diminish with decreasing dose rate. We propose a larger version of a previous experiment that was reported only in abstract form (Shellabarger and Brown 1972). Here, the mammary neoplastic response of female Sprague-Dawley rats was studied for 336 days after a single exposure to 88 R or 265 R at a dose rate of either 0.03 or 10 R/min. After 265 R, at 0.03 R/min, 4 of 35 rats (11.4%) developed one or more mammary adenocarcinomas, and in 10 R/min, the response was 7 of 20 (35%). A chi-square value, with Yates correction, of 3.01 ($P < 08$) was obtained. However, if the time of appearance was taken into account, by using the Cox test or K-W analysis (Thomas et al. 1977), then the response to 265 R at 0.03 R/min was less than the response to 265 R at 10 R/min at $P < 04$ and $P < 02$, respectively (Fig. 1). These data do not establish whether or not a dose-rate-sparing effect obtains for radiation-induced mammary carcinogenesis in the rat, but they do suggest that additional study of dose rate in this system might be worthwhile.

As noted earlier, we believe that the rat mammary adenocarcinoma response to irradiation can serve as a model system for mammary carcinogenesis in the human. In addition, I would now like to interject a brief discussion on the rat mammary fibroadenoma response to irradiation. First, because radiation exposure tends to increase nonmalignant breast tumors in the human female (Shore et al. 1977), the study of radiation-induced mammary fibroadenomas in irradiated female rats may serve as a model system for this situation. Second, although X-ray exposure of female Sprague-Dawley rats does increase the incidence of rats with one or more mammary fibroadenomas (Fig. 2), lowering the dose rate did not change the mammary fibroadenoma response. Third, the

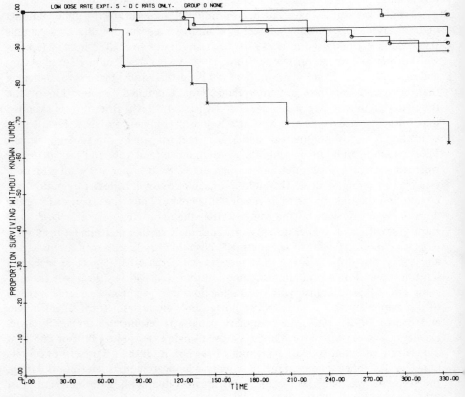

Figure 1
A plot of the proportion of rats without a mammary adenocarcinoma against days after irradiation. Significant comparisons of irradiated vs nonirradiated and 10 R/min vs .03 R/min at the same total dose are given below for each test along with the P value. 265 R at 10 R/min vs no radiation; chi-square = .0001, Cox = .001, K/W = .001. 265 R at 0.03 R/min vs no radiation; K/W = .0387. 265 R at 10 R/min vs 265 R at 0.03 R/min; Cox = .0384, K/W = .0111. (3) Group 0, no radiation; (○) group 1, 88 R at 0.03 R/min; (△) group 2, 88 R at 10 R/min; (+) group 3, 265 R at 0.03 R/min; (×) group 4, 265 R at 10 R/min.

data on 149 irradiated rats show that 13 rats developed only adenocarcinomas, 49 developed only fibroadenomas, 6 rats developed both adenocarcinomas and fibroadenomas, and 81 rats developed no mammary neoplasms of either kind. Analysis of these data (Brown and Hollander 1977) disclosed that the development of mammary adenocarcinomas and mammary fibroadenomas are ($P < 001$) likely to be independent processes. Similar findings have been reported for DMBA and procarbazine (Shellabarger et al. 1979), indicating that perhaps some

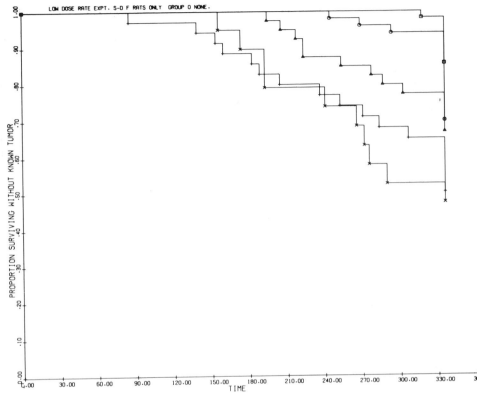

Figure 2
A plot of the proportion of rats without a mammary fibroadenoma against days after irradiation. Significant comparisons of irradiated vs nonirradiated are given below. There were no significant comparisons between dose rates at either dose. 265 R at 10 R/min vs no radiation; chi-square = .0021, Cox .001, K/W .001. 265 R at 0.03 R/min vs no radiation; chi-square = .005, Cox = .0001, K/W .001. 88 R at 10 R/min vs no radiation; chi-square = .0409, Cox = .0238, K/W = .0088. 85 R at 0.03 R/min vs no radiation; K/W .0445. See Fig. 1 legend for explanation of symbols.

rats are programmed to develop adenocarcinomas and others are programmed to develop fibroadenomas in response to carcinogens. If so, it might be worthwhile to compare, endocrinologically, the rats that develop only adenocarcinomas to those that develop only fibroadenomas. Russo et al. (1977) present morphological evidence for two independent processes when they state, "Adenocarcinomas result when the target of the carcinogenic stimulus is the terminal end bud. Benign lesions . . . are derived from more differentiated portions of the gland, namely, the alveolar buds and lobules."

CHEMICALLY-INDUCED CARCINOGENESIS

The fact that both radiation and certain chemicals induce mammary carcinogenesis in rats allows one to compare the mechanisms of chemical carcinogenesis and radiation carcinogenesis. There have been many more studies of chemical carcinogenesis than of radiation carcinogenesis (Dr. Huggins often refers to 7,12-dimethylbenz[a]anthracene [DMBA] as the poor man's radiation). When both carcinogens have been compared, the results have often been similar. Some of these comparisons have included the following:

1. the enhancement of chemically induced mammary carcinogenesis and radiation-induced mammary carcinogenesis by diets with a high fat content (Silverman et al. 1980);
2. the inhibition of both chemically induced (Yamura et al. 1978) and radiation-induced (Troll et al. 1980) mammary carcinogenesis by diets containing large amounts of protease inhibitors;
3. a synergistic interaction of both radiation (Segaloff and Maxfield 1971) and DMBA (Shellabarger et al. 1980b) with diethylstilbestrol (DES) on mammary adenocarcinoma formation in ACI rats;
4. the stimulation of both chemically induced and radiation-induced mammary carcinogenesis by prolactin-secreting transplantable pituitary tumors (Yokoro et al. 1977);
5. a correlation of strain-related sensitivity to both chemicals and radiation (Shellabarger 1972).

Additional evidence that chemically induced mammary carcinogenesis and radiation-induced mammary carcinogenesis are similar was the finding of additivity when the two carcinogens were given in combination (Shellabarger 1967). The similarities between the chemical and physical carcinogens can be extended further in terms of their scopal mechanism of action. Either carcinogen is effective when applied directly to the mammary gland (Dao 1970; Shellabarger 1971). If it is true that the rat X-ray-induced rat mammary carcinogenesis model is a good model for human breast cancer and if both chemically induced and radiation-induced mammary carcinogenesis share a common scopal mechanism, then it is only a matter of time before it can be demonstrated that chemical carcinogens (including environmental pollutants?) are associated with human breast cancer. Some authors who have studied hair dye use and breast cancer incidence (Shore et al. 1979) have expressed this view.

There are of course known differences between chemically induced mammary carcinogenesis and radiation-induced rat mammary carcinogenesis. One of these differences concerns the regional, anatomical distribution of the tumors. When rats are given total-body X-rays, the mammary adenocarcinomas and mammary fibroadenomas tend to occur at random in the four quadrants of breast tissue, but when either DMBA or procarbazine is given by stomach tube, more of these tumors tend to occur in the anterior quadrants (Shellabarger et al. 1979). We argued that the random distribution of tumors following total-body X-irradiation indicates that the amount of breast tissue in the anterior and posterior halves of the animal must be essentially equal. This led us to conclude that the chemical carcinogens were delivered, perhaps because of different clearance rates or other vascular differences, in larger amounts to the anterior quadrants.

A more troublesome difference between mammary carcinogenesis induced by chemicals and that induced by radiation concerns age-related sensitivity. Dao (1969) showed conclusively that 120-175-day-old rats gave a smaller adenocarcinoma response to DMBA than 50-day-old rats. Previously, Huggins et al. (1961) had indicated that 50-66-day-old rats gave a larger mammary adenocarcinoma response than did younger or older rats. On the other hand, we found rats of 42, 84, or 225 days about equally sensitive to total body X-irradiation (Shellabarger 1974), as did Huggins and Fukuniski (1963) for rats of 52 and 162 days of age. It is tempting to correlate the age-related sensitivity to chemical carcinogens with the age-related developmental structure of the mammary gland, as so elegantly described by the Russos (Russo and Russo 1978a,b).

We have no explanation for the mechanism that allows age-related sensitivity for chemical carcinogens and no such age-related sensitivity for radiation other than to suggest that the target cell for radiation might be a "stem cell" that does not change its numbers with age, whereas more highly differentiated cells that do change their numbers are the targets for chemicals. From our literature review, we have been unable to answer the question of whether or not the age-related sensitivity for chemical carcinogens is specific for polycyclic hydrocarbons, because we have found no references to water-soluble carcinogens and age-related sensitivity. It should also be pointed out that the human female, in contrast to the female rat, does indeed show an age-related sensitivity to radiation exposure, as the risk "was heavily dependent on age at exposure" (Land et al. 1980).

Another large difference in mammary carcinogenesis following either X-irradiation or administration of chemical carcinogens concerns the physiological state of the mammary gland at the time of carcinogen administration. Dao (1971) showed clearly that pregnant rats and lactating rats give a much smaller response than virgin rats to 3-methylcholanthrene (3-MC). This is not true for X-rays (Shellabarger 1976; S. Holtzman et al., unpubl.), as virgin, pregnant, and lactating rats all give essentially the same response to X-irradiation. In irradiated women, the risk per rad was not very different for lactating women than for nonlactating women (Land et al. 1980), suggesting that the lactating breast and the nonlactating breast are about equally sensitive. The mechanism that allows radiation carcinogenesis to be independent of and chemical carcinogenesis to be dependent on the physiological state of the mammary gland at the time of carcinogen is not obvious to me, although the clearance of the chemical carcinogen (Dao 1971), the morphology of the gland

(Russo and Russo 1980), and the cell kinetics of the gland (Russo and Russo 1978a,b) probably all play interacting roles.

I think that mammary carcinogenesis (adenocarcinoma formation) and mammary tumorigenesis (fibroadenoma formation) are independent processes, at least in noninbred Sprague-Dawley rats. Further, if one counts the number of tumors per rat, one is struck by the finding that many rats have 2-10 or more tumors per individual rat. If the distribution of the number of tumors per rat is tested against a Poisson distribution, the departure from a Poisson distribution is obvious: There is an "overdispersion." An interpretation of these findings is that the development of multiple tumors in a Sprague-Dawley rat is not an independent process. Clifton and Crowley (1978) recognized this: "multiple mammary tumors do not occur independently, i.e., a first mammary neoplasm significantly increases the probability of development of another neoplasm." We pointed out that "there may be inherent differences in the tumor rate between animals" (Shellabarger et al. 1980a) and that "this does not necessarily mean that the presence of a mammary adenocarcinoma predisposes the animal to the development of an additional mammary adenocarcinoma. Rather, it may mean that there are inherent differences among rats as to their capacity to develop multiple mammary adenocarcinomas" (Shellabarger et al. 1980b). Human breast cancer has been discussed in terms of a multicentric disease.

ESTROGEN SYNERGISM IN MAMMARY CARCINOGENESIS

The first and major discovery about estrogen synergism in mammary carcinogenesis was Segaloff's and Maxfield's (1971) demonstration that the interaction between DES and X-irradiation is synergistic in regard to adenocarcinoma formation in ACI rats. They also showed that the synergism between DES and X-rays occurs only in irradiated mammary tissue, that is, by a scopal mechanism. It was then shown (Segaloff 1973) that progesterone protects against the DES-radiation synergism and that the synergism is radiation dose-dependent (Segaloff and Pettigrew 1978). Segaloff (1974) also showed that an intact ovary is required for the mammary adenocarcinoma response to DES. (I am aware that Dr. Segaloff has been studying the effect of prior pregnancy on this synergism, but I do not know the results.)

In a group of papers from Brookhaven, we have shown the following: the synergism between X-radiation and DES could be extended to neutron radiation and DES (Shellabarger et al. 1976); the synergism between radiation and DES could not be extended to Sprague-Dawley rats (Shellabarger et al. 1978) or to Fischer rats (Holtzman et al. 1979a); the synergism between radiation and DES could be extended to include radiation and ethinyl-estradiol (Holtzman et al. 1979b); the synergism between radiation and DES could be extended to DMBA and DES (Shellabarger et al. 1980b); and the synergism between radiation and DES is DES dose-dependent (Stone et al. 1980). Because the synergism between radiation and DES in ACI rats was accompanied by a huge prolactin response to DES, and because the lack of synergism between radiation and DES was accompanied by a very modest prolactin response in Sprague-Dawley rats, we have suggested (Stone et al. 1979; Holtzman et al. 1979c) that the synergism between radiation and DES is, at least in part, a synergism between radiation and prolactin.

The synergistic interaction between DES and radiation in ACI rats pertains mostly to the number of adenocarcinomas per rat. Often, so many tumors appear that they cannot be counted accurately. Segaloff (Segaloff and Maxfield 1971) have termed this "essentially total carcinogenesis" and this is illustrated in Figure 3. I am not sure how this system can be used as a model for human mammary carcinogenesis. However, in terms of general principles of carcinogenesis, this system has made one contribution. We have found Stone et al. 1980) that DES given as much as 200 days after X-irradiation still results in synergism. Following the reasoning of Yokoro (Yokoro et al. 1977), we suggest that DES can "rescue" long-dormant initiated cells and turn them into tumors. This could mean, in terms of the initiation-promotion hypothesis, that there are

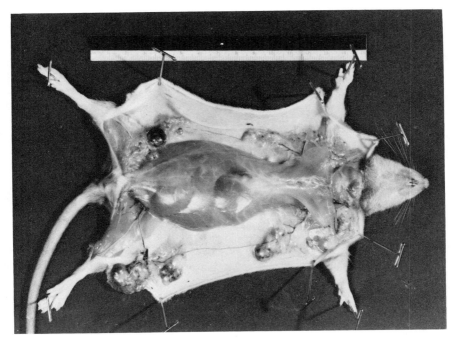

Figure 3
Female ACI rat given a 20-mg pellet of 25% DES and 75% cholesterol on the 60th day of age, and 9.6 rad of 0.43 MeV neutrons on the 62nd day of age, and killed on the 200th day of age.

"initiated" women who will develop breast cancer if they are "promoted," even if the promotion occurs years after initiation. This suggestion is, I believe, compatible with the estrogen-window hypothesis of Korenman (1980).

ACKNOWLEDGMENTS

Portions of this research were supported by the National Cancer Institute (contract nos. Y01-CP-3021, Y01-CP-30213, and Y01-CP-60219). Brookhaven National Laboratory is operated by Associated Universities, Inc., under contract no. DE-AC02-76-CH00016 with the U.S. Department of Energy. Excellent technical assistance has been provided by John P. Shanley, Elizabeth M. Jellett, Mary R. Snead, Lindora Boyd, and Robert A. Brown. Computer programming and computer operation were done by Howard R. Pate. Many of the experiments discussed herein were done with the participation of Victor P. Bond, Eugene Cronkite, Seymour Holtzman, and J. Patrick Stone. Portions of the text reflect helpful discussions with Seymour Holtzman, J. Patrick Stone, and V. P. Bond.

REFERENCES

Bond, V.P. 1979. Quantitative risk in radiation protection standards. *Radiat. Environ. Biophys.* 17:1.

Bond, V.P., E.P. Cronkite, S.W. Lippincott, and C.J. Shellabarger. 1960a. Studies on radiation-induced mammary gland neoplasia in the rat. III. Relation of the neoplastic response to dose of total-body radiation. *Radiat. Res.* 12:276.

Bond, V.P., C.J. Shellabarger, E.P. Cronkite, and T.M. Fliedner. 1960b. Studies on radiation-induced mammary gland neoplasia in the rat. V. Induction by localized radiation. *Radiat. Res.* 13:318.

Brown, W.B., Jr. and M. Hollander. 1977. Comparing two success probabilities. In *Statistics, a biomedical introduction,* p. 173. John Wiley and Sons, Inc., New York.

Clifton, K.H. 1978. Discussion of research approaches relevant to mammography. *J. Natl. Cancer Inst.* 61:1544.

Clifton, K.H. and J.J. Crowley. 1978. Effects of radiation type and dose and the role of glucocorticoids, gonadectomy, and thyroidectomy in mammary tumor induction in mammotropin-secreting pituitary tumor-grafted rats. *Cancer Res.* 38:1507.

Dao, T.L. 1969. Mammary cancer induction by 7,12-dimethylbenzanthracene. Relation to age. *Science* 165:810.

————. 1970. Induction of mammary cancer after in vitro exposure to 7,12-dimethylbenz(a)anthracene. *Proc. Soc. Exp. Biol. Med.* 133:416.

————. 1971. Inhibition of tumor induction in chemical carcinogenesis in the mammary gland. *Prog. Exp. Tumor Res.* 14:59.

Dethlefsen, L.A., J.M. Brown, A.V. Carrano, and S. Nandi. 1978. Can animal and in vitro studies give new relevant answers to questions concerning mammographic screening for human breast cancer? *J. Natl Cancer Inst.* 61:1537.

Furth, J. and O.B. Furth. 1936. Neoplastic disease produced in mice by general irradiation with x-rays. I. Incidence and types of neoplasms. *Am. J. Cancer* 28:54.

Holtzman, S., J.P. Stone, and C.J. Shellabarger. 1979a. Synergism of diethylstilbestrol and radiation in female Fischer 344 rats. *J. Natl. Cancer Inst.* 63:1071.

_____. 1979b. Synergistic interactions of estrogens and x-rays on mammary carcinogenesis in female ACI rats. *Cancer Treat. Rep.* 63:1180.

_____. 1979c. Influence of diethylstilbestrol treatment on prolactin cells of female ACI and Sprague-Dawley rats. *Cancer Res.* 39:779.

Huggins, C. and R. Fukuniski. 1963. Cancer in the rat after single exposures to irradiation or hydrocarbons. *Radiat. Res.* 20:493.

Huggins, C., L.C. Grand, and F.P. Brillantes. 1961. Mammary cancer induced by a single feeding of polynuclear hydrocarbons, and its suppression. *Nature* 189:204.

Korenman, S.G. 1980. Oestrogen window hypothesis of the aetiology of breast cancer. *Lancet* i:700.

Land, C.E., J.D. Boice, Jr., R.E. Shore, J.E. Normal, and M. Tokunaga. 1980. Breast cancer risk from low-dose exposures to ionizing radiation. Results of parallel analysis of three exposed populations of women. *J. Natl. Cancer Inst.* 65:353.

MacKenzie, I. 1965. Breast cancer following multiple fluoroscopies. *Br. J. Cancer* 19:1.

Mettler, F.A., Jr., L.H. Hempelmann, A.M. Dutton, J.W. Pifer, E.T. Toyooka, and W.R. Ames. 1969. Breast neoplasms in women treated with x-rays for acute postpartum mastitis. A pilot study. *J. Natl. Cancer Inst.* 43:803.

National Academy of Sciences (NAS). 1980. The effects on populations of exposure to low levels of ionizing radiation. *Report of the Advisory Committee on the Biological Effects of Ionizing Radiation.* National Research Council, Washington, D.C.

National Council on Radiation Protection and Measurements (NCRP 64). 1980. *Influence of dose and its distribution in time on dose-response relationships for low-LET radiations.* NCRP, Washington, D.C.

_____ (NCRP 66). 1980. *Mammography.* NCRP, Washington, D.C.

Russo, I.H. and J. Russo. 1978a. Developmental stage of the rat mammary gland as determinant of its susceptibility to 7,12-dimethylbenz(a)anthracene. *J. Natl. Cancer Inst.* 61:1439.

Russo, J. and I.H. Russo. 1978b. DNA labeling index and structure of the rat mammary gland as determinants of its susceptibility to carcinogenesis. *J. Natl. Cancer Inst.* 61:1451.

_____. 1980. Influence of differentiation and cell kinetics on the susceptibility of the rat mammary gland to carcinogenesis. *Cancer Res.* 40:2677.

Russo, J., J. Saby, W.M. Isenberg, and I.H. Russo. 1977. Pathogenesis of mammary carcinomas induced in rats by 7,12-dimethylbenz(a)anthracene. *J. Natl. Cancer Inst.* 435:1977.

Segaloff, A. 1973. Inhibition by progesterone of radiation-estrogen-induced mammary cancer in the rat. *Cancer Res.* 33:1136.

―――――. 1974. The role of the ovary in estrogen production of mammary cancer in the rat. *Cancer Res.* **34**:2708.

―――――. 1978. Discussion of research approaches relevant to mammography. *J. Natl. Cancer Inst.* **61**:1544.

Segaloff, A. and W.S. Maxfield. 1971. The synergism between radiation and estrogen in the production of mammary cancer in the rat. *Cancer Res.* **31**:1661.

Segaloff, A. and H.M. Pettigrew. 1978. Effect of radiation dosage on the synergism between radition and estrogen in the production of mammary cancer in the rat. *Cancer Res.* **38**:3445.

Shellabarger, C.J. 1967. Effect of 3-methylcholanthrene and x-irradiation, given singly or combined on rat mammary carcinogenesis. *J. Natl. Cancer Inst.* **38**:73.

―――――. 1971. Induction of mammary neoplasia after in vitro exposure to x-rays. *Proc. Soc. Exp. Biol. Med.* **136**:1103.

―――――. 1972. Mammary neoplastic response of Lewis and Sprague-Dawley female rats to 7,12-dimethylbenz(a)anthracene or x-ray. *Cancer Res.* **32**: 883.

―――――. 1974. A comparison of rat mammary carcinogenesis following total-body irradiation at different ages. *5th Int. Cong. Rad. Res.* (Abstr. 103).

―――――. 1976. Modifying factors in rat mammary carcinogenesis. In *Biology of radiation carcinogenesis* (ed. J.M. Yuhas et al.), p. 31. Raven Press, New York.

―――――. 1978. Discussion of research approaches relevant to mammography. *J. Natl. Cancer Inst.* **61**:1545.

Shellabarger, C.J. and R.D. Brown. 1972. Rat mammary neoplasia following ^{60}Co irradiation at 0.03R or 10R per minute. *Radiat. Res.* **51**:493. (Abstr.)

Shellabarger, C.J., J.P. Stone, and S. Holtzman. 1976. The synergism between neutron radiation and diethylstilbestrol in the production of mammary adenocarcinomas in the rat. *Cancer Res.* **36**:1019.

―――――. 1978. Rat strain differences in mammary tumor induction with estrogen and neutron radiation. *J. Natl. Cancer Inst.* **61**:1505.

Shellabarger, C.J., S. Holtzman, and J.P. Stone. 1979. Apparent rat strain-related sensitivity to phorbol promotion of mammary carcinogenesis. *Cancer Res.* **39**:3345.

Shellabarger, C.J., D. Chmelevsky, and A.M. Kellerer. 1980a. Induction of mammary neoplasms in the Sprague-Dawley rat by 430 keV neutrons and x-rays. *J. Natl. Cancer Inst.* **64**:821.

Shellabarger, C.J., E.P. Cronkite, V.P. Bond, and S.W. Lippincott. 1957. The occurrence of mammary tumors in the rat after sublethal whole-body irradiation. *Radiat. Res.* **6**:501.

Shellabarger, C.J., V.P. Bond, E.P. Cronkite, and G.E. Aponte. 1969. Relationship of dose of total-body ^{60}Co radiation to incidence of mammary neoplasia in female rats. In *Radiation-induced cancer*, p. 161. International Atomic Energy Agency, Vienna.

Shellabarger, C.J., B. McKnight, J.P. Stone, and S. Holtzman. 1980b. Interaction of dimethylbenzanthracene and diethylstilbestrol on mammary adenocarcinoma formation in female ACI rats. *Cancer Res.* **40**:1808.

Shore, R.E., B.S. Pasternack, E.U. Thiessen, M. Sadow, R. Forbes, and R.E. Albert. 1979. A case-control study of hair dye use and breast cancer. *J. Natl. Cancer Inst.* **62**:277.

Shore, R.E., L.H. Hempelmann, E. Kowaluk, P.S. Mansur, B.S. Pasternack, R.E. Albert, and G.E. Haughie. 1977. Breast neoplasms in women with x-rays for acute postpartum mastitis. *J. Natl. Cancer Inst.* **59**:813.

Silverman, J., C.J. Shellabarger, S. Holtzman, J.P. Stone, and J.H. Weisburger. 1980. Effect of dietary fat on x-ray-induced mammary cancer in Sprague-Dawley rats. *J. Natl. Cancer Inst.* **64**:634.

Stone, J.P., S. Holtzman, and C.J. Shellabarger. 1979. Neoplastic responses and correlated plasma prolactin levels in diethylstilbestrol-treated ACI and Sprague-Dawley rats. *Cancer Res.* **39**:773.

_____. 1980. Synergistic interactions of various doses of DES and x-irradiation on mammary neoplasia in female ACI rats. *Cancer Res.* **40**:396.

Thomas, D.G., N. Breslow, and J.J. Gart. 1977. Trend and homogenity analyses of proportions and life table data. *Comp. Biomed. Res.* **10**:373.

Troll, W., R. Wiesner, C.J. Shellabarger, S. Holtzman, and J.P. Stone. 1980. Soybean diet lowers breast tumor incidence in irradiated rats. *Carcinogenesis* **1**:469.

United Nations Scientific Committee on the Effects of Atomic Radiation (UNSCEAR). 1977. Sources and Effects of Ionizing Radiation. *Report to the General Assembly, with Annexes Publ. E77IX1.* United Nations, New York.

Upton, A.C., G.W. Beebe, J.M. Brown, E.H. Quimby, and C.J. Shellabarger. 1977. Report of NCI ad hoc working group on the risks associated with mammography in mass screening for the detection of breast cancer. *J. Natl. Cancer Inst.* **59**:479.

Yamura, M., N. Nakamura, Y. Fukui, C. Takamura, M. Yamamoto, Y. Minato, Y. Tamura, and S. Fujui. 1978. Inhibition of 7,12-dimethylbenz(a)anthracene induced mammary tumorigenesis in rats by a synthetic protease inhibitor, *N, N*-dimethyl-(*p* (*p* guani-dinobenzoyloxy)) benzie-carbonyloxyglycolate. *Gann* **69**:749.

Yokoro, K., M. Nakano, A. Ito, K. Nagao, Y. Kodama, and K. Hamada. 1977. Role of prolactin in rat mammary carcinogenesis: Detection of carcinogenicity of low-dose carcinogens and of persisting dormant cancer cells. *J. Natl. Cancer Inst.* **58**:1777.

Influence of Pregnancy and Lactation on Experimental Mammary Carcinogenesis

RICHARD C. MOON
Life Sciences Division
IIT Research Institute
Chicago, Illinois 60616

There is general agreement that mammary carcinoma occurs with the greatest frequency in women after the reproductive years. Haagensen (1956) has estimated that approximately 75% of all breast cancers in women are evident clinically beyond the childbearing years. The estimate of Lewison (1962) is somewhat less, being on the order of 60-65%. Although several factors undoubtedly are involved in the etiology of cancer of the breast, most of the statistics available indicate that mammary carcinoma occurs more frequently in nulliparous than in multiparous women (Wynder et al. 1960; Lewison 1962).

It is equally well established that chemically induced mammary cancer in the rat is also affected by pregnancy and lactation. Dao and Sunderland (1959), using 3-methylcholanthrene (3-MC), observed an increase in induction rate during pregnancy followed by a regression of all tumors during the subsequent lactation. Huggins et al. (1962) observed that rats mated 15 days after the administration of 7,12-dimethylbenz[a]anthracene (DMBA) exhibited an increased number of tumors per animal and a decrease in the latent period of tumor appearance. However, tumor growth patterns in the subsequent lactation were not reported.

McCormick and myself (1965) have also shown that pregnancy accelerates the appearance of DMBA-induced mammary cancer, irrespective of whether it ensues prior to or after the appearance of palpable tumors. In animals mated after tumor appearance, well-established tumors grew at a faster rate and new cancers appeared at a relatively rapid rate. During lactation, however, many tumor growth patterns were observed. The majority of DMBA-induced mammary tumors regressed during lactation to one-half their size at parturition, but some maintained a constant size and others continued to grow rapidly. Furthermore, it was shown (McCormick and Moon 1967a) that maintenance of tumor size or continued growth during lactation was highly dependent on the suckling stimulus, as virtually all tumors regressed when the young were removed from the dam at birth. Moreover, a greater number of growing tumors were observed in dams nursing larger litters, indicating that the frequency and intensity of the suckling stimulus was involved intimately in continued tumor growth during the postpartum period.

In a subsequent study of the endocrine factors affecting postpartum growth of mammary tumors, we (McCormick and Moon 1967b) found that ovariectomy performed on day 2 of lactation abolished the tumor growth stimulating effect of suckling. Although prolactin maintained postpartum tumor growth in the nonnursed rat, it was ineffective in maintaining tumor growth in the ovariectomized lactating rat. Progesterone, on the other hand, stimulated growth of tumors during the postpartum period in the ovariectomized lactator. Thus, the maintenance of tumor size and growth during lactation probably was due to the effect of progestin released as a result of the suckling stimulus. It is apparent, therefore, that both pregnancy and lactation have a profound effect on mammary cancer induced with chemical carcinogens.

I have also investigated the relationship between previous reproductive history of the Sprague-Dawley rat and DMBA-induced mammary carcinogenesis (Moon 1969). In these studies, virgin animals receiving DMBA at 190 days old exhibited a 39% incidence of mammary cancer. Rats undergoing a single pregnancy or a single pregnancy followed by a subsequent nursing period exhibited a decrease in mammary cancer incidence and an increase in the tumor latent period. Animals subjected to two pregnancies or lactations exhibited a significant decrease in mammary cancer incidence and a prolonged tumor latent period when compared with virgin control animals, although tumor incidence did not vary greatly from that of animals undergoing a single pregnancy and lactation. Thus, the effect of previous pregnancies and lactations on mammary cancer incidence in rats appeared to be similar to that found in the human female.

Although increased parity is associated with a decreased risk for breast cancer in women, the protective effect is limited essentially to the age at which the woman bears her first full-term child. Since DMBA-induced mammary carcinogenesis in the rat is also influenced by parity, studies were initiated to determine whether or not the age at which the first litter is borne has an effect upon DMBA-induced mammary carcinogenesis when initiated at a subsequent period in the life of the animal.

METHODS

Mammary Tumor Incidence

Sprague-Dawley female rats were received from the dealer 3 weeks prior to mating. At either 50, 145, or 235 days of age, females were placed with males of the same strain and from the same source for 5 days. Pregnant rats were housed separately in cages so constructed that the offspring fell away from the dams at parturition, thus preventing suckling. At age 300 days, each primiparous rat received 20 mg DMBA by intragastric instillation. Animals that received the carcinogen were palpated twice each week and were maintained until sacrificed at 525-565 days of age. Virgin control rats received either no

DMBA or 20 mg DMBA at 300 days old, and were sacrificed at the time that the primiparous rats were killed.

Another group of virgin animals and a group of primiparous rats mated at 50 days of age received DMBA at age 91 days and were maintained until 340-345 days of age. At sacrifice, all tumors were removed and processed for histopathologic evaluation.

DMBA Binding

The binding of DMBA to mammary parenchymal cell DNA was determined in groups of primiparous rats mated at 50, 145, or 235 days of age. At age 300 days, each primiparous rat received 20 mg DMBA containing 2.5 mCi [^{3}H]DMBA. At 3, 16, 24, and 48 hours following DMBA administration, groups of rats were killed, mammary glands removed, and the parenchymal cells isolated according to the procedure of Moon et al. (1969). The mammary parenchymal cells were homogenized in 0.15% NaCl:0.015 M sodium citrate (pH 7.0) containing 1% SDS. DNA was extracted from the homogenate with water-saturated phenol followed by another extraction with chloroform:isoamyl alcohol (10:1, v/v) and then precipitated with 2 volumes of cold ethanol. The purified DNA was dissolved in deionized water and hydrolyzed with hot 0.5 N perchloric acid. [^{3}H]DMBA radioactivity in an aliquot of hydrolysate was determined using Searle Mark III liquid scintillation spectrometer. DNA content was measured by the diphenylamine procedure.

Virgin animals receiving [^{3}H]DMBA at either 50 or 300 days of age served as controls and were sacrificed at the time points indicated for the primiparous rats.

Hormone Responsiveness

Primiparous rats mated at 50, 145, or 235 days of age received 20 mg DMBA by stomach tube at 300 days of age. When the first palpable tumor attained a diameter of 1 cm, the rat was ovariectomized. Tumors were measured with vernier calipers three times each week and the number of tumors regressing significantly was recorded. The rats bearing tumors that regressed to one-third the size at ovariectomy were injected with 5 μg estradiol benzoate for 10 days followed by 5 μg estradiol benzoate and 6 mg progesterone for another 10 days if the tumor had not attained its original size in response to estradiol alone. Virgin animals served as controls.

RESULTS

Mammary Tumor Incidence

The incidence of mammary tumors of primiparous rats bearing their first litter at different ages is shown in Figure 1. As shown, virgin animals fed DMBA at age 300 days and sacrificed at age 531 days exhibited a tumor incidence of 79%.

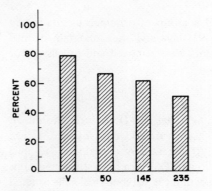

Figure 1
Percentage of mammary tumor incidence in virgin (V) rats and primiparous rats mated at 50, 145, and 235 days of age. All rats received 20 mg DMBA at age 300 days and were sacrificed at approximately age 525 days.

The tumor incidence in primiparous rats mated at 50 days of age was reduced to 67% when compared with that of virgin controls. A further decrease in tumor incidence was evident in animals mated at ages 145 and 235 days; these animals exhibited a tumor incidence of 62% and 52%, respectively. Furthermore, it appeared that the differences in tumor incidence between rats bearing their first litter at different ages was due primarily to a difference in the incidence of benign tumors. As indicated in Table 1, there was a progressive decrease in benign tumor incidence and tumor number from that exhibited by virgin animals

Table 1
Effect of Age at First Litter on Incidence of Benign Mammary Tumors Induced with DMBA

Reproductive history	Age at administration of DMBA (days)	Number rats	Number rats with tumors	Tumor incidence (%)	Total number tumors
Virgin	no DMBA	37	8	22.0	10
Virgin	91	15	15	100	19
Mated-50 days[a]	91	30	17	54.8	26
Virgin	300	89	35	39.3	63
Mated-50 days[a]	300	109	37	34.0	94
Mated-145 days[a]	300	92	28	30.4	67
Mated-235 days[a]	300	118	24	20.3	53

[a]One male caged with three females for 5 days beginning at the indicated age of the female.

to that of primiparous animals bearing their first litter at the later ages. Although mammary cancer incidence was reduced in animals bearing a single litter, as evidenced by a reduction in cancer incidence from 52% in virgin animals to approximately 30% in primiparous rats (Table 2), no difference was evident in cancer incidence between animals mated and bearing their first litter at different ages.

In another experiment, in which animals were mated at age 50 days, bore their litter, and then received DMBA at age 91 days, a decrease in incidence of mammary cancer was evident between virgin controls and primiparous rats. Mammary cancer incidence was reduced from 73% to 23%, respectively. A similar effect was noted between these groups of animals relative to the decrease in benign mammary tumors (Tables 1 and 2). Furthermore, the effect of bearing the first litter at an early age on mammary cancer incidence as well as tumor number is more pronounced in animals receiving the carcinogen shortly following parturition (91 days of age) than in animals receiving the carcinogen at a later date (Table 2).

DMBA Binding

As indicated in Figure 2, the age at which the animal bears its first litter has little effect on either the pattern of uptake and binding of DMBA to parenchymal cell DNA or the quantity of DMBA that is bound. No differences were found in the amount of DMBA bound at any time point between the groups of animals mated at different ages. Furthermore, the 300-day-old virgin control animals exhibited a degree of DMBA binding similar to that of the primiparous rats. However, parenchymal cell DNA binding of DMBA in 50-

Table 2
Effect of Age at First Litter on Incidence of Mammary Cancer Induced with DMBA

Reproductive history	Age at administration of DMBA (days)	Number rats	Number rats with cancer	Cancer incidence (%)	Total number tumors
Virgin	no DMBA	37	1	2.7	1
Virgin	91	15	11	73.3	16
Mated-50 days[a]	91	30	7	23.3	8
Virgin	300	89	46	51.7	69
Mated-50 days[a]	300	109	36	33.0	58
Mated-145 days[a]	300	92	29	31.5	35
Mated-235 days[a]	300	118	38	32.2	45

[a]One male caged with three females for 5 days beginning at the indicated age of the female.

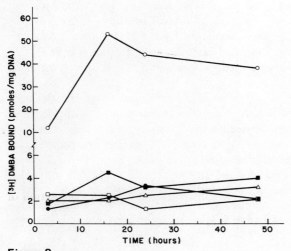

Figure 2
Pattern of radioactivity bound to DNA isolated from mammary parenchymal cells following the intragastric instillation of [^{3}H]DMBA to virgin rats mated at 50 (O) and 300 (●) days of age and primiparous rats mated at 50 (■), 145 (△), and 235 (□) days of age.

day-old virgin rats was approximately 15 times greater than that which occurred in the 300-day-old virgin animal.

Hormone Responsiveness

There was no difference in the percentage of ovarian-hormone-dependent cancers of animals mated at different ages (Fig. 3). In all cases, hormone-dependent

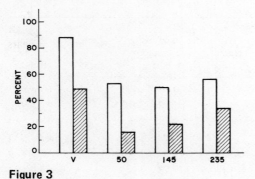

Figure 3
Percentage of mammary cancers regressing (□) following ovariectomy and percentage of regressed cancers responding (▨) to ovarian steroids in virgin (V) and primiparous rats mated at 50, 145, and 235 days of age.

tumors (those that regress after ovariectomy) were approximately 50%. However, this differed considerably from the hormone-dependent tumors of virgin animals, in which approximately 89% of the cancers were hormone-dependent. Furthermore, 17 of 35 cancers of virgin animals responded to the ovarian steroids by renewed growth. The percentage of hormone-responsive of primiparous rats mated at 50, 145, and 235 days of age was 16%, 22%, and 33%, respectively.

DISCUSSION

Although considerable information is available concerning the induction and growth of DMBA-induced mammary cancer in the rat, only a few studies regarding the effect of previous pregnancies and lactations on chemical induction of mammary cancer in this species have been reported. Elsewhere (Moon 1969), I have presented data clearly demonstrating that a previous history of pregnancy or nursing resulted in a significant reduction in mammary cancer induced by DMBA. Subsequent studies by Russo et al. (1977) have confirmed these observations. Such a relationship between parity and mammary cancer in the rat closely paralleled that of the human female. However, a review of the epidemiological evidence by MacMahon et al. (1973) indicated that the risk for breast cancer increases with an increase in age at first full-term pregnancy and that the protective effect of parity is essentially limited to the first birth.

In the present study, a single pregnancy without a subsequent nursing period afforded protection against DMBA-induced mammary tumorigenesis as evidenced by a reduction in tumor incidence (Fig. 1) and average number of tumors per animal (Table 1 and 2). However, as indicated in Figure 1, it would appear that an inverse relationship exists between tumor incidence and age at which the first litter is borne. If such is the case, then the situation is opposite to that of the human female; in humans the earlier the age at first birth the lesser the risk for breast cancer. Although tumor incidence apparently decreases with an increase in age at which the first litter is borne, the incidence in mammary cancer (Table 2) was not affected by age at which pregnancy ensues, for all groups of parous animals exhibited a similar incidence of cancer. Thus, it appears that parity affords protection against DMBA-induced mammary carcinogenesis, but the age at which pregnancy ensues bears little relationship to the incidence of mammary cancer. However, in the experiment in which animals were mated at 50 days of age, bore the litter, and then received DMBA at 91 days of age, the incidence of mammary cancer was less than that observed in similar animals receiving DMBA at 300 days of age. This would seem to indicate that the degree of protection afforded by an early pregnancy decreases somewhat from the time of first litter until the carcinogenic insult, although the protection afforded by pregnancy is still existent even late in the animal's life.

We previously suggested that the effect of parity on mammary carcinogenesis may result from a reduction in the susceptibility of the mammary parenchymal cell to DMBA (Moon 1969). This does not seem to be the case. As shown in Figure 2, no differences were evident in parenchymal cell DNA binding of the carcinogen among animals undergoing pregnancy at different ages. Furthermore, the 300-day-old virgin control animals exhibit a degree of DMBA binding similar to that of the primiparous rats, whereas parenchymal cell DNA binding of DMBA in 50-day-old virgin rats was approximately 15 times greater than that which occurred in the 300-day-old virgin animal. The data derived from the 50-day-old virgin animals agree well with a previous study (Janss et al. 1972) and indicate that DMBA binding to parenchymal cell DNA is age-related and is not affected by a single pregnancy, irrespective of the time at which pregnancy ensues. Thus, it would appear that the decrease in cancer incidence in animals exposed to a carcinogen following a single pregnancy is due to factors other than the interaction of the carcinogen with mammary parenchymal DNA.

It is possible that fluctuations in hormone secretion concomitant with pregnancy may result in an alteration in the sensitivity of neoplastic cells to hormones that influence tumor growth, and this in turn may be reflected in the hormone dependency or responsiveness of the cancers that subsequently develop. As shown in Figure 3, parity results in a reduction in the percentage of ovarian-hormone-dependent cancers, although the effect is not related to the age at which pregnancy ensued. Also in primiparous animals, the percentage of cancers that respond to the ovarian steroids by renewed growth is considerably less than the percentage in virgin animals. However, in primiparous rats, the percentage of hormone-responsive cancers increases with an increase in age at which pregnancy occurs. These data suggest that the number of hormone-dependent cancers decreases with pregnancy, and that the earlier in life that the pregnancy ensues, the lesser the degree of hormone responsiveness of these cancers.

It is evident from these studies as well as others that mammary carcinoma in the rat behaves much like mammary carcinoma in the human female. However, the two species do not parallel each other. Although parity in both species protects against the development of mammary cancer, the age at which pregnancy ensues does not appear critical in the rat. That tumor hormone responsiveness in primiparous rats appears to be related to the age at which pregnancy occurs suggests that pregnancy may in some manner alter the sensitivity of mammary cells to stimulatory hormones. Further experiments into the mechanisms by which parity protects against mammary cancer should serve to delineate more precisely the similarities and differences between the two species.

ACKNOWLEDGMENTS

I am indebted to Ms. Cathy Fricks for her expert technical assistance and to Mrs. Margaret Collins for invaluable aid in preparation of the manuscript. This investigation was supported in part by Public Health Service Grant CA-18968 from the National Cancer Institute.

REFERENCES

Dao, T.L. and H. Sunderland. 1959. Mammary carcinogenesis by 3-methylcholanthrene. I. Hormonal aspects in tumor induction and growth. *J. Natl. Cancer Inst.* 23:567.

Haagensen, C.D. 1956. The frequency and age distribution of mammary carcinoma. In *Diseases of the breast,* p. 331. W.B. Saunders Co., Philadelphia.

Huggins, C., R.C. Moon, and S. Morii. 1962. Extinction of experimental mammary cancer. I. Estradiol-17β and progesterone. *Proc. Natl. Acad. Sci.* 48: 379.

Janss, D.H., R.C. Moon, and C.C. Irving. 1972. The binding of 7,12-dimethylbenz(a)anthracene to mammary parenchymal DNA and protein in vivo. *Cancer Res.* 32:254.

Lewison, E.F. 1962. Prophylactic versus therapeutic castration in the total treatment of breast cancer. A collective review. *Obstet. Gynecol. Surv.* 17:769.

MacMahon, B., P. Cole, and J. Brown. 1973. Etiology of human breast cancer: A review. *J. Natl. Cancer Inst.* 50:21.

McCormick, G.M. and R.C. Moon. 1965. Effect of pregnancy and lactation on growth of mammary tumors induced by 7,12-dimethylbenz(a)anthracene (DMBA). *Br. J. Cancer* 19:160.

_____. 1967a. Effect of nursing and litter size on growth of 7,12-dimethylbenz(a)anthracene (DMBA)-induced rat mammary tumors. *Br. J. Cancer* 21:586.

_____. 1967b. Hormones influencing postpartum growth of 7,12-dimethylbenz(a)anthracene-induced rat mammary tumors. *Cancer Res.* 27:626.

Moon, R.C. 1969. Relationship between previous reproductive history and chemically induced mammary cancer in rats. *Int. J. Cancer* 4:312.

Moon, R.C., D.H. Janss, and S. Young. 1969. Preparation of fat cell-"free" rat mammary gland. *J. Histochem. Cytochem.* 17:182.

Russo, I.H. and J. Russo. 1980. Pregnancy interruption as a risk factor in mammary carcinogenesis. *Proc. Am. Assoc. Cancer Res.* 21:67.

Russo, J., I.H. Russo, M. Ireland, and J. Saby. 1977. Increased resistance of multiparous rat mammary gland to neoplastic transformation by 7,12-dimethylbenz(a)anthracene. *Proc. Am. Assoc. Cancer Res.* 18:38.

Wynder, E.L., I.J. Bross, and T.A. Hirayama. 1960. A study of the epidemiology of cancer of the breast. *Cancer* 13:559.

COMMENTS

SHELLABARGER: I understood Russ [Hilf] to say that, in a single animal, he could find tumors that were growing and regressing, maybe even static. Dick [Moon], do you find the same thing with your hormones?

MOON: Yes I do, particularly during lactation or after pregnancy. Even if you isolate the litter from the dam, they will continue to show different patterns of tumor growth. Some will continue to regress very slowly and they are present at the time of autopsy. But there is also an increase and some will remain static.

HENDERSON: In humans, there is information suggesting that there are two effects of pregnancy. If the first pregnancy is of less than 3 months duration, then the risk of breast cancer is increased (Pike et al. 1981). If the first pregnancy is a completed pregnancy, then the risk goes down, as you showed. I wonder if you have information on whether such different effects occur in your system.

Second, it would seem to me that you could look at the effect of parity on prolactin levels in your system. This would complement the human data we have obtained.

MOON: I have the serum and I have the tumors, but I haven't done the work. I believe Russo (Russo and Russo 1980) reported the interruption of pregnancy and found that there is really no discernible difference between the tumor incidence in such a case and the controls. So I think it follows the human situation quite readily. There is not much change in tumor incidence caused by an interrupted pregnancy.

PIKE: In women there is an increased risk if the first pregnancy is 12 weeks or less. A 15- or 16-week pregnancy appears to be as protective as a full-term pregnancy.

MOON: Russo interpreted it at 12 days in the rat.

DAO: Dick, you showed that you are giving DMBA at 190 days and that you get about 35% tumor incidence.

MOON: Actually, we had about 39-40% incidence.

DAO: And you have a slight increase in the pregnant rat.

MOON: I believe in that first study that we had about a 28% incidence in the first pregnancy, as compared to 39%. But if the rats undergo multiple pregnancies—up to two pregnancies and two lactations—there was approximately a 13% incidence.

DAO: Can you reconcile the fact that the rats you used in your experiment were at the age that they would not develop tumors after carcinogen treatment? In our laboraotry, as well as in others, we cannot induce tumors in 190-day-old rats.

MOON: I think it depends on how long you let them go afterwards, Tom [Dao]. Even if we give the carcinogen in 300 days, tumors develop—let's say, at 500 and some days. We have observed a 50% incidence in the number of adenocarcinomas with a 20-mg dose of DMBA. But I am talking about 300 days. Haslam (1979) administered DMBA at a late date also, and she found that if you observe the animals long enough, a high percentage of mammary adenocarcinomas develop.

DAO: In my opinion, your data shows that pregnancy enhances mammary tumorigenesis rather than inhibiting it. It is vary hard for me to believe that you can get so high a tumor incidence in 190-day-old rats. You are using Sprague-Dawley rats. I was just curious how you would reconcile this type of data.

MEITES: Just a very brief comment. I think it should be mentioned that there very well may be different forms of prolactin, growth hormone, and other pituitary hormones. I would submit to all of you that the physiological data and the radioimmunoassays, on the whole, fit very well with what we know about the physiology of the animal. We may not be assaying, all of the prolactin, for example. But, by golly, it goes up if you stimulate the nipples; it goes down if you ovariectomize the rat; it goes up if you give estrogen; it goes up if you give tranquilizing drugs; it goes down if you give L-dopa. Show me one situation where the physiology does not fit, at least in a general way, with the hormone levels in the blood.

SINHA: Dr. Meites, there are several instances when prolactin levels do not fit with the physiological manifestations of prolactin's action. Pregnancy in the rat and mouse is one instance where prolactin levels do not parallel the increment in mammary gland growth. Other instances include idiopathic galactorrhea, where 86% of the patients have normal plasma prolactin (Kleinberg et al. 1977). There is little correlation between milk yield and serum prolactin in cows (Koprowski and Tucker 1973). And in mice, as I pointed out in my talk, the C3H strain has only one-half to one-third as much prolactin as the C57BL strain; yet it has larger mammary glands and it produces more milk than the latter.

References

Haslam, S.Z. 1979. Age as a modifying factor of 7,12-dimethylbenz(a)anthracene-induced mammary carcinogenesis in the Lewis rat. *Int. J. Cancer* 23: 374.

Kleinberg, D.L., G.L. Noel, and A.G. Frantz. 1977. Galactorrhea: A study of 235 cases including 48 with pituitary tumors. *N. Engl. J. Med.* 296:589.

Koprowski, J.A. and H.A. Tucker. 1973. Serum prolactin during various physiological states and its relationship to milk products in the bovine. *Endocrinology* 92:1480.

Pike, M.C., B.E. Henderson, J.T. Casagrande, I. Rosario, and G.E. Gray. 1981. Oral contraceptive use and early abortion as risk factors for breast cancer in young women. *Br. J. Cancer* 43:72.

Russo, I.H. and J. Russo. 1980. Pregnancy interruption as a risk factor in mammary carcinogenesis. *Proc. Am. Assoc. Cancer Res.* 21:67.

Relation of Neuroleptic Drugs to Development and Growth of Mammary Tumors

JOSEPH MEITES AND CHARLES F. AYLSWORTH
Department of Physiology
Neuroendocrine Research Laboratory
Michigan State University
East Lansing, Michigan 48824

Prolactin and estrogen are believed to be the two most important hormones involved in mammary tumorigenesis in the rat and mouse (Meites 1972; Welsch and Nagasawa 1977; Welsch and Meites 1978). Other hormones, including progesterone, insulin, thyroid hormones, and adrenal cortical steroids, can influence mammary tumorigenesis in these species but are not essential for this process. Prolactin and estrogen also are necessary for growth of established mammary tumors in rats, but they have little or no influence on growth of established mammary tumors in mice that are largely hormone independent (Welsch and Nagasawa 1977; Welsch and Meites 1978).

Of the two hormones, prolactin appears to be more important than estrogen for mammary tumor development and growth in the rat, and probably for mammary tumorigenesis in the mouse as well. This is based on several observations. Thus, in carcinogen-treated rats, ovariectomy prevented induction of mammary tumors; treatment of such ovariectomized rats with prolactin or a prolactin-growth hormone (GH) combination was equally or even more effective than estrogen in promoting mammary tumorigenesis (Talwalker et al. 1964). Prolonged administration of estrogens to rats or mice can induce mammary tumorigenesis, but there is reason to doubt that this treatment is effective in hypophysectomized animals. Chronic treatment of female C3H mice with estrogens increased the incidence of mammary tumors, but concurrent treatment with an ergot drug (bromoergocryptine) to inhibit prolactin secretion prevented this increase in tumors by estrogen (Welsch and Meites 1978). Prolonged administration of prolactin, grafting of pituitaries to the kidney capsule or other sites, lesions placed in the hypothalamus, or administration of reserpine, all of which are known to enhance blood prolactin levels, increased mammary tumor incidence in mice (see Welsch and Nagasawa 1977). Similar treatment of female rats with pituitary grafts or lesions placed in the median eminence (ME) hastened development and increased the incidence of spontaneous benign mammary tumors in rats (Welsch et al. 1970, 1978). In rats with established mammary tumors, hypophysectomy resulted in regression of these tumors;

estrogen treatment of these rats was ineffective for inducing resumption of mammary tumor growth (Sterental et al. 1963). In rats with established mammary tumors, ovariectomy or ovariectomy and andrenalectomy resulted in mammary tumor regression; treatment of such rats with perphenazine (Pearson et al. 1969) or placement of a lesion in the ME (Welsch et al. 1969), both of which promote prolactin secretion, resulted in maintenance of mammary tumor growth for variable periods of time.

The observations described above do not mean that estrogen does not participate in mammary tumorigenesis and growth; they do signify, however, that estrogen's importance is secondary to that of prolactin in murine species. Additional reasons for believing this are related to the mode of action of estrogen on the mammary gland. Thus, although both estrogen and prolactin receptors have been shown to be present in mammary tumor tissue (DeSombre et al. 1976), estrogen alone cannot promote growth of rat mammary tumor tissue in vitro without the presence of prolactin (Welsch and Nagasawa 1977). Also, and of equal importance, estrogen acts to stimulate prolactin secretion by the pituitary, both by a direct action on the pituitary and also via the hypothalamus (Meites et al. 1972). This may be its major mechanism for promoting mammary tumor development and growth in murine species.

Development and growth of mammary tumors in rats does not require greater than normal blood levels of prolactin or estrogen. It has been shown in rats that the serum levels of prolactin, collected at monthly intervals after development of carcinogen-induced mammary tumors, remains unaltered and the rats continue to cycle normally (Nagasawa et al. 1973). On the other hand, an increase or deficiency of prolactin secretion prior to development of carcinogen-induced mammary tumors inhibits development of tumors. Inhibition of carcinogen-induced mammary tumorigenesis by high prolactin secretion may be effected by marked stimulation of lobulo alveolar growth, rendering the mammary gland refractory to the carcinogen. On the other hand, high prolactin secretion favors development of spontaneous benign mammary tumors. In rats with established mammary tumors, either benign or malignant, an excess of prolactin in the blood promotes mammary tumor growth, whereas a deficiency of prolactin depresses it. A deficiency or an excess of estrogen is inhibitory to both development and growth of mammary tumors in rats.

No definite role for prolactin has yet been found in human breast cancer, although prolactin receptors, as well as estrogen ones, are present in human breast cancer tissue. Although there have been a few exceptions, treatment of breast cancer patients with drugs that inhibit prolactin secretion has not produced cancer regression. Unfortunately, none of the treatments (ergot drugs, L-dopa) inhibit secretion of human GH, which has inherent prolactin activity. On the contrary, these drugs stimulate secretion of GH. Estrogen appears to be of much greater importance than prolactin in human breast cancer (for fuller discussion of this topic, see Pearson et al. 1980).

EFFECTS OF NEUROLEPTIC DRUGS ON NEUROENDOCRINE FUNCTIONS

Neuroleptics are generally classified into three major classes: the rauwolfian alkaloids (of which reserpine is the prototype), the phenothiazines (of which chlorpromazine is the prototype), and the butyrophenomes (of which haloperidol is the prototype) (Byck 1975). Blockade of dopaminergic neurons in the central nervous system is believed to be essential to the pharmacological action of neuroleptic drugs and is probably the most important factor in producing their effects on neuroendocrine function (Sacher et al. 1977).

Effects of Secretion of Anterior Pituitary Hormones and Target Gland Hormones

Secretion of most anterior pituitary hormones is influenced by neuroleptic drugs. The stimulatory effects of neuroleptic agents on prolactin secretion are the best understood of their effects on anterior pituitary hormones. Reserpine elevates serum prolactin levels in rats (Lu et al. 1970) and in humans (Lal and Nair 1980). Chlorpromazine also stimulates prolactin in rats (Clemens et al. 1974) and humans (Kato et al. 1975). Clemens et al. (1974) reported that the increase in serum prolactin levels induced by neuroleptic agents such as pimozide and chlorpromazine is greater in female than in male or ovariectomized female rats. Meltzer et al. (1977) reported that the elevation of plasma prolactin by chlorpromazine was not different between the men and women tested and that the increase in prolactin could be antagonized by dopamine. Haloperidol also stimulated serum prolactin levels in rats (Dickerman et al. 1972; Mueller et al. 1976) and humans (Sacher et al. 1977). A relatively new neuroleptic agent, sulpiride, also causes elevation of serum prolactin levels in rats (MacLeod and Robyn 1977). Iwasaki et al. (1976) reported that sulpiride increased plasma prolactin levels in urethane anesthetized rats, and that this effect could be blunted by simultaneous administration of L-dopa. Both acute and chronic administration of sulpiride stimulate secretion of prolactin in rats (Debeljuk et al. 1975) and in humans (Kato et al. 1975).

The effects of neuroleptics on GH secretion are not as conclusive as those on prolactin. Chlorpromazine has been reported to increase GH in both the rat (Kato et al. 1973; Chihara et al. 1975) and the rhesus monkey (Meyer and Knobil 1967). However, Müller et al. (1967) reported that chlorpromazine suppressed the release of GH induced by insulin. Similar results were reported for the human; Sherman et al. (1971) found that chlorpromazine suppressed fasting serum GH levels and GH levels elevated by insulin. Chlorpromazine also has been shown to have no consistent suppressive effect on GH secretion elevated in acromegaly (Dimond et al. 1973; Singh et al. 1973). Reserpine appears to have little effect on pituitary somatotropic function, as reported by Ruedi et al. (1969). However, studies by Cavagnini and Peracchi (1971) showed that reserpine reduced the release of GH induced by insulin hypoglycemia. Mueller et al. (1976) reported tht basal GH secretion was decreased in haloperidol-treated rats. In the same study, it was shown that haloperidol could block the release of GH induced by apomorphine. Sulpiride does not appear to alter basal GH secretion, but it can reduce the increase in GH induced by L-dopa in humans (Mori et al. 1973). Inasmuch as dopamine stimulates GH secretion in humans and rats and the neuroleptic drugs inhibit hypothalamic dopamine activity, most of the evidence favors the idea that neuroleptics are inhibitory to GH secretion.

Most evidence suggests that neuroleptics suppress thyroid-stimulating hormone (TSH) secretion by the pituitary. Haloperidol (Müller et al. 1976) and pimozide (Collu et al. 1975) reduced serum TSH levels in rats. Reserpine also blocked accumulation of intrathyroid colloid droplets induced by cold stress (Kotani et al. 1973). Sulpiride, however, was shown to have no effect either on basal serum TSH values or TSH levels elevated by thyrotropin-releasing hormone (TRH) (Mori et al. 1973).

Neuroleptic drugs appear to suppress the secretion of thyroid hormones, possibly by a direct mechanism independent of TSH. Reserpine and chlorpromazine were shown to interfere directly with thyroid hormone synthesis in vitro (Meyer et al. 1956). In this study, chlorpromazine was incubated with thyroid slices, resulting in a decrease in ^{131}I trapped by the gland. Chronic chlorpromazine treatment inhibited ^{131}I uptake by the thyroid in vivo (Arvay et al. 1960). High doses of chlorpromazine also appeared to decrease the release of ^{131}I by the thyroid (George and Lomax 1965). These reports indicate that chlorpromazine treatment effected a depression of thyroid activity.

Adrenocorticotropin (ACTH) secretion appears to be stimulated by acute administration of neuroleptic drugs. Reserpine depleted pituitary ACTH content in rats, reflecting increased release of ACTH (Saffran and Vogt 1960). Increased serum ACTH levels after reserpine treatment was reported in rats (Bhatlacharya and Marks 1969) and humans (Ruedi et al. 1969). Similarly, chlorpromazine increased serum ACTH levels in rats (Bhatlacharya and Marks 1969). Conversely, Hamburger et al. (1955) showed that chlorpromazine inhibited the stress-induced increase in ACTH.

Adrenal glucocorticoid secretion is increased by neuroleptic drug treatment, presumably as the result of increased ACTH secretion. Klein and Sigg (1977) reported that haloperidol elevated basal plasma corticosterone levels in rats. The same study, however, also showed that treatment with haloperidol prior to application of restraint stress inhibited the stress-induced increase in corticosterone secretion. It is possible that the tranquilizing effect of haloperidol may have decreased the perception of stress, resulting in an attenuated corticosterone response. Reserpine also was reported to stimulate adrenal glucocorticoid secretion in rats (Maickel et al. 1961). Reserpine increased the adrenal glucocorticoid response to cold stress (Maickel et al. 1961). Chlorpromazine also has been reported to increase basal corticosterone secretion, and like haloperidol, decreased the corticosterone response to stresses such as a strange environment or ether (de Wied et al. 1967). Gonadotropin secretion appears to be inhibited by administration of neuroleptic drugs. Dickerman et al. (1974) reported that haloperidol reduced both luteinizing hormone (LH) and follicle-stimulating hormone (FSH) serum levels in rats. Pimozide and reserpine also were reported to reduce gonadotropin levels (Khazan et al. 1960; Ojeda et al. 1974; Collu et al. 1975). Chlorpromazine and reserpine inhibited the preovulatory surge of LH on the afternoon of proestrus when administered on the morning of proestrus (Barraclough and Sawyer 1957). Debeljuk et al. (1975) reported that acute and chronic sulpiride treatment had no effect on gonadotropin secretion.

The effects of neuroleptic drugs on gonadotropin secretion are reflected on reproductive functions. Chlorpromazine treatment delayed gonadal development in female rats (Nagata et al. 1957) and mice (Jarrett 1963). Numerous reports have described the ability of chlorpromazine, haloperidol, reserpine, and other neuroleptic drugs to block spontaneous and induced ovulation in rats (Barraclough and Sawyer 1957; Dickerman et al. 1974) and mice (Jarrett 1963; Bhargava and Jaitley 1964). Chlorpromazine was reported to interfere with menstrual cycles in women (Ayd 1959). Haloperidol was shown to induce a permanent state of diestrus when administered to normal cycling rats (Tuchmann-Duplessis 1966). Ovarian atrophy (Jarret 1963) and decreases in testicular and accessory male sex organs weights (Khazan et al. 1960) following prolonged administration of chlorpromazine and reserpine, respectively, have been observed. Moreover, Khazan et al. (1960) have reported that reserpine inhibited gonadal secretion of estrogens in women. Decreased gonadal sex steroid secretion also was observed in women treated with sulpiride (Robyn et al. 1976). Prolonged treatment with sulpiride and other neuroleptic agents induced galactorrhea and amenorrhea in humans, presumably as a result of stimulation of prolactin secretion and inhibition of gonadotropin secretion (Chimones et al. 1970).

Mechanisms by Which Neuroleptic Drugs Influence Anterior Pituitary Function

The effects of neuroleptic drugs on neuroendocrine function are believed to be mediated by specific blockade of dopaminergic nerve transmission and subsequent stimulation or inhibition of release of hypothalamic hormones into the pituitary portal vessels. Reserpine and haloperidol were reported to decrease hypothalamic prolactin-inhibiting factor (PIF) activity (Ratner et al. 1965; Dickerman et al. 1972). Ojeda et al. (1974) showed that when implants of pimozide were implanted into the ME of the hypothalamus, serum prolactin levels were elevated. Smaller increases in prolactin secretion were observed when pimozide implants were placed directly into the pituitary. This indicates that pimozide can increase prolactin secretion by depressing PIF release, by increasing prolactin-releasing factor (PRF) release, or by directly blocking the action of PIF (DA) on the adenohypophysis. Sulpiride was able to antagonize inhibition of prolactin secretion from anterior pituitaries in vitro by dopamine, but it could not stimulate prolactin secretion from untreated anterior pituitaries (MacLeod and Robyn 1977). Clemens et al. (1974) reported that antipsychotic neuroleptic drugs, including pimozide, haloperidol, chlorpromazine, sulpiride, and fluphenazine, stimulated prolactin release, whereas nonantipsychotic phenothiazines, such as promethazine, methdilazine, and ethopropazine, had no such effect. Therefore, the dopamine receptor involved in the antipsychotic action of neuroleptics may be similar to the dopamine receptor that inhibits prolactin release.

Hypothalamic peptide hormones also appear to be involved in the inhibitory action of neuroleptics on gonadotropin secretion. Haloperidol has been shown to decrease hypothalamic luteinizing hormone releasing factor (LRF) content in rats (Dickerman 1974). When implanted in the ME area of the hypothalamus, pimozide reduced LH secretion. However, when pimozide was implanted in the pituitary, no change in LH secretion was observed (Ojeda et al. 1974). These results indicate that pimozide inhibits gonadotropin secretion by depressing release of LRF, rather than by a direct action on the pituitary.

Reserpine decreased corticotropin-releasing factor (CRF) content in the ME area of the hypothalamus, which was interpreted to indicate an increase in CRF release that resulted in stimulation of ACTH release (Bhatlacharya and Marks 1969). Lengvari and Halasz (1972) demonstrated by selective hypothalamic deafferentation that reserpine influences on CRF release were not exerted directly on the medial basal hypothalamus. Furthermore, they showed that anterior afferents to the hypothalamus were critical for the manifestation of the ACTH response to reserpine and that hippocampal and mesencephalic structures were not involved.

EFFECTS ON DEVELOPMENT AND GROWTH OF MAMMARY TUMORS

The effects of neuroleptic drugs on the development and growth of mammary tumors appears to be largely mediated by their effect on pituitary prolactin secretion. Neuroleptic drugs have been shown to stimulate profoundly growth of established mammary tumors in the rat. An influence on the induction and growth of breast cancer in women has not been demonstrated.

Murine Species

Lacassagne and Duplan (1959) reported that reserpine hastened development of spontaneous mammary tumors in C3H mice. Welsch and Meites (1970) showed that reserpine decreased the incidence of 7,12-dimethylbenz[a]anthracene (DMBA)-induced mammary tumors in rats when administered prior to carcinogen administration but increased growth of the tumors when given after they appeared. Reserpine and chlorpromazine were reported to have no effect on the growth of established spontaneous mammary tumors in mice (Cranston 1958). This is not surprising, because mammary tumors in mice are largely autonomous and uninfluenced by hormone treatment (Welsch and Nagasawa 1977).

Other neuroleptic drugs, such as haloperidol, perphenazine, and sulpiride, have been reported to stimulate the growth of DMBA-induced mammary tumors markedly (Quadri et al. 1973; Bodgen et al. 1974; Pass and Meites 1976). Sulpiride also has been shown to increase growth of transplanted mammary tumors in mice (Anton and Rozados 1976).

Human Subjects

The evidence on the possible effects of neuroleptic drugs on human breast cancer is not so conclusive, but on the whole it indicates that neuroleptics have little or no effect. In a retrospective study, Heinomen et al. (1975) found a positive correlation between reserpine use and breast cancer incidence. Also, in England, a significant association was found between breast cancer occurrence and use of rauwolfia derivatives, whereas no association was found between breast cancer incidence and use of other hypotensive agents (Armstrong et al. 1974). Therefore, it was concluded that the hypotensive action of reserpenoids was not responsible for the association found between reserpine use and breast cancer incidence. It also was noted that no relationship could be found between other agents that increased plasma prolactin levels and breast cancer incidence. Jick et al. (1974) compared reserpine use in patients with and without breast cancer and found a higher risk (over threefold) of breast cancer in women exposed to reserpine than in women not exposed to the drug. On the other hand, just as many studies have been reported in which no association was found between use of neuroleptics and breast cancer occurrence. Laska et al. (1975) matched 55 female psychiatric patients having breast cancer with psychiatric patients not having breast cancer, all of whom were on reserpine treatment. They found no significant increase in relative risk among the breast cancer women on reserpine. Likewise, O'Fallon et al. (1975) found the use of reserpine to be identical among women with breast cancer and age-matched women without breast cancer. Mack et al. (1975) reported a low risk ratio for reserpine between women with and without breast cancer who lived in a retirement facility. More recently, Wagner and Mantel (1978) compared the 15 years preceding the introduction of neuroleptics into medical practice (1940-1954) with the second decade after their introduction (1965-1974) at a psychiatric hospital. They found that although the use of neuroleptics during the second period was more extensive, there was no statistically or medically significant change in the incidence of breast cancer between the two periods. It can, therefore, be concluded that no definite relationship has been established between use of neuroleptic drugs and breast cancer.

CONCLUSIONS

Neuroleptic drugs stimulate prolactin and generally inhibit gonadotropin secretion in animals and humans. Because of the overriding importance of prolactin on mammary tumorigenesis in the rat and mouse and on growth of established mammary tumors in rats, administration of neuroleptic drugs can profoundly influence mammary tumors in these species. In humans, a definite role for prolactin in breast cancer development and growth has not been demonstrated, whereas estrogen has been shown to be of primary importance. Most of the evidence to date indicates that neuroleptic drugs do not increase the incidence or promote growth of breast cancers in humans.

ACKNOWLEDGMENTS

Research on mammary tumors in our laboratory has been supported by National Institutes of Health grants CA10771 from the National Cancer Institute and AM04784 from the National Institute of Arthritis, Metabolism and Digestive Diseases.

REFERENCES

Anton, E.B. and R. Rozados. 1976. The effect of sulpiride on mammary tumor growth. *Tumor* 62:123.

Armstrong, B., N. Stevens, and R. Doll. 1974. Retrospective study of the association between use of rauwolfia derivatives and breast cancer in English women. *Lancet* ii:672.

Arvay, E., L. Lampe, L. Kertesz, and L. Medveczky. 1960. Changes of thyroid function in response to severe nervous stimulation. *Acta Endocrinol.* 35: 469.

Ayd, R.J. 1959. Prolonged administration of chlorpromazine (thorazine) hydrochloride. *J. Am. Med. Assoc.* 169:1296.

Barraclough, C.A. and C.H. Sawyer. 1957. Blockade of the release of pituitary ovulatory hormone in the rat by chlorpromazine and reserpine: Possible mechanisms of action. *Endocrinology* 61:341.

Bhargava, K.P. and K.D. Jaitly. 1964. The effect of some phenothiazine tranquilizers on the oestrus cycle of albino mice. *Br. J. Pharmacol.* 22:162.

Bhatlacharya, A.M. and B.H. Marks. 1969. Reserpine and chlorpromazine-induced changes in hypothalamo-hypophyseal-adrenal system in rats in the presence or absence of hypothermia. *J. Pharmacol. Exp. Ther.* 165: 108.

Bodgen, E.E., E.J. Taylor, E.Y.H. Kuo, M.M. Mason, and A. Speropoulos. 1974. The effect of perphenazine-induced serum prolactin response on estrogen-primed mammary tumor-host systems, 13762 and R-35 mammary adenocarcinomas. *Cancer Res.* 34:3018.

Byck, R. 1975. Drugs and treatment of psychiatric disorders. In *The pharmacological basis of therapeutics*, 4th edition (ed. L.S. Goodman and E. Gilman), p. 152. MacMillan Publishing Co., New York.

Cavagnini, F. and M. Peracchi. 1971. Effect of reserpine on growth hormone response to insulin hypoglycemia and to arginine infusion in normal subjects and hypothyroid patients. *J. Endocrinol.* 51:851.

Chihara, K., Y. Kato, S. Ohgo, and H. Imura. 1975. Studies on the mechanism controlling growth hormone release induced by chlorpromazine in the anesthetized rat. *Endocrinol. JPN.* 22:105.

Chimones, H. 1970. Syndrome amenorrhee-galactorrhee par sulpiride. *Presse Med.* 78:1844.

Clemens, J.A., E.B. Smalstig, and B.D. Sawyer. 1974. Antipsychotic drugs stimulate prolactin release. *Psychopharmacologia* 40:123.

Collu, R., L.G. Jequier, J. Letarte, and J.R. Ducharme. 1975. Endocrine effects of pimozide, a specific dopaminergic blocker. *J. Clin. Endocrinol. Metab.* 41:981.

Cranston, E.M. 1958. Effects of some tranquilizers on a mammary adenocarcinoma in mice. *Cancer Res.* 18:897.

Debeljuk, L., D.H. Rozados, C. Villegas Belez, and A.M. Mancini. 1975. Acute and chronic effects of sulpiride on serum prolactin and gonadotropin levels in castrated male rats. *Proc. Soc. Exp. Biol. Med.* 148:550.

DeSombre, E.R., G. Kledzik, S. Marshall, and J. Meites. 1976. Estrogen and prolactin receptor concentrations in rat mammary tumors and response to endocrine ablation. *Cancer Res.* 36:354.

de Wied, D. 1967. Chlorpromazine and endocrine function. *Pharmacol. Rev.* 19: 251.

Dickerman, S., J. Clark, E. Dickerman, and J. Meites. 1972. Effect of haloperidol on serum and pituitary prolactin and hypothalamic PIF in rats. *Neuroendocrinology* 9:332.

Dickerman, S., G. Kledzik, M. Gelato, H.J. Chen, and J. Meites. 1974. Effects of haloperiidol on serum and pituitary prolactin, LH and FSH, and hypothalamic PIF and LRF. *Neuroendocrinology* 15:10.

Dimond, R.C., S.R. Brammer, R.L. Atkinson, Jr., W.J. Howard, and J.M. Earll. 1973. Chlorpromazine treatment and growth hormone secretory responses in acromegaly. *J. Clin. Endocrinol. Metab.* 36:1189.

George, R. and P. Lomax. 1965. The effects of morphine, chlorpromazine, and reserpine on pituitary-thyroid activity in rats. *J. Pharmacol. Exp. Ther.* 150:129.

Hamburger, C. 1955. Substitution of hypophysectomy by the administration of chlorpromazine in the assay of corticotrophin. *Acta Endocrinol.* 20:383.

Heinomen, O.P., S. Shapiro, L. Tuominen, and M.I. Turunen. 1975. Reserpine use in relation to breast cancer. *Lancet* ii:675.

Iwasaki, Y., Y. Kato, K. Chihara, S. Ohgo, K. Maeda, and H. Imura. 1976. Effect of sulpiride on plasma prolactin in rats. *Neuroendocrinology* 21: 267.

Jarrett, R.J. 1963. Some endocrine effects of two phenothiazine derivatives, chlorpromazine and perphenazine in the female mouse. *Br. J. Pharmacol.* 20:497.

Jick, H., D. Sloan, S. Shapiro, S. Heinomen, O.P. Hartz, S.C. Miettinen, M.P. Vessey, D.H. Lawson, and R.R. Miller. 1974. Reserpine and breast cancer. *Lancet* ii:669.

Kato, Y., J. Dupre, and J.C. Beck. 1973. Plasma GH in the anesthetized rat: Effects of dibutyryl cAMP, prostaglancin E_1 adrenergic agents, vasopressin, chlorpromazine, amphetamine and L-dopa. Endocrinology 93:135.

Kato, Y., S. Ohgo, K. Chihara, and H. Imura. 1975. Stimulation of human prolactin secretion by sulpiride. Endocrinol. JPN. 22:457.

Khazan, N., F.G. Sulman, and H.Z. Winnik. 1960. Effects of reserpine on the pituitary-gonadal axis. Proc. Soc. Exp. Biol. Med. 105:201.

Klein, K.L. and E.B. Sigg. 1977. Plasma corticosterone and brain catecholamines in stress effect of psychotropic drugs. Pharmacol. Biochem. Behav. 6:79.

Kotani, M., T. Onaya, and T. Yamada. 1973. Acute increase of thyroid hormone secretion in response to cold and its inhibition by drugs which act on the autonomic or central nervous system. Endocrinology 92:288.

Lacassagne, A. and J.F. Duplan. 1959. Le mecanisme de la cancerisation de la mamelle chez la souris, considere d'aprés les resultats d'experiences au mojen de la reserpine. Comptes. Rendus. Academy of Science (Paris) 249:810.

Lal, S. and N.P.V. Nair. 1980. Effects of neuroleptics on prolactin and growth hormone secretion in man. In Neuroactive drugs in endocrinology (ed. E.E. Müller), p. 223. Elsevier/North-Holland Biomedical Press, Amsterdam.

Laska, E.M., C. Siegel, M. Meisner, S. Fischer, and J. Wanderling. 1975. Matched-pairs study of reserpine use and breast cancer. Lancet ii:296.

Lengvari, I. and B. Halasz. 1972. On the site of action of reserpine on ACTH secretion. J. Neural Transm. 33:289.

Lu, K.H., Y. Koch, Y. Amenomori, C.L. Chen, and J. Meites. 1970. Effects of central acting drugs on serum and pituitary prolactin levels in rats. Endocrinology 87:667.

Mack, T.M., B.E. Henderson, V.R. Gerkins, M. Arthur, J. Baptista, and M.C. Pike. 1975. Reserpine and breast cancer in a retirement community. N. Engl. J. Med. 292:1366.

MacLeod, R.M. and C. Robyn. 1977. Mechanism of increased prolactin secretion by sulpiride. J. Endocrinol. 72:273.

Maickel, R.F., E.O. Westermann, and B.B. Brodie. 1961. Effects of reserpine and cold exposure on pituitary adrenocortical function in rats. J. Pharmacol. Exp. Ther. 134:167.

Meites, J. 1972. Relation of prolactin and estrogen to mammary tumorigenesis in the rat. J. Natl. Cancer Inst. 48:1217.

Meites, J., K.H. Lu, W. Wuttle, C.W. Welsch, H. Nagasawa, and S.K. Quadri. 1972. Recent studies on functions and control of prolactin secretion in rats. Recent Progr. Horm. Res. 28:471.

Meltzer, H.Y., D.J. Goode, and V.S. Fang. 1977. Effects of chlorpromazine on plasma prolactin and chlorpromazine levels. Psychopharmacol. Bull. 13:59.

Meyer, S.W., F.H. Kelly, and M.E. Morton. 1956. The direct anti-thyroid action of reserpine, chlorpromazine, and other drugs. J. Pharmacol. Exp. Ther. 117:197.

Meyer, V. and E. Knobil. 1967. Growth hormone secretion in the unanesthetized rhesus monkey in response to noxious stimuli. Endocrinology 80:163.

Mori, M., I. Kobayashi, S. Shimoyama, T. Uchara, T. Nemoto, H. Fukuda, and N. Kamio. 1973. Effect of sulpiride on serum growth hormone and prolactin concentrations following L-dopa administration in man. *Endocrinol. JPN.* 24:149.

Mueller, G.P., J. Simpkins, J. Meites, and K.E. Moore. 1976. Differential effects of dopamine agonists and haloperidol on release of prolactin, thyroid stimulating hormone, growth hormone, and luteinizing hormone in rats. *Neuroendocrinology* 20:121.

Müller, E.E., T. Saito, A. Arimura, and A.V. Schalley. 1967. Hypoglycemia, stress and growth hormone release: Blockade of growth hormone release by drugs acting on the central nervous system. *Endocrinology* 80:109.

Nagasawa, H., C. Chen, and J. Meites. 1973. Relation between growth of carcinogen-induced mammary cancers and serum prolactin values in rats. *Proc. Soc. Exp. Biol. Med.* 142:625.

Nagata, G. 1957. Influence of chlorpromazine upon the pituitary function, especially corticotropine and gonadotropin secretion. *Annual Report Shionogi Research Laboratory* 7:71.

O'Fallon, W.M., D.R. Labarthe, and L.T. Kurland. 1975. Rauwolfia derivatives and breast cancer. *Lancet* ii:292.

Ojeda, S.R., P.G. Harms, and S.M. McCann. 1974. Effect of blockade of dopaminergic receptors on prolactin and LH release: Median eminence and pituitary sites of action. *Endocrinology* 4:1650.

Pass, K.A. and J. Meites. 1977. Enhanced growth of carcinogen-induced mammary tumors in rats by sulpiride. *IRCS Med. Sci.* 5:241.

Pearson, O.H., B. Arafah, and A. Manni. 1980. Prolactin and mammary cancer. In *Central and peripheral regulation of prolactin function* (ed. R.M. MacLeod and M. Scapagnini), p. 237. Raven Press, New York.

Pearson, O.H., O. Llerena, L. Llerena, A. Molina, and T. Butler. 1969. Prolactin-dependent rat mammary cancer: A model for man? *Transactions of the Association of American Physicians* 82:255.

Quadri, S.K., J.L. Clark, and J. Meites. 1973. Effects of LSD, pargyline and haloperidol on mammary tumor growth. *Proc. Soc. Exp. Biol. Med.* 142:22.

Ratner, A., P.K. Talwalker, and J. Meites. 1965. Effect of reserpine on prolactin-inhibiting activity of rat hypothalamus. *Endocrinology* 77:315.

Robyn, C., M. Vekemans, A. Caufriez, and M. L'Hermite. 1976. Effects of sulpiride-induced hyperprolactinemia on circulating gonadotropins and sex steroids during the menstrual cycle. *IRCS Med. Sci.* 4:14.

Ruedi, B., M. Aubert, C. Mieville, P. Benuzzi, J. Wertheimer, and J.P. Felber. 1969. Action de quelques medicaments psycotropes sur les responses hypophysaires somatotrope et adrenocorticotrope a l'hypoglycemie. *Schweiz. Med. Wochenschr.* 99:1128.

Sacher, E.J., P.H. Green, N. Altman, G. Langer, F.S. Halpern, and M. Liefer. 1977. Prolactin responses to neuroleptic drugs: An approach to the study of brain dopamine blockade in humans. In *Neuroregulators and psychiatric disorders* (ed. E. Usdin et al.), p. 242. Oxford University Press, New York.

Saffran, M. and M. Vogt. 1960. Depletion of pituitary corticotrophin by reserpine and a nitrogen mustard. *Br. J. Pharmacol.* 15:165.

Sherman, L., S. Kim, F. Benjamin, and H.D.C. Kolodny. 1971. Effects of chlorpromazine on serum growth hormone concentrations in man. *N. Engl. J. Med.* 284:72.

Singh, P., D.G. McDivitt, J. Mackay, and D.R. Hadden. 1973. Effects of L-dopa and chlorpromazine on human growth hormone and TSH secretion in normal subjects and acromegalics. *Hormone Research* 4:293.

Sterental, A., J.M. Dominguez, C. Weissman, and O.H. Pearson. 1963. Pituitary role in the estrogen dependency of experimental mammary cancer. *Cancer Res.* 23:481.

Talwalker, P.K., J. Meites, and H. Mizuno. 1964. Mammary tumor induction by estrogen or anterior pituitary hormones in ovariectomized rats given 7,12-dimethyl-1,2 benzanthracene. *Proc. Soc. Exp. Biol. Med.* 116:531.

Tuchmann-Duplessis, H. and L. Mercier-Parot. 1966. Action d'un neuroleptique le R1625 (Haloperidol) sur l'activite genitale de la ratte. *Comptes Rendus Academy Sciences* (Paris) 236:1493.

Wagner, S. and N. Mantel. 1978. Breast cancer at a psychiatric hospital before and after the introduction of neuroleptic agents. *Cancer Res.* 38:2703.

Welsch, C.W. and J. Meites. 1970. Effects of reserpine on development of 7,12-dimethylbenz(a)anthracene-induced mammary tumors in female rats. *Experientia* 26:1133.

Welsch, C.W. and H. Nagasawa. 1977. Prolactin and murine mammary tumorigenesis. A review. *Cancer Res.* 37:951.

Welsch, C.W. and J. Meites. 1978. Prolactin and mammary carcinogenesis. In *Endocrine control in neoplasia* (ed. R.K. Sharma and W.E. Criss), vol. 9, p. 71. Raven Press, New York.

Welsch, C.W., J.A. Clemens, and J. Meites. 1969. Effects of hypothalamic and amygdaloid lesions on development and growth of carcinogen induced mammary tumors in the female rat. *Cancer Res.* 29:1541.

Plasma Prolactin Analysis as a Potential Predictor of Murine Mammary Tumorigenesis

Y. N. SINHA
Lutcher Brown Center for Diabetes and Endocrinology
Scripps Clinic and Research Foundation
La Jolla, California 92037

The importance of prolactin in the mammary tumorigenesis of mice and rats is overwhelmingly supported by experimental evidence (Meites 1972; van der Gugten and Verstraeten 1973; Kim and Furth 1976; Welsch and Nagasawa 1977). Nevertheless, there has been little success in correlating plasma levels of prolactin with the incidence of breast cancer in either rodents or humans. Most studies have found either a lack of correlation or a poor correlation at best. This paradoxical situation has led to the suggestion that mammary tumors can develop even when the amount of prolactin in plasma is normal, perhaps as a result of alterations in the sensitivity of the mammary gland to prolactin (Welsch and Nagasawa 1977). This, of course, may be true. However, a very important aspect of this question is generally overlooked. That pertains to the chemical heterogeneity of prolactin and the problems of quantitation associated with it. In this paper, I discuss some of the chemical and methodological factors that may be responsible for the apparent lack of correlation between plasma prolactin and breast cancer development, and I attempt to give an idea of the work that lies ahead in resolving this issue.

CORRELATION BETWEEN PLASMA PROLACTIN AND BREAST CANCER

Since the advent of radioimmunoassays (RIAs) for prolactin in humans (Hwang et al. 1971; Sinha et al. 1973), rats (Niswender et al. 1969), and mice (Sinha et al. 1972) during the early 1970s, many researchers have attempted to demonstrate a correlation between plasma prolactin and the incidence of breast cancer.

Humans

Studies in humans have yielded conflicting reports. Murray et al. (1972) and Rolandi et al. (1974) initially reported higher levels of plasma prolactin in women with metastatic breast carcinoma than in patients without the disease.

However, other authors (Dickey and Minton 1972; Boyns et al. 1973b; Franks et al. 1974; Sheth et al. 1975; Hill et al. 1976; McFayden et al. 1976; Cole et al. 1977) failed to correlate serum prolactin levels and the presence or absence of breast cancer. Kwa et al. (1974, 1976) and Henderson et al. (1975) found no correlation in serum prolactin levels of patients with or without the disease, but prolactin levels were high in patients with family histories of the disease. In one study (Mittra et al. 1974), serum prolactin levels were similar in patients with and without the disease, but there was a greater pituitary reserve of prolactin in women with advanced breast cancer than in women without the disease. Several reports (Kwa and Wang 1977; Malarkey et al. 1977; Tarquini et al. 1978) have noted higher nocturnal levels of plasma prolactin in high-risk women and women with benign or malignant breast diseases. However, the differences are much too small to be of clinical significance.

Rats

Boyns et al. (1973a) and Hawkins et al. (1976) reported higher levels of plasma prolactin in strains of rats having greater than usual susceptibility to carcinogen-induced mammary tumors. However, neither Gala and Loginsky (1973) nor Nagasawa et al. (1973) found any correlation between serum prolactin and the induction or growth rate of 7,12-dimethylbenz[a]anthracene (DMBA)-induced mammary tumors.

Mice

The mouse has been investigated more extensively than other species in this respect, but the same problem remains. That is, mice carrying spontaneous mammary tumors have no higher levels of prolactin than those without tumors (Sinha et al. 1976). Induction of mammary tumors with chemical carcinogens does not involve increases in serum or pituitary prolactin (Medina et al. 1977). Similarly, comparisons of the basal levels of prolactin in mouse strains with high or low incidences of mammary tumors (Table 1) have yielded inconsistent results (Sinha et al. 1975, 1979b; Nagasawa et al. 1976). However, measurement of resting hormone levels may not reveal subtle abnormalities in hormone secretion. For this reason, we have compared prolactin levels after a provocative stimulus, such as acute nursing or perphenazine injection. Early works (Sinha et al. 1974, 1975), which included few strains of mice, seemed to indicate that there was a negative correlation between nursing- or perphenazine-induced serum prolactin concentrations and the incidence of mammary tumors (Fig. 1A), but when more strains were included (Sinha et al. 1979b), this pattern did not hold up (Fig. 1B).

What did remain constant was the tremendous difference among mouse strains in the amount of prolactin detectable in blood after the provocative stimulus. What caused this difference? Do mice of different strains release

Table 1

Basal Levels of Prolactin (mean + s.E.) in Female Mice of Several Strains with Varying Incidences of Mammary Tumors

Strain	Mammary tumor incidence (%)	Number of mice	Body weight (g)	Serum prolactin (ng/ml)	Pituitary prolactin (µg/mg)
			Experiment 1		
C3H/St	high	12	23 ± 0.7	92 ± 16	11.6 ± 0.8
CBA/St	high	12	22 ± 0.6	151 ± 28	9.3 ± 0.6
DBA/2St	medium	9	20 ± 0.6	47 ± 10	6.8 ± 0.3
Balb/cSt	low	13	19 ± 0.5	68 ± 13	5.9 ± 0.2
C57BL/St	low	15	19 ± 0.5	182 ± 33	8.3 ± 0.5
			Experiment 2		
C3H/He	99	9	26 ± 1.1	87 ± 21	10.3 ± 0.4
C3H-A^{vy}/He	100	8	30 ± 0.9	80 ± 19	11.7 ± 0.5
GR/Hf	100	9	20 ± 0.4	19 ± 4	7.4 ± 0.5
C3H-A^{vy}fB/He*	90	8	30 ± 0.9	33 ± 6	8.7 ± 0.4
DD/He	84	9	22 ± 0.3	26 ± 10	10.3 ± 0.5
C3HfB/He	40	8	23 ± 0.6	27 ± 6	11.1 ± 0.5
Balb/cHe	20	9	24 ± 0.2	7 ± 2	8.3 ± 0.4
C57BL/He	<1	9	20 ± 0.3	90 ± 23	6.1 ± 0.6

Data from Sinha et al. (1975, 1979b).

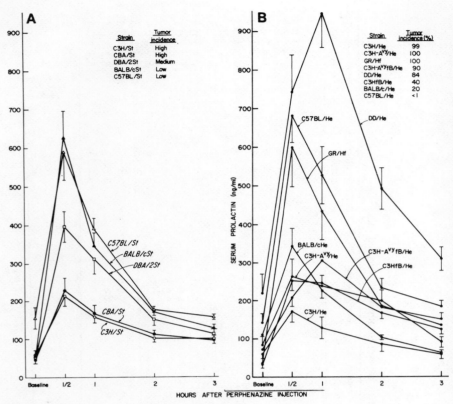

Figure 1
Serum prolactin concentrations after challenge with perphenazine (1 μg/g body weight) in female mice of several strains with varying incidences of mammary tumors. Vertical lines represent mean ± S.E. There were 10 mice in each group. The ages of the mice ranged from 70 to 80 days. (Data redrawn from Sinha et al. 1975, 1979b.)

different amounts of prolactin in response to the perphenazine challenge? In clinical work, differences in plasma hormone levels after a provocative test are interpreted to indicate differences in the pituitary reserve of the hormone or secretory capacity of the pituitary. An examination of the mouse pituitaries, however, revealed that such was not the case. Strains that showed the least prolactin in blood did not have the least hormone in their pituitaries and vice versa (Table 1). Furthermore, the amounts of prolactin depleted from the pituitary in response to the challenge were more or less equivalent in most strains tested (Table 2). Certainly, there was no strong evidence of a difference in pituitary reserve or release that matched the difference seen in plasma.

Table 2
Amount of Prolactin Depleted from the Pituitary and Detected in Serum in Response to Perphenazine Administration

Strain	Mammary tumor incidence (%)	Prolactin depleted from pituitary (μg)[a]	Prolactin measured in serum (ng)[b]
	Experiment 1		
C3H/St	high	3.2 ± 1.6	659 ± 84
CBA/St	high	2.6 ± 1.0	693 ± 130
DBA/2St	medium	2.6 ± 0.5	1204 ± 140
Balb/cSt	low	4.4 ± 0.8	1594 ± 187
C57BL/St	low	2.7 ± 0.4	1085 ± 110
	Experiment 2		
C3H/He	99	5.8 ± 1.3	437 ± 61
C3H-A^{vy}/He	100	7.9 ± 2.1	1233 ± 175
GR/Hf	100	5.2 ± 1.2	1622 ± 267
C3H-A^{vy}fB/He	90	5.7 ± 1.4	1247 ± 234
DD/He	84	10.0 ± 1.3	2857 ± 303
C3HfB/He	40	6.2 ± 1.3	1081 ± 119
Balb/cHe	20	5.7 ± 0.7	905 ± 130
C57BL/He	<1	6.5 ± 0.9	1546 ± 286

Data from Sinha et al. (1975, 1979b).
[a]Estimated by injecting mice with saline or perphenazine (1 $\mu g/g$ body weight) and calculating the difference in the pituitary prolactin contents of the 2 groups.
[b]Calculated from the area under the prolactin response curves of Fig. 1. The values under experiment 2 differ slightly from those published, because of an error in the original calculation.

POSSIBLE REASONS FOR THE LACK OF CORRELATION BETWEEN PLASMA PROLACTIN AND BREAST CANCER

Metabolic Clearance Rate of Prolactin

One factor that could account for this discrepancy between amounts of prolactin in the plasma and pituitary is the clearance rate of the hormone. If the hormone released from the pituitary is cleared from plasma more rapidly in one strain than in another, the plasma levels can differ even though equal amounts of hormone are released. Comparing the metabolic clearance rate (MCR) of prolactin in the C3H/St and C57BL/St strains of mice showed that the clearance rate was indeed higher in the C3H/St strain (with its low serum prolactin level) than in the C57BL/St strain (with its high serum prolactin levels) (Fig. 2). Females in both the virgin and pregnant states manifested this difference, but not lactating mice (Sinha et al. 1979a).

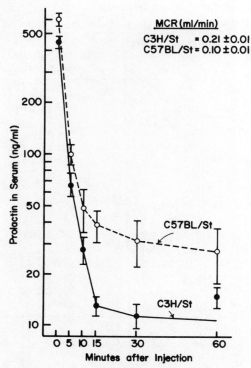

MCR (ml/min)

C3H/St = 0.21 ±0.01
C57BL/St = 0.10 ±0.01

Figure 2
Disappearance of immunoreactive prolactin from the sera of female mice after a single i.v. injection of mouse prolactin (~20 ng/g body weight). Note that the ordinate is plotted on a logarithmic scale. Vertical lines represent mean ± S.E. There were 10 mice in each group. Each of the mice was approximately 75 days old. (Data redrawn from Sinha et al. 1979 a.)

Conversion of Prolactin into Nonimmunodectable Forms

The MCR of a hormone is a function of several factors. Tissue uptake, excretion into body fluids, and metabolic degradation are some of the well-known avenues of hormone loss from the plasma. Generally, what is not recognized is the fact that conversion of the hormone into a nonimmunoreactive but still bioactive form could also significantly influence the MCR estimates, if RIA or other immunological techniques were used in its estimation. The following experiment illustrates this point: A dose of monomeric mouse prolactin containing an ^{125}I label was injected into female mice of the C3H/St and C57BL/St strains. Their sera were collected and fractionated on a Sephadex G-100 column. Prolactin in the fractions was estimated by two methods—by RIA and by counting radio-activity directly. At 15 min after injection, direct counting revealed that almost 80% of the injected prolactin was in the monomeric form in mice of both strains

(Fig. 3). However, according to RIA, the monomeric peak constituted only 51% of the total prolactin in the C3H/St strain and only 69% in the C57BL/St strain. The values further dropped to 25% in the C3H/St and to 55% in the

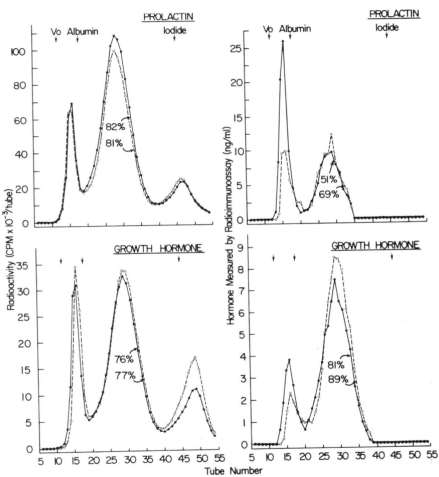

Figure 3

Chromatographic profile on Sephadex G-100 of prolactin and GH in mouse sera 15 min after injection, as determined by radioactivity counting (*left panels*) and by radioimmunoassay (*right panels*). A dose of mouse prolactin or GH containing ^{125}I-labeled hormone was injected i.p. into female mice, and sera were collected by decapitation at various time intervals. Sera were fractionated immediately on a column 1.5 × 30 cm long in volumes of 1 ml. (———) The C3H/St strain; (– – –) the C57BL/St strain. (→) The positions of the void volume (Vo), peaks of human serum albumin, and free [125]I. The percentages given indicate the relative size of the monomeric peak. (Data redrawn from Sinha and Baxter 1979 b.)

C57BL/St strain at 60 min after injection (Sinha and Baxter 1979b). In an identical experiment with mouse growth hormone (GH), both methods gave similar estimates for the two components at each interval examined. Clearly, soon after injection some of the injected monomeric mouse prolactin assumed a form that was undetectable with RIA. This observation is corroborated by the fact that the immunological estimates of prolactin's clearance in the rat (Koch et al. 1971) are higher than those by bioassay (Grosvenor 1967). Whether the converted form of prolactin is still biologically active has not been determined, but it is a strong possibility. Physiological parameters of prolactin activity show that the low prolactin-containing C3H mice actually have larger mammary glands and better milk-producing ability than the high prolactin-containing C57BL mice (Nagasawa et al. 1967a,b).

Size Heterogeneity of Circulating Prolactin

There is evidence to suggest that endogenous prolactin also is modified similarly when released from the pituitary into circulation. Since the immunoinactivation of exogenously administered monomeric prolactin was greater in the C3H/St strain than in the C57BL/St strain, the monomeric prolactin would be expected to constitute a smaller proportion in the plasma of the former than it does in the plasma of the latter if such a modification did occur in the endogenously secreted hormone. Figure 4 shows that when sera and pituitary extracts from intact, virgin females of the two strains were fractionated on a Sephadex G-100 column, there was no difference in the proportions of the so-called big and little forms in the pituitary extracts. However, the pattern in sera from the two strains differed dramatically: As expected, the C3H/St strain had very little monomeric prolactin and mostly big prolactin whereas the C57BL/St strain had mostly monomeric prolactin and very little big prolactin. The proportions of the two GH peaks were identical in the two strains under similar circumstances (Sinha 1980).

This molecular-size heterogeneity for circulating prolactin has been found in every species examined thus far, including the human being (Suh and Frantz 1974), cow (Gala and Hart 1980), goat (Gala and Hart 1980), rat (Lawson and Stevens 1980), and mouse (Sinha 1980). Generally, two or three forms are seen; in some cases even four. Their proportions change with changes in physiological states. However, more relevant to our discussion is the fact that the current RIAs measure only a fraction of the total amount of each of the size forms present. Although no estimates for the different size forms of human or rat prolactin are available presently, Moore and Jin (1978) have reported that the polymeric form of human GH isolated from clinical grade human GH has only 3% immunoreactivity in RIA; Lewis et al. (1977) find only 50% immunoreactivity for the dimeric GH from human pituitaries. Our estimate in mice is that, under steady-state conditions, as much as 30-70% of the monomeric prolactin in plasma is not detected with RIA. As for the big form, there is no quantitative estimate,

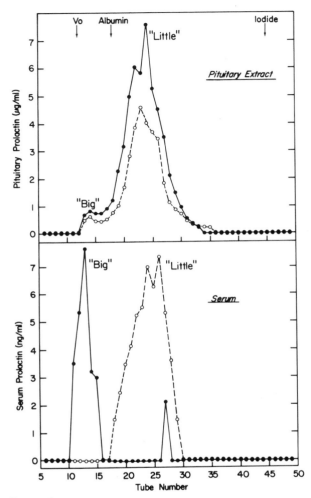

Figure 4
Chromatographic profile on Sephadex G-100 of endogenous immunoreactive prolactin in the sera and pituitary extracts of adult, virgin female mice. A column of 1.5 × 30 cm was used, and fractions were collected in volumes of 1 ml. (———) the C3H/St strain; (– – –) the C57BL/St strain. (→) The positions of the void volume (Vo), peaks of human serum albumin, and free [125]I. (Data from Sinha and Baxter 1979b.)

but the addition of an excess of mouse prolactin antiserum failed to precipitate completely the big prolactin peak, indicating the existence of a nonimmunoreactive component (Sinha and Baxter 1979b). Thus, it is safe to assume that for every nanogram of so-called big or little prolactin detected in plasma with the current RIA, perhaps several nanograms go undetected.

An Immunologically Unreactive Form of Prolactin in the Pituitary

In addition to these immunodetectable and nonimmunodectable size forms of prolactin, we have recently discovered that there is another form of prolactin in the mouse pituitary that is not detectable with RIA (Sinha and Baxter 1979a). This molecular variant is also present in the rat pituitary gland, but because it migrates with the same mobility as the main prolactin band in 7.5% acrylamide, the gel concentration generally used for the disc electrophoretic analysis of rat pituitary, it has easily gone unnoticed. Examination of the rat pituitary in different concentrations of acrylamide gel has enabled us to identify this new protein (Sinha and Gilligan 1981). Figure 5 shows the location of this new band (designated PRL 3) in the mouse and rat pituitary extracts electrophoresed in 10% and 12% gels, respectively. Table 3 shows its biological and immunological potencies in relation to the main pituitary prolactin designated PRL 1). Although highly active in the pigeon crop-sac bioassay, the new protein fails to cross-react in the current RIA for mouse and rat prolactin. The variant constitutes only a small proportion of total prolactin in the pituitary, but its turnover rate is rapid and it is approximately 35% greater in molecular weight (m.w.) than the main pituitary prolactin. Whether or not this nonimmunoreactive prolactin is released into circulation is not known, but is is released in vitro. That such a prolactin may indeed be present in plasma is also suggested by the experiments of Leung and Nicoll (1978), who have shown that the bio-

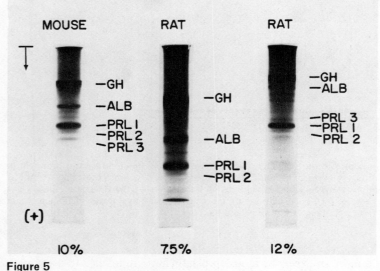

Figure 5
Disc electrophoretic patterns of mouse and rat anterior pituitary extracts. Pituitary extracts (100 μl) containing 1 mg (mouse) or 2 mg (rat) equivalents of wet pituitary tissue were applied on a 0.5 × 5.5-cm gel column. PRL 1 is the main prolactin, PRL 2 is believed to be a deamidated form, and PRL 3 is the new form. (Data redrawn from Sinha and Gilligan 1981.)

Table 3
Biological and Immunological Potencies of the Three Electrophoretic Bands
of Mouse and Rat Prolactins

Band number	Pigeon crop-sac activity[a] (IU/mg protein)	Activity in RIA (IU/mg protein)
	Mouse	
PRL 1	7.0 (0.9-17.1)	12.8
PRL 2	5.3 (1.8-10.0)	9.0
PRL 3	14.8 (2.3-33.1)	2.2
	Rat	
PRL 1	47.4 (25.3-105.0)	41.7
PRL 2	18.1 (3.8-41.9)	45.0
PRL 3	19.1 (4.8-38.5)	5.3

Data from Sinha and Baxter (1979a) and Sinha and Gilligan (1981).
[a] Values in parentheses indicate 95% confidence interval of the potency estimate.

assay estimates of prolactin in rat plasma are threefold higher than the radio-immunoassay estimates.

CONCLUSION

It is obvious that we are dealing with several forms of the prolactin hormone (Fig. 6). The pituitary gland contains, first, the monomeric prolactin of 23K m.w., some of which is detected with RIA and some of which is not. Second, there are the polymeric forms—dimers and larger aggregates. We can detect only a fraction of these with the radioimmunoassay. Finally, we find the new 31K-m.w. nonimmunoreactive form. Whether any of these nondetectable forms is released into circulation and in what quantities we do not know.

We do know that one of the forms that is released into circulation in vast quantities is the 23K-m.w. monomeric prolactin. However, when released, some 20% of this type converts into the larger forms—part of which is detected with our RIA and part of which is not. Still another important modification takes place in the remaining 23K-m.w. monomeric prolactin released into circulation: A good portion of it (as much as 70% in the case of the high-mammary-tumor C3H/St strain) becomes undectable with our RIA.

Thus, what we are measuring today with the RIA represents only a fraction of the total prolactin circulating in blood. It is not surprising then that

PITUITARY GLAND

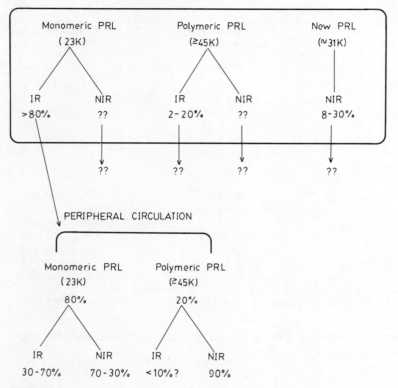

Figure 6

A summary of the different molecular forms of prolactin found in the pituitary gland and plasma. (IR) Immunoreactive; (NIR) nonimmunoreactive.

most of the studies conducted so far have failed to uncover a strong, clinically useful correlation between plasma prolactin and the incidence of breast cancer in humans and experimental animals. We need to develop methods to quantitate all the different molecular forms of prolactin present in blood. Only then can we hope to learn whether or not there is an actual relationship.

ACKNOWLEDGMENTS

This work is supported by grant CA-18664 from the National Institutes of Health. The reagents for rat prolactin RIA were kindly provided by the Pituitary Hormone Distribution Program of the NIH. This is Publication No. 41 from the Lutcher Brown Center for Diabetes and Endocrinology.

REFERENCES

Boyns, A.R., R. Buchan, E.N. Cole, A.P.M. Forrest, and K. Griffiths. 1973a. Basal prolactin blood levels in 3 strains of rat with differing incidence of 7,12-dimethylbenz(a)anthracene induced mammary tumors. *Eur. J. Cancer* 9:169.

Boyns, A.R., E.N. Cole, K. Griffiths, M.M. Roberts, R. Buchan, R.G. Wilson, and A.P.M. Forrest. 1973b. Plasma prolactin in breast cancer. *Eur. J. Cancer* 9:99.

Cole, E.N., P.C. England, R.A. Sellwood, and K. Griffiths. 1977. Serum prolactin concentrations throughout the menstrual cycle of normal women and patients with recent breast cancer. *Eur. J. Cancer* 13:677.

Dickey, R.P. and J.P. Minto. 1972. L-dopa effect on prolactin, follicle-stimulating hormone, and luteinizing hormone in women with advanced breast cancer: A preliminary report. *Am. J. Obstet. Gynecol.* 114:267.

Franks, S., D.N.L. Ralphs, V. Seagroatt, and H.S. Jacobs. 1974. Prolactin concentrations in patients with breast cancer. *Br. Med. J.* 4:320.

Gala, R.R. and S.J. Loginsky. 1973. Correlation between serum prolactin levels and incidence of mammary tumors induced by 7,12-dimethylbenz(a)-anthracene in the rat. *J. Natl. Cancer Inst.* 51:593.

Gala, R.R. and I.C. Hart. 1980. Serum prolactin heterogeneity in the cow and goat. *Life Sci.* 27:723.

Grosvenor, C.E. 1967. Disappearance rate of exogenous prolactin from serum of female rats. *Endocrinology* 80:195.

Hawkins, R.A., D. Drewitt, B. Freedman, E. Killin, D.A. Jenner, and E.H.D. Cameron. 1976. Plasma hormone levels and the incidence of carcinogen-induced mammary tumours in two strains of rat. *Br. J. Cancer* 34:546.

Henderson, B.E., V. Gerkins, I. Rosario, J. Casagrande, and M.C. Pike. 1975. Elevated serum levels of estrogens and prolactin in daughters of patients with breast cancer. *N. Engl. J. Med.* 293:790.

Hill, P., E.L. Wynder, H. Kumar, P. Helman, G. Rona, and K. Kuno. 1976. Prolactin levels in populations at risk for breast cancer. *Cancer Res.* 36:4102.

Hwang, P., H. Guyda, and H. Friesen. 1971. A radioimmunoassay for human prolactin. *Proc. Natl. Acad. Sci.* 68:1902.

Kim, U. and J. Furth. 1976. The role of prolactin in carcinogenesis. In *Vitamins and hormones* (ed. P.L. Munson et al.), vol. 34, p. 107. Academic Press, New York.

Koch, Y., Y.F. Chow, and J. Meites. 1971. Metabolic clearance and secretion rates of prolactin in the rat. *Endocrinology* 89:1303.

Kwa, H.G. and D.Y. Wang. 1977. An abnormal luteal-phase evening peak of plasma prolactin in women with a family history of breast cancer. *Int. J. Cancer* 20:12.

Kwa, H.G., M. De Jong-Bakker, E. Engelsman, and F.J. Cleton. 1974. Plasma prolactin in human breast cancer. *Lancet* i:433.

Kwa, H.G., F. Cleton, M. De Jong-Bakker, R.D. Bulbrook, J.L. Hayward, and D.Y. Wang. 1976. Plasma prolactin and its relationship to risk factors in human breast cancer. *Int. J. Cancer* 17:441.

Lawson, D.M. and R.W. Stevens. 1980. Size heterogeneity of pituitary and plasma prolactin: Effect of chronic estrogen treatment. *Life Sciences* 27:1489.

Leung, F.C., S.M. Russell, and C.S. Nicoll. 1978. Relationship between bioassay and radioimmunoassay estimates of prolactin in rat serum. *Endocrinology* 103:1619.

Lewis, U.J., S.M. Peterson, L.F. Bonewald, B.K. Seavey, and W.P. VanderLaan. 1977. An interchain disulfide dimer of human growth hormone. *J. Biol. Chem.* 252:3697.

McFayden, I.J., A.P.M. Forrest, R.J. Prescott, M.P. Golder, G.V. Groom, D.R. Fahmy, and K. Griffiths. 1976. Circulating hormone concentrations in women with breast cancer. *Lancet* i:1100.

Malarkey, W.B., L.L. Schroeder, V.C. Stevens, A.G. James, and R.R. Lanese. 1977. Disordered nocturnal prolactin regulation in women with breast cancer. *Cancer Res.* 37:4650.

Medina, D., S.B. O'Bryan, M.R. Warner, Y.N. Sinha, W.P. VanderLaan, S. McCormack, and P. Hahn. 1977. Mammary tumorigenesis in chemical carcinogen-treated mice. VII. Prolactin and progesterone levels in BALB/c mice. *J. Natl. Cancer Inst.* 59:213.

Meites, J. 1972. Relation of prolactin and estrogen to mammary tumorigenesis in the rat. *J. Natl. Cancer Inst.* 48:1217.

Mittra, I., J.L. Hayward, and A.S. McNeilly. 1974. Hypothalamic-pituitary-prolactin axis in breast cancer. *Lancet* i:889.

Moore, W.V. and D. Jin. 1978. Polymeric and monomeric human growth hormone binding to rat liver plasma membranes. *J. Clin. Endocrinol. Metab.* 46:374.

Murray, R.M.L., G. Mozaffarian, and O.H. Pearson. 1972. Prolactin levels with L-dopa treatment in metastatic breast carcinoma. In *Prolactin and carcinogenesis* (ed. A.R. Boyns and K. Griffiths), p. 158. Alpha Omega Alpha Publishing, Cardiff, Wales.

Niswender, G.D., C.L. Chen, A.R. Midgley, Jr., J. Meites, and S. Ellis. 1969. Radioimmunoassay for rat prolactin. *Proc. Soc. Exp. Biol. Med.* 130:793.

Nagasawa, H., C.L. Chen, and J. Meites. 1973. Relation between growth of carcinogen-induced mammary cancers and serum prolactin values in rats. *Proc. Soc. Exp. Biol. Med.* 142:625.

Nagasawa, H., F. Kanzawa and K. Kuretani. 1967a. Lactation performance of the high and low mammary tumor strains of mice. *Gann* 58:331.

Nagasawa, H., H. Iwashi, F. Kanzawa, M. Fujimoto, and K. Kuretani. 1967b. A comparative study on the normal mammary gland development in high and low mammary tumor strains of virgin mice. *Gann* 58:45.

Nagasawa, H., R. Yanai, H. Taniguchi, R. Tokuzen, and W. Nakahara. 1976. Two-way selection of a stock of swiss albino mice for mammary tumorigenesis: Establishment of two new strains (SHN and SLN). *J. Natl. Cancer Inst.* 57:425.

Rolandi, E., T. Barreca, P. Masturzo, A. Polleri, F. Indiveri, and A. Barabino. 1974. Plasma prolactin in breast cancer. *Lancet* ii:845.

Sheth, N.A., K.J. Ranadive, J.N. Suraiya, and A.R. Sheth. 1975. Circulating levels of prolactin in human breast cancer. *Br. J. Cancer* 32:160.

Sinha, Y.N. 1980. Molecular size variants of prolactin and growth hormone in mouse serum: Strain differences and alterations of concentrations by physiological and pharmacological stimuli. *Endocrinology* **107**:1959.

Sinha, Y.N. and S.R. Baxter. 1979a. Identification of a non-immunoreactive but highly bioactive form of prolactin in the mouse pituitary by gel electrophoresis. *Biochem. Biophys. Res. Commun.* **86**:325.

————. 1979b. Metabolism of prolactin in mice with high incidence of mammary tumours: Evidence for greater conversion into a non-immunoassayable form. *J. Endocrinol.* **81**:299.

Sinha, Y.N. and T.A. Gilligan. 1981. Identification of a less immunoreactive form of prolactin in the rat pituitary. *Endocrinology* **108**:1091.

Sinha, Y.N., C.B. Salocks, and W.P. VanderLaan. 1975. Prolactin and growth hormone levels in different inbred strains of mice: Patterns in association with estrous cycle, time of day, and perphenazine stimulation. *Endocrinology* **97**:1112.

————. 1976. Circulating levels of prolactin and growth hormone and natural incidence of mammary tumors in mice. *J. Toxicol. Environ. Health* (Suppl.) **1**:131.

Sinha, Y.N., S.R. Baxter, and W.P. VanderLaan. 1979a. Metabolic clearance rate of prolactin during various physiological states in mice with high and low incidence of mammary tumors. *Endocrinology* **105**:680.

Sinha, Y.N., G. Vlahakis, and W.P. VanderLaan. 1979b. Serum, pituitary and urine concentrations of prolactin and growth hormone in eight strains of mice with varying incidence of mammary tumors. *Int. J. Cancer* **24**:430.

Sinha, Y.N., F.W. Selby, U.J. Lewis, and W.P. VanderLaan. 1972. Studies of prolactin secretion in mice by a homologous radioimmunoassay. *Endocrinology* **91**:1045.

————. 1973. A homologous radioimmunoassay for human prolactin. *J. Clin. Endocrinol. Metab.* **36**:509.

Sinha, Y.N., C.B. Salocks, U.J. Lewis, and W.P. Vanderlaan. 1974. Influence of nursing on the release of prolactin and GH in mice with high and low incidence of mammary tumors. *Endocrinology* **95**:947.

Suh, H.K. and A.G. Frantz. 1974. Size heterogeneity of human prolactin in plasma and pituitary extracts. *J. Clin. Endocrinol. Metab.* **39**:928.

Tarquini, A., L. di Martino, A. Malloci, H.G. Kwa, A.A. van der Gugten, R.D. Bulbrook, and D.Y. Wang. 1978. Abnormalities in evening plasma prolactin levels in nulliparous women with benign or malignant breast disease. *Int. J. Cancer* **22**:687.

van der Gugten, A.A. and A.A. Verstraeten. 1973. The relation of prolactin and mammary gland carcinogenesis. In *Methods in cancer research* (ed. H. Busch), vol. 10, p. 161. Academic Press, New York.

Welsch, C.W. and H. Nagasawa. 1977. Prolactin and murine mammary tumorigenesis: A review. *Cancer Res.* **37**:951.

COMMENTS

SIITERI: I would like to thank Dr. Sinha for his presentation, because it was a marvelous piece of work and because it points out something that we should all remember—that is, that the production rate of a hormone is equal to its MCR times the concentration. When you measure the concentration, it tells you nothing about its clearance rate or its production rate.

If you have a system in which the production rate doesn't necessarily change, that is, it doesn't respond to an ordinary kind of feedback system, then the clearance rate is the primary determinant of the concentration.

Dr. Sinha showed differences in clearance rates of prolactin among mouse strains. Therefore, a strain that clears the hormone more rapidly will have a lower serum concentration, and that is exactly what he observed in the high-tumor-incidence strain. So clearly, then, MCR, which depends on rates of target tissue uptake of the hormone as well as metabolism, will determine the serum concentration.

This is a lesson to those of us who measure steroid hormones also. If you have a system in which there is no feedback, such as extraglandular estrogen production in postmenopausal women, you can imagine a situation in which the concentration of the hormone is lower than normal because there is more going to the target tissue and having a bigger effect than if the serum concentration were normal or, in fact, elevated.

Dr. Sinha's studies tie in beautifully with the idea that I was trying to get across yesterday. Our gut instinct is to look for higher hormone levels and then conclude that there is more effect. The fact of the matter is, you can have a lower level and, at the target level, have a bigger effect.

DAO: Is the MCR reported for progesterone and estrogen in the premenopausal very similar?

SIITERI: There is only one study I know of that has been done in breast cancer and that is by Marv Kirschner (Kirschner et al. 1978). He obtained extraordinarily interesting results, which are difficult to understand. He measured the MCR of estrone in 46 women with breast cancer and two-thirds of the values clustered at about 1800 liters per day, which was the same as the controls. The other third had clearance rates that were much higher, with a mean value of about 3500 and some values as high as 5000-6000 liters per day.

MEITES: Finn [Siiteri], isn't it true that it is not so easy to change the MCR? As I recall, work that was done in human subjects with luteinizing hormone (LH), follicle-stimulating hormone (FSH), and testosterone during pregnancy, for example, did not show any change as compared to nonpregnancy (Koch et al. 1970).

Incidentally, regarding prolactin, we compared the MCR in hypophysectomized and castrated rats in males versus females, and in pregnant and nonpregnant animals, and found no difference in MCR.

SIITERI: Dr. Sinha just showed you a twofold difference for prolactin. In the case of testosterone, the MCR is increased in hyperandrogenic states.

SINHA: Even in rats, the clearance rate of prolactin increases during lactation, as shown by Grosvenor et al. (1977).

ROSEN: In the case of adrenocorticotropin (ACTH), there is a larger precursor containing melancyte-stimulation hormone (MSH) and β-endorphin that is synthesized as a single precursor and then processed. But the data for prolactin, where they have isolated mRNA and translated it in cell-free systems, suggest that it is synthesized as a 24K-m.w. moiety. Except for the single peptide in preprolactin, they don't find a very much larger form.

Have you taken and run on an SDS gel your larger forms to see if they really run as intact molecules? Have you done any tryptic mapping to see their relationship to the 24K-m.w. form?

SINHA: We are in the process of doing those studies. These molecular weight estimates are preliminary at this time.

ROSEN: So those are nondenaturing gels that you showed.

SINHA: Yes. The data I have shown are from nondenaturing polyacetylamide gels.

ROSEN: Okay. So, most likely, these represent some sort of intermolecular associations rather than actually a larger precursor polypeptide for prolactin.

SINHA: We have to experiment further to tell for sure what the actual molecular weight is.

KORENMAN: Have you studied the effects of hormonal stimulation of prolactin secretion?

SINHA: No, we have not progressed that far in our work yet.

SHIU: In reference to Dr. Sinha's demonstration of a different form of prolactin, we also have a lot of evidence for that in our lab, even in just the ordinary rat. We have been switching to the lymphoma cell bioassay system. In the old days, the bioassay was not sensitive enough to pick up low levels of prolactin, but now everything has changed around. When your RIA is not accurate enough, you use the lymphoma cell line, which is sensitive to 10 pg/ml of prolactin.

However, we have also observed that if you take sera from animals, especially under different physiological situations, for example, during pregnancy in the rat, you do find discrepancies between the two assays. The RIA will pick up a certain amount of RIA prolactin; but you pick up a lot more by using a bioassay.

There are some people who are beginning to use these sorts of tests to screen human sera under different conditions. For example, a lot of sera has been screened for patients with renal failure. Now we are trying to collect human sera from breast cancer patients, using this assay, and trying to see whether something different shows up.

SINHA: I did not have time to review the literature on this matter. But Dr. Nicoll's laboratory has been doing studies for a number of years trying to demonstrate discrepancies among RIA, bioassay, and disc electrophoretic assay for prolactin. He has shown that if you measure prolactin in the rat with bioassay, you detect three- to fivefold more prolactin than you detect with RIA (Leung et al. 1978). Of course in the case of GH, there is even more data on the discrepancies between bioassay and RIA. We have to be very cautious at this point as to what we are talking about when we are discussing correlations.

SIRBASKU: Is it possible to dissociate the big form in the plasma to the other forms? That is, can you dissociate the big form back to little form by any specific treatment?

SINHA: Yes you can. We have not done these studies with mouse hormones yet, but it has been done by others with human prolactin and human GH. You take the big form and then treat it with dissociating agents, such as mercaptoethanol and urea. There is a proportion that reverts back to the monomeric form, but not all of it. Some of it does not dissociate.

SIRBASKU: So you mean it is disulfide rich.

SINHA: Yes, some of the big form is disulfide-bonded.

References

Grosvenor, C.E., S. Mena, and M.S. Whitworch. 1977. Metabolic clearance of rat prolactin in the lactating and nonlactating rat. *J. Endocrinol.* 73:1.

Kirschner, M.A., F.B. Cohen, and C. Ryan. 1978. Androgen-estrogen production rates in postmenopausal women with breast cancer. *Cancer Res.* 38:4029.

Koch, Y., K.H. Lu, and J. Meites. 1970. Biphasic effect of catecholamines on pituitary prolactin release in vitro. *Endocrinology* 87:673.

Leung, F.C., S.M. Russell, and C.S. Nicoll. 1978. Relationship between bioassay and radioimmunal assay estimates of prolactin in rat serum. *Endocrinology* 103:1619.

SESSION 8:
Mechanism of Hormone Action

Regulation of Casein Gene Expression in Hormone-dependent Mammary Cancer

JEFFREY M. ROSEN, SCOTT C. SUPOWIT, PRABHAKAR GUPTA,
LI-YUAN YU, AND ANDREW A. HOBBS
Department of Cell Biology
Baylor College of Medicine
Houston, Texas 77030

The preceding presentations at this conference have focused on the epidemiology of breast cancer and studies concerned with the endocrine physiology and cell biology of normal and neoplastic mammary tissue. In the past few years, however, the mammary gland also has provided an attractive model system of increasing interest to molecular biologists. The principal reason that our laboratory became interested in studying the regulation of gene expression in normal and transformed mammary cells is the existence of a family of hormone-inducible genes. This is the casein gene family that is composed principally of three major proteins in the rat (α-, β-, and γ-caseins). In addition, there is a fourth major milk protein, α-lactalbumin, that is also under hormonal regulation. These four milk protein genes are regulated by the interaction of several peptide and steroid hormones (Topper 1970).

An additional advantage of the mammary gland system is that the multihormonal regulation of gene expression can be studied in organ culture using a chemically defined, serum-free medium (Elias 1957). Although there may be differences in the endocrine physiology and genetic backgrounds of various species, the mechanism of hormone action at the molecular level should be similar in all cases. However, the interpretation of homonal effects observed, even using a chemically defined medium, may be complicated by the prior exposure of explants to hormones both in vivo and during preincubation periods in culture (Bolander et al. 1979; Bolander and Topper 1980). As hormonally responsive cell culture systems are developed, it will be possible to extend the studies described in this chapter to primary cell cultures grown on collagen matrices (as described by Nandi, this volume). Ideally, cloned cell lines should be employed because cell heterogeneity, especially as observed in tumor cell populations (Supowit et al. 1981), may present a problem in the interpretation of the results obtained using whole tumor samples and explant or primary cell cultures.

A final reason for studying gene expression in the mammary gland is that hormone-dependent mammary tumor cells provide a series of genetic variants that may contain defects at levels other than that of the hormone receptor. As discussed by Lippman (this volume) and previously reported by Tomkins and coworkers (Sibley and Tomkins 1974), the majority of hormone-resistant cell lines either contain altered hormone receptors or lack receptors. Hormone-dependent tumor cells provide another type of variant, which presumably maintains an active receptor, as evidenced by hormone-dependent growth properties; yet these cells may contain other altered hormonal responses. Thus, a major objective in our laboratory has been to elucidate the mechanisms by which hormones regulate growth and the expression of differentiation in the normal mammary gland, and how these regulatory mechanisms have deviated in hormone-dependent breast cancer.

In this presentation, I will summarize briefly what we have learned about the structure, organization, and expression of the casein gene family and the α-lactalbumin gene in the normal mammary gland. In addition, I will discuss the altered regulation of casein gene expression, and gene expression in general, in hormone-dependent mammary cancer.

THE MILK PROTEIN STRUCTURAL GENES

The milk protein genes provide a group of well-defined molecular markers for studying the mechanism by which hormones regulate gene expression in normal and neoplastic mammary tissue. Unfortunately for molecular biologists, cell growth is not a satisfactory end point for elucidating regulatory mechanisms, because the many and complex processes involved in DNA replication are not really well understood, even in the simplest prokaryotic system. As the milk protein mRNAs are highly abundant mRNAs (i.e., they represent 60-80% of the mRNA in an 8-day lactating rat mammary gland), they are purified easily from the bulk of other mRNAs (Fig. 1). In the rat and mouse, there are three principal casein mRNAs coding for the α-, β-, and γ-caseins. In addition to these three major caseins, there may be other minor caseins, such as κ-casein, and other expressed genes and pseudogenes related to the three major caseins. The casein genes appear to comprise a family of nonidentical but related genes that may have arisen from the duplication and divergence of a common ancestral gene (Taborsky 1974; Rosen and Shields 1980). However, the precise evolutionary and functional relations between the members of the casein gene family have yet to be elucidated. The fourth major milk protein gene, α-lactalbumin, is also under hormonal regulation, although its expression may be regulated differentially compared to the casein genes (Nakhasi and Qasba 1979; Ono and Oka 1980).

As shown in Figure 1C, the milk protein mRNAs are the predominant mRNAs observed in a total poly(A) RNA preparation isolated from an 8-day lactating mouse mammary gland. The comparative migration of partially purified rat α- and β-casein mRNAs is shown in Figure 1B, and in Figure 1D is shown a bovine total poly(A) RNA preparation. Although the α-casein mRNAs and their

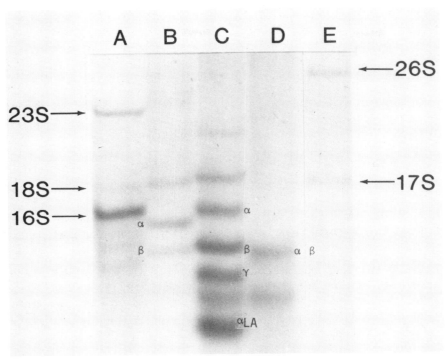

Figure 1
Characterization of milk protein mRNAs on a 1.5% agarose, 10 mM CH₃HgOH gel (Richards et al. 1981a). In all, 5–10 μg of RNA were loaded on each track. Lane A, *E. coli* rRNA standards; B, rat casein Sepharose 4B fraction containing α- and β-casein mRNAs; C, mouse poly(A) RNA isolated from 8-day lactating tissue; D, bovine poly(A) RNA isolated from lactating Holstein cow; E, yeast rRNA standards.

respective proteins are significantly larger than the β-caseins in the rat and mouse, the α- and β-caseins and their mRNAs appear to be quite similar in size in the cow and other species. Because these mRNAs are highly abundant, it is possible to separate them from other nonmilk protein mRNAs and to synthesize specific casein and α-lactalbumin cDNA probes with which to quantitate the levels of these mRNAs (Rosen and Barker 1976; Nakahasi and Qasba 1979). Most of our earlier studies were performed using a cDNA probe synthesized from a mixture of predominantly α- and β-casein mRNAs, as it was difficult to completely resolve these two mRNAs from each other (Matusik and Rosen 1978).

With the advent of recombinant DNA technology, it has been possible to generate specific probes for each of the casein mRNAs—α, β, and γ, and α-lactalbumin mRNA (Richards et al. 1981a,b). The construction and analysis of the rat cDNA clones are described in detail in Richards et al. (1981a,b).

Recently, we also have constructed and isolated cDNA clones for the corresponding mouse milk protein mRNAs (Gupta et al. 1981). Analysis of both sets of clones indicates that there has been sufficient divergence of the casein genes at both the inter- and intraspecies levels, with the β-casein gene being the most highly conserved between different species. Thus, it is possible to generate specific hybridization probes for each of the casein genes, as well as α-lactalbumin. Furthermore, divergence between species requires the use of homologous probes in hybridization experiments. These cloned probes have been used to quantitate the levels of the four milk protein mRNAs after hormonal manipulation in organ culture, so as to determine the structure, organization, and chromosomal localization of these genes and to identify putative RNA precursors for each of these mRNAs. These studies will be reviewed briefly in the following sections.

HORMONAL REGULATION OF MILK PROTEIN mRNA ACCUMULATION IN RAT MAMMARY GLAND ORGAN CULTURE

Previously, we have reported the acute effects of hormones on milk protein mRNA accumulation in rat mammary gland organ culture (Matusik and Rosen 1978). In these studies, mammary glands were removed from 14-day-pregnant animals and cultured for 48 hr, either in the presence of insulin alone or insulin and hydrocortisone. Following prolactin addition, a rapid induction of casein mRNA accumulation was observed, with an increased level detectable by at least 4 hr and a 10-fold induction after 24 hr. In the absence of prolactin, with insulin and hydrocortisone alone, a basal level of casein mRNA was attained and no net accumulation was observed. The continuous presence of hydrocortisone in the culture medium also resulted in potentiation of the effect of the peptide hormone and increased casein mRNA levels (Matusik and Rosen 1978; Guyette et al. 1979).

Using individual cDNA probes prepared from the cloned milk protein structural genes, we recently have reinvestigated the induction of each of the four milk protein mRNAs in organ culture (Fig. 2). Although it had been expected a priori that the three casein mRNAs might display similar induction kinetics, instead, differential rates of accumulation for each of these mRNAs were observed (Fig. 2). During the initial 48-hr incubation period with insulin and hydrocortisone alone, all four mRNAs (α-, β-, and γ-casein and α-lactalbumin) decreased to, respectively, 1.3%, 0.7%, 0.07%, and 2.1% of the levels of each mRNA observed in the maximally induced 8-day lactating gland. The basal level of γ-casein mRNA was, therefore, almost 20-fold lower than that of α-casein mRNA. Addition of prolactin then resulted in the rapid induction of the casein mRNAs reaching levels 7-, 32-, and 240-fold (for α-, β-, and γ-casein mRNAs, respectively) greater than that with insulin and hydrocortisone alone after 24 hr. In contrast, little change was observed in α-lactalbumin mRNA levels during the first 12 hr after prolactin addition with a 5-fold induction

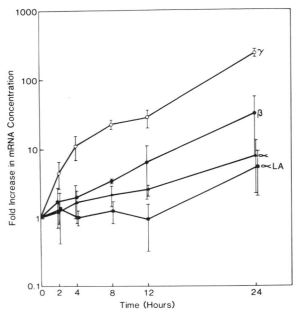

Figure 2
Differential induction of milk protein mRNA accumulation in mammary gland organ culture. Cultures were performed as described by Matusik and Rosen (1978) and Guyette et al. (1979). Following the initial 48-hr preincubation containing insulin (I) and hydrocortisone (F), prolactin was added at a concentration of 1 μg/ml for the times indicated. The concentration of each mRNA (expressed as the fold induction over the respective IF basal level) was determined in total RNA extracts by cDNA excess hybridization using individual cDNAs prepared from cloned DNA probes.

achieved by 24 hr. Omission of hydrocortisone during both the initial 48-hr incubation and the 24-hr induction period resulted in a reduction in mRNA levels with differential effects observed on both the basal and induced levels of each of these four mRNAs.

One of the critical questions inherent in these studies is, at what level do hormones regulate the differential accumulation of these mRNAs? The milk protein mRNAs are somewhat unique in that they constitute superprevalent mRNAs, i.e., those mRNAs present at a level of greater than 10,000 copies per cell. Clearly, selective mRNA accumulation is one of the principal mechanisms that regulates the expression of the cellular phenotype in both normal and transformed cells (Jacobs and Birnie 1980; Supowit and Rosen 1980). In our previous studies of casein gene expression, we had attempted to dissociate effects of hormones at the transcriptional level from those at the posttranscriptional level, i.e., mRNA processing and turnover (Guyette et al. 1979). The conclusions of these earlier studies were that prolactin regulated casein gene expression by increasing both the rate of transcription of the casein genes (α and β) 2- to 4-fold, as well as by increasing the half-life of their individual mRNAs 17- to 25-fold. Although we do not understand the mechanism by which prolactin elicits these changes, it is apparent that there are coordinated effects of hormones on both the rates of synthesis and either the processing or turnover of these mRNAs.

This type of coordinated response to a single hormone explains the complexity of understanding the multihormonal regulation of gene expression. For example, we have demonstrated that in the presence of maximally effective concentrations of prolactin, the addition of hydrocortisone to the culture medium did not increase further the rate of transcription, but it did act posttranscriptionally to affect casein mRNA accumulation (Guyette et al. 1979). In these experiments the initial 48-hr incubation was performed in the presence of insulin and hydrocortisone, and the subsequent induction performed with insulin and prolactin or with insulin, hydrocortisone, and prolactin. Because of the possibility of retention of some residual hydrocortisone in the explants during the subsequent induction period (Bolander et al. 1979), it is not possible to ascertain in our experiments if a small amount of hydrocortisone is required for prolactin induction of casein mRNA (Ganguly et al. 1980). Both prolactin and hydrocortisone are required for the maximal expression of the casein genes (Matusik and Rosen 1978), and hydrocortisone has significant effects on the development of the mammary gland (Topper 1970). At present, however, there is no definitive evidence that hydrocortisone acts to increase the rate of casein gene transcription.

Using pulse-labeling and pulse-chase studies and specific cloned DNA probes, it now should be possible to examine the interaction of these hormones at the transcriptional and posttranscriptional levels in greater detail. In particular, it will be possible to determine if the differential rates of accumulation of the four milk protein mRNAs (Fig. 2) are the results of their different rates of synthesis, processing, or turnover. Furthermore, because hydrocortisone differentially affects both the basal and induced levels of these mRNAs, similar studies can be performed in cultures incubated in the presence of insulin and prolactin or of insulin, prolactin, and hydrocortisone in which a 48-hr preincubation will be performed with insulin alone. An analysis of the effects of hormones on milk protein gene expression as compared with the expression of constitutively synthesized housekeeping genes and hormone-regulated ribosomal RNA genes (Teysott and Houdebine 1980) may also help define the mechanisms responsible for the selective accumulation of these specialized, abundant mRNAs. For example, a recent comparison of prolactin effects on the transcription and accumulation of both β-casein mRNA and 28S rRNA in the rabbit mammary gland indicated that the transcription rate of both genes was increased. However, although there was a good correlation between changes in the transcription rate and 28S rRNA accumulation, the increase in β-casein gene transcription was unable to account for the simultaneous accumulation of its mRNA (Teyssot and Houdebine 1980). These experiments help confirm the selective posttranscriptional effect of prolactin on casein mRNA accumulation reported in our earlier studies (Guyette et al. 1979).

MILK PROTEIN GENE ORGANIZATION
AND CHROMOSOMAL LOCALIZATION

A necessary prerequisite to understanding the regulation of the milk protein genes is the elucidation of their structure, organization, and chromosomal localization. In particular, it is important to determine if these genes are regulated in a *cis* or *trans* fashion in analogy to the α- and β-globin gene families (Leder et al. 1980). Initially, we wanted to establish the chromosomal localization of the casein and the α-lactalbumin genes. This was accomplished by analyzing a series of mouse-hamster somatic cell hybrids (kindly provided by Drs. Peter D'Eustachio and Frank Ruddle at Yale University) that selectively exclude mouse chromosomes. The DNA extracted from different cloned cells is analyzed by nucleic acid hybridization and, following their karyotype determination, it is possible to map the chromosomal localization of specific genes. For example, such an approach has been employed recently to determine the chromosomal assignment of the mouse κ-light-chain genes (Swan et al. 1979). In this technique, each DNA sample is digested with a restriction endonuclease and, following agarose gel electrophoresis and Southern transfer to a nitrocellulose filter, the specific genes are mapped by hybridization with a cloned cDNA probe.

As illuatrated in Figure 3, a panel of hybrid DNAs (lanes 3-13), as well as the parental mouse (lane 1) and hamster (lane 2) DNAs, were screened by the above technique using both α- (Fig. 3A) and β-mouse casein (Fig. 3B) cDNA clones. Three positive lines were identified (Fig. 3, lanes 5, 6, and 11) using both the α- and β-casein probes. Note that a rearrangement was observed in one cell line in both the α- and β-casein genes or their flanking DNA sequences (Fig. 3, lane 5). No cross hybridization was detected between the mouse α-casein cDNA and hamster DNA (Fig. 3A, lane 2), but the more highly conserved mouse β-casein probe showed a specific 3.1-kb *Eco*RI band present in the parental hamster line and all the hybrid lines containing hamster chromosomes. The weak signal observed in lane 11 was the result of an incomplete digest of that DNA sample as was evidenced also by the weak 3.1-kb hamster DNA band (Fig. 3B, lane 11).

Karyotype analysis of the mouse-hamster hybrids indicated that all the positive lines contained mouse chromosome 5, while all the negative lines had excluded this chromosome. This tentative assignment of the α- and β-casein genes to mouse chromosome 5 has been confirmed as well for the γ-casein gene and a fourth gene designated "β-like," which codes for an abundant mRNA of unknown function. This gene may represent another member of the casein gene family that has diverged recently from the mouse β-casein gene.

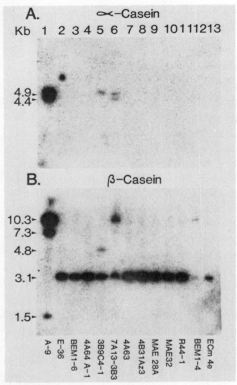

Figure 3
Chromosomal localization of the α-casein (*A*) and β-casein (*B*) genes in somatic cell hybrids. Here, 30 μg of *Eco*RI-digested DNAs were electrophoresed on a 1% agarose gel as described by Swan et al. (1979). Hybridization was performed using homologous mouse α- and β-casein cDNA clones (Gupta et al. 1981). Lane 1, parental mouse A-9 L-cell line; 2, parental hamster E-36 cell line; 3–13, individual hybrid cell clones.

To establish definitively the localization of the casein genes, we have utilized a mouse albumin cDNA probe (kindly provided by Dr. Shirley Tilghman at the Institute of Cancer Research, Fox Chase, Pa.) to screen the original set, and another independently constructed panel of somatic cell hybrids. Albumin has been mapped previously by both genetic and biochemical technique to chromosome 5. In all cases, albumin and the four caseins hybridized to the same hybrid cell lines. Similar experiments were performed with an α-lactalbumin gene probe. However, a different set of somatic cell hybrid DNAs hybridized with this probe. Thus, although the caseins are present most likely as a gene cluster on chromosome 5 and should be regulated in *cis*, another hormone-regulated gene in the mammary gland, α-lactalbumin, is present on a different chromosome and should be regulated in *trans*. More precise chromosomal localization of these genes may be possible by in situ hybridization and by the analysis of various translocations of chromosome 5 (Meo et al. 1980). Possible rearrangements of these genes following transformation by chemical and viral agents also can be analyzed and may be correlated with specific altered banding patterns in tumor chromosomes.

In addition to elucidating the chromosomal localization of the milk protein genes, it was important to determine their primary structures and the linkage arrangements, if present, among the casein genes. These studies are a necessary prerequisite for future transcriptional analyses and might help define common control regions adjacent to these genes. To determine the primary structures of these genes, it was necessary first to isolated them from a DNA library containing large, random DNA fragments cloned in a phage λ vector (Maniatis et al. 1978). The partial *Eco*RI rat DNA library employed in our studies was kindly provided by Drs. Tom Sargent, R. Bruce Wallace, and James Bonner at the California Institute of Technology.

Initial screening was performed with a mixed hybridization probe consisting of three rat casein cDNA clones (Richards et al. 1981b). Following plaque purification of individual phage DNAs, the DNAs then were screened with the individual α-, β-, or γ-casein cDNA probes. In this manner, it was hoped that it might be possible to localize two casein genes on a single DNA fragment. However, we have yet to find any individual DNA fragments ranging in size up to 22 kb and containing more than a single casein gene. In fact, most of the large, cloned *Eco*RI DNA fragments contain only a portion of each of the individual casein genes. The reason for this is that these genes are extremely large, ranging in size from 17 kb to 25 kb. They are much larger than their respective mRNAs, which, as illustated in Figure 1, ranged in size from 900 to 1330 nucleotides in the rat.

The structure of the casein genes has been studied by both restriction mapping and R-loop analysis. An electron micrograph showing an R-loop analysis of the γ-casein gene (kindly provided by Dr. Myles L. Mace at Baylor) is presented in Figure 4. In this technique, hybridization of the γ-casein mRNA to the genomic DNA was performed under conditions of formamide, with ionic strength and temperature such that the DNA-RNA hybrids are more stable than the corresponding DNA-DNA duplex. The presence of loops in the electron micrograph illustrates that the γ-casein gene is divided into noncontiguous pieces, i.e., it is interrupted by intervening sequences, or introns. This is not unusual, because intervening sequences are characteristic of almost all mammalian genes that have been studied to date, with just a few exceptions (Crick 1979). One interesting feature of the γ-casein gene is that it is a 17-kb gene, almost 18 times larger than the mature γ-casein mRNA, and interrupted by a minimum of nine intervening sequences. The particular clone illustrated in Figure 4 appears to be missing a small portion of its 5′ end, as demonstrated by more detailed restriction mapping studies.

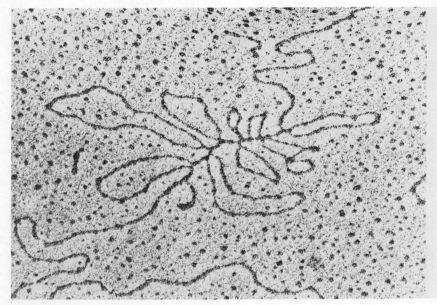

Figure 4
Electron microscopic analysis of a γ-casein genomic DNA clone. Here, 250 ng phage DNA containing the γ-casein gene (10 μg/ml) was hybridized to 750 ng of a Sepharose 4B fraction containing γ-casein mRNA (30 μg/ml) under R-loop conditions, i.e., 70% formide, 0.3 M NaCl, 10 mM Tris-HCl (pH 7.6), 10 mM EDTA in a reaction volume of 25 μl. The samples were denatured for 2 min at 80°C, hybridized for 3 hr at 52°C and cooled to room temperature prior to EM spreading (Richards et al. 1981a.)

Similar complex genes have been isolated for the α- and β-caseins, but their precise structures have not yet been determined. Because these genes are quite large, it was not unexpected that we did not isolate a single DNA fragment containing more than one casein gene. The maximum size of DNA that can be cloned into the Charon 4A vector used to construct the rat DNA library was only 20-22 kb in size. Therefore, to determine the precise arrangement of the casein genes, it will be necessary to perform gene walking experiments, in which adjacent DNA fragments progressively are isolated until the neighboring gene of interest is isolated. Overlapping fragments then can be ordered to define the structure of larger DNA regions, as, for example, the entire β-gene cluster present in 65 kb of human DNA (Fritsch et al. 1980).

The complexity of the milk protein genes provides another potential site of hormonal regulation of gene expression, i.e., at the level of RNA processing. In addition to the regulation of transcription and mRNA turnover, efficient γ-casein mRNA synthesis requires the splicing out of a minimum of nine intervening sequences. As a first step in studying the role of hormones at the level of RNA processing, we have analyzed the size of the steady-state pre-mRNA intermediates that are present in nuclear RNA isolated from lactating tissue. A series of unique, poly(A), putative mRNA precursors for each of the milk protein mRNAs have been identified, ranging in size up to 10 kb (Rodgers et al. 1980). However, within the limitations of our present technology, we have not been able to isolate RNA transcripts representative of the entire length of the respective milk protein genes. Thus, processing is most likely a rapid event, and the concentrations of these transcripts are extremely low. At present, we have no evidence for the existence of a common primary transcript containing more than a single casein mRNA. Each of the casein mRNAs appears to have a series of unique, higher-molecular-weight-processing intermediates, which may be representative of the multiple intervening sequences in these genes.

CASEIN GENE EXPRESSION IN HORMONE-DEPENDENT MAMMARY CANCER

As this conference is focused on breast cancer, I would like to devote the remainder of this presentation to a discussion of our studies of gene expression as they relate to hormone-dependent breast cancer. Previously in our laboratory, molecular hybridization and cell-free translation were employed to compare total poly(A$^+$) RNA populations from hormone-dependent 7,12-dimethyl[a]-benzanthracene (DMBA)-induced mammary tumors and normal midpregnant rat mammary tissue (Supowit and Rosen 1980). Quantitative rather than qualitative differences were observed between these two RNA populations with the most striking difference being a 100-fold reduction in the expression of the milk protein mRNA sequences in the tumors. Although these tumors displayed hormone-dependent growth, quantitation of casein mRNA levels in tumors grown either in virgin animals (Supowit and Rosen 1980) or in ovariectomized animals, which had received hormone replacement (Rosen and Socher 1977), revealed that usually only 1% of the levels of casein mRNA were present in the tumors as compared to 8-day-lactating mammary tissue. In addition, both DMBA-induced tumors and another hormone-dependent mammary carcinoma induced by the carcinogen, N-nitrosomethylurea (NMU) (Gullino et al. 1975), . have been reported to contain α-lactalbumin at levels that are less than 10% of those found in a 5-day-lactating mammary gland (Qasba and Gullino 1977). As these tumors retain hormone-dependent growth, the defect in hormonally regulated milk protein gene expression is apparently not due to a receptor-minus phenotype observed in most hormone-resistant cell lines and tumors (Sibley and Tomkins 1974).

To determine whether milk protein gene expression can be hormonally induced in both types of tumors, we have measured casein mRNA levels in DMBA-induced tumors growing in 14-day-pregnant animals and in NMU-induced tumors from animals treated with thioproperazine, a drug that increases serum prolactin levels. Localization of the tumor epithelial cells that were actively synthesizing casein also was accomplished by use of an antirat casein antiserum in conjunction with a peroxidase-antiperoxidase (PAP) staining technique. Finally, we have examined the methylation patterns of the hormonally-responsive milk protein genes in DMBA- and NMU-induced mammary tumors, lactating mammary gland, and liver DNAs. These studies were performed utilizing three cloned gene probes for the α-, β- and γ-casein structural genes (Richards et al. 1981a).

To study the relationship between hormonally regulated growth and the induction of differentiated function, we measured both the basal and induced casein mRNA levels in two different carcinogen-induced mammary carcinomas. Casein mRNA levels were compared in DMBA-induced mammary tumors growing in either 14-day-pregnant or virgin animals and in NMU-induced tumors from untreated or ovariectomized rats, or in animals treated with thioproperazine. Titration hybridizations were performed using a 15S (α- and β-) casein cDNA probe and total tumor RNA. A 3.4-fold increase in casein mRNA levels was observed in DMBA-induced tumors grown in pregnant animals when compared to those from virgin animals (Table 1). The levels of casein mRNA were $1.2 \pm .4\%$ and $0.35 \pm .05\%$ of those found in RNA isolated from 8-day-lactating mammary tissue for the tumors grown in the pregnant and virgin animals, respectively. The 8-day-lactating RNA represents a maximally induced state of casein gene expression (Rosen and Barker 1976). Thus, even in an identical hormonal environment, the casein mRNA sequences are expressed at 40-fold

Table 1
Effects of Hormones on DMBA- and NMU-induced Mammary Tumors

Tissue	Casein mRNA[a] (% of 8-day lactating)		Fold change
DMBA tumor			
14-Day-midpregnant	1.2 ± 0.4	$(N = 4)$	$3.4^d (p < 0.05)$
Virgin	0.35 ± 0.05	$(N = 2)$	—
14-Day-midpregnant gland			
Treated	51.0	$(N = 1)$	$42.5^e (p < 0.001)$
Untreated	44.0	$(N = 1)$	$36.7 (p < 0.001)$
NMU tumor			
Control	0.135 ± 0.01	$(N = 2)$	—
Ovariectomized[b]	0.08 ± 0.014	$(N = 2)$	$-.41^f (p < 0.01)$
Thioproperazine[c]	0.28 ± 0.06	$(N = 3)$	$2.1^f (p < 0.05)$

Values are listed ± S.D.; N = number of samples analyzed; p values were calculated by the student's t test.
[a] Calculated from slope of 15S casein mRNA-cDNA back hybrid.
[b] Ovariectomized 36 hr before sacrifice.
[c] Thioproperazine (10 mg/kg, twice daily, for 3 days before sacrifice).
[d] Compared to DMBA tumors grown in virgin animals.
[e] Compared to DMBA tumors grown in 14-day-midpregnant animals.
[f] Compared to NMU control tumors.

lower levels in the tumors as compared to the normal 14-day-pregnant mammary gland that was taken from the tumor-bearing animal (40-50% of 8-day lactating, Table 1). Tumors grown in pregnant animals displayed enhanced growth rates compared to those grown in virgin animals (data not shown), probably in response to the elevated serum placental lactogen, prolactin, and steroid hormone levels during pregnancy. However, only a 3.4-fold induction of casein mRNA sequences was observed in these tumors. Thus, they have retained an attenuated ability to express these mammary gland-specific gene products.

Casein mRNA levels were also measured by cDNA titration hybridization in primary, NMU-induced mammary tumors, another type of hormonally dependent mammary adenocarcinoma. As shown in Table 1 the casein mRNA levels from control tumors were .135 ± 0.01% of the 8-day-lactating level. This low level of expression is comparable to that found in the DMBA-induced tumors grown in virgin animals. Tumors from ovariectomized animals contained a slightly decreased level of casein mRNA as compared to the control tumors, while a 2.1-fold induction of casein mRNA was observed in the tumors from the thioproperazine-treated animals. Thus, for both types of hormonally dependent mammary tumors, a limited induction of casein mRNA was observed, but maximally induced levels were usually only 0.2-2% of the levels found in the 8-day-lactating rat mammary gland.

Casein Localization of Mammary Cell Populations by PAP Staining

Titration hybridization using a specific casein cDNA probe revealed that both the DMBA and NMU-induced mammary tumors synthesize very low levels of casein mRNA, which can be increased by hormonal manipulation of the tumor-bearing animal. Because casein inducibility appears to be a marker for hormone responsiveness in these tumors, we wanted to determine if the induction of casein synthesis was due to a low level of increased synthesis throughout the entire tumor cell population or the response of only a few maximally induced cells. Immunocytochemical studies were performed using a specific anticasein antiserum and PAP staining to localize casein in fixed sections of DMBA-induced mammary tumors grown in either pregnant or virgin animals.

A trichome-stained section of hormone-stimulated midpregnant gland is shown in Figure 5A. Secretory alveolar and ductal cells, as well as fat cells and connective tissue, can be seen in the photograph. PAP staining with the antirat casein antiserum revealed intense staining of the secretory epithelial cells in the midpregnant gland (Fig. 5C). Negatively reacting controls stained with normal rabbit serum are shown in Figure 5B. The vast majority of the secretory epithelial cells displayed intense staining, and a uniform response was evident (Fig. 5C).

The photograph in Figure 5D shows a hematoxalin and eosin (H & E)-stained section of a DMBA-induced mammary tumor grown in a virgin animal.

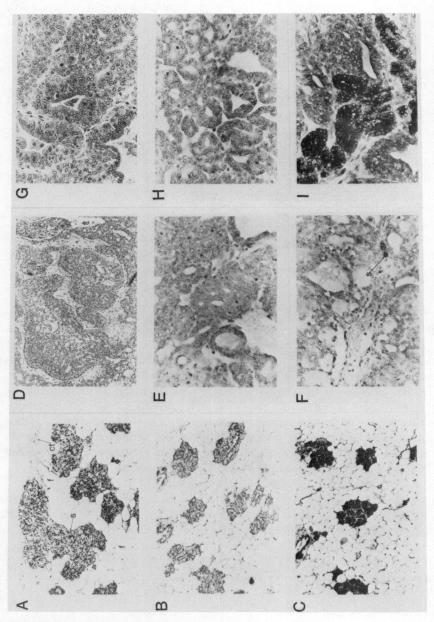

Figure 5 *(See facing page for legend.)*

The tumor epithelial cells are not arranged into secretory units as found in the normal midpregnant gland, but rather are found in a random arrangement that is more typical of mammary adenocarcinoma. In addition, very few fat cells and an increase in connective tissue are observed in these tumors. When casein localization was analyzed in these tumors. only a few cells were positively stained (shown by arrow in Fig. 5F), whereas the great majority of the epithelial cells contained no detectable casein. The negatively stained control is shown in Figure 5E.

In the mammary tumors taken from 14-day-pregnant animals, a different pattern of casein localization was seen. Instead of single cells containing casein, as in the tumors grown in virgin animals, there were clusters of positively stained cells containing large quantities of casein randomly located throughout the tumor (Fig. 5I). The negatively stained control is shown in Figure 5H. In tumors grown in pregnant animals >95% of the cells appear to have lost their ability to synthesize casein, even though the hormonal milieu of pregnancy resulted in an enhanced growth response of the tumors. It is interesting to note that in the H & E-stained section of these tumors (Fig. 5G) the epithelial cells appear to have more of a tubular or secretory arrangement than is found in tumors growing in virgin animals. Thus, the attenuated ability of the DMBA-induced mammary tumors to synthesize casein is due to a very small percentage of the transformed epithelial cells that retain their ability to synthesize casein and not to a very low level of synthesis by the entire tumor cell population. The hormonal induction of casein mRNA sequences is presumably a result of both an increase in the number of cells that are actively synthesizing casein mRNA as well as an increase in casein mRNA levels in these cells.

METHYLATION PATTERNS OF THE CASEIN GENES

Based on the observation that the low levels of casein synthesis in the DMBA-induced mammary tumors result from a defect in hormonally regulated casein gene expression in the vast majority (>95%) of the tumor cells, the possible role

Figure 5
Casein localization in DMBA-induced mammary tumors and 14-day midpregnant mammary gland by PAP staining. (A) A 5-μm thick section of 14-day-midpregnant gland, which was fixed in Telley's solution and stained with trichrome. Secretory cells are designated as (s), fat cells (f), and connective tissue (ct). (B) A 14-day-midpregnant gland tissue section in which preimmune rabbit serum was utilized in the PAP staining procedure. (C) A similar tissue section in which a specific antirat casein antibody was employed in the PAP staining procedure. The dark staining material is the casein in the secretory cells. (D) A 5-μm-thick section of fixed, DMBA-induced mammary tumor from virgin animals which was stained with H & E. (E) Negative control of a DMBA-induced tumor section as described previously. (F) PAP-stained tumor section utilizing the antirat casein antibody. The arrow indicates a representative single cell that is synthesizing casein. (G) An H & E-stained section of hormonally stimulated DMBA-induced tumor. (H) The negative control as described previously. (I) Positively PAP-stained tumor section. The dark staining material identifies the cluster of casein-synthesizing cells. Magnification for all photographs is 250X. All PAP-stained sections were counterstained with Gill's hematoxalin.

of altered casein gene organization and, specifically, cytosine base methylation was examined. Recently, several laboratories have reported an apparent correlation of DNA hypomethylation at certain DNA loci with the expression of specific viral and eukaryotic genes (for a recent review, see Razin and Riggs 1980). The restriction endonucleases HpaII and HhaI were employed to analyze the 5-methycytosine content of the three casein genes (α, β, γ), as well as the methylation pattern of the 18S ribosomal RNA gene, in DNA isolated from tumors, lactating mammary gland, and liver. These enzymes require the dinucleotide CpG as part of their recognition sequence and will not cleave at this position if the cytosine is methylated. For this study we used the enzymes HpaII and its isoschizomer MspI (recognition site, 5′ CCGG), and HhaI (recognition site, 5′ GCGC). HpaII will cleave the sequence CCGG and not cleave C^{m}CGG, while MspI cleaves CCGG and C^{m}CGG but will not cleave ^{m}CCGG. In addition, HhaI cleaves the sequence GCGC but not G^{m}CGC.

Analyses with MspI and HpaII were performed initially using DNA extracted from DMBA- and NMU-induced mammary tumors, lactating mammary gland, and liver, and a ^{32}P-labeled β-casein cloned cDNA probe. As shown in Figure 6, each of the DNAs yielded up to five specific fragments ranging in size from 16 kb to 1.1 kb. Tissue-specific changes are seen in the HpaII digests of tumor and liver DNA samples (lanes 2 and 6). For the DMBA tumor DNA, β-casein sequences are found in the area of the gel where the fragment size is >10 kb. There appear to be unique fragments at 18 kb and 13 kb as well as an intense signal at 7.5 kb, which is not found in any other lanes. The most striking difference is the marked reduction of the 1.1-kb fragment, which is predominant in the MspI digest. Figure 6, panel B, contains an enlargement of this region of the autoradiogram (deliberately overexposed) from a separate experiment. A faint signal is observed consistently in this location for the HpaII digest of DMBA DNA. One possibility is that the few cells in the tumors that are capable of synthesizing casein contain DNA which is hypomethylated at this particular site or sites. The absence of distinct 16.0-kb, 11.5-kb, 6.3-kb, and 5.0-kb fragments suggests the possibility of hypermethylation of the internal cytosine at the MspI-HpaII recognition sites, because the HpaII digest of lactating DNA displayed these specific fragments. The HpaII digest of liver DNA contained fragments at 11.5 kb and at 6.3 kb that were common to all of the samples. There also appear to be 13-kb and 7.5-kb fragments, which also are found in the HpaII tumor DNA digest. Again, the most striking difference is the absence of the 1.1-kb fragment. This fragment appeared to be totally absent in the HpaII liver DNA digest, whereas a faint signal was observed for the HpaII DMBA DNA digest (Fig. 6, panel B). Of interest is the recent observation in our laboratory of the localization of the 1.1-kb fragment at the 5′ end of the β-casein gene. These data suggest that both DMBA tumor and liver DNA have a similar modification of the MspI-HpaII recognition site, which is not found in the lactating DNA for the β-casein gene. Thus, hypermethylation of specific CpG sites in the casein genes may play a regulatory

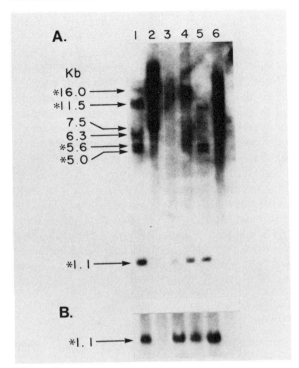

Figure 6
Methylation patterns of the β-casein gene in DMBA tumor, lactating mammary gland and liver DNA digested with *Msp*I (*A*) lanes 1, 3, 5 and *Hpa*II (*A*) lanes 2, 4, 6. (*B*) An enlargement of the 1.5-kb fragment for each sample obtained in a separate experiment. The autoradiogram has been slightly overexposed to detect the minor DMBA-*Hpa*II 1.5-kb fragment.

role in the repression of these genes in hormone-dependent mammary tumors. As previously mentioned, many of these sites appear to be localized preferentially at the 5′ end of these genes. However, we cannot determine at present if the specific increase in casein gene methylation observed in the tumors is a result of carcinogen-induced alterations of the DNA in the normal cell population or clonal selection of pre-existing cells containing hypermethylation of the casein gene. An understanding of the origin and the hormonal responsiveness of the subpopulation of casein-synthesizing cells, as well as the majority of cells that have lost the ability to regulate casein gene expression, will require methods both to separate and identify individual cell types within the DMBA tumors. Such studies are in progress in our laboratory.

DNA REARRANGEMENT IN MAMMARY TUMORS

In addition to identifying an altered methylation pattern of the casein genes in tumor DNA, we have noticed occasionally the presence of both rearrangements in and amplification of the casein genes in certain mammary tumors. Initially, such changes were observed during the screening of several DNAs isolated from somatic cell hybrid clones derived from primary cultures of GR mammary tumor cells fused with hamster cells (provided by Drs. A. Sonnenberg and J. Hilgers at the Netherlands Cancer Institute). These experiments are analogous to those previously mentioned, in which the chromosomal localization of the milk protein genes was determined in somatic cell hybrids. However, in this case, the mouse cell lines were derived from mouse mammary tumor virus (MMTV)-positive primary cultures of mammary tumor cells. In the experiment illustrated in Figure 7, it did not appear that any of these hybrid cells have lost mouse chromosome 5, i.e., they all displayed positive hybridization with the α- and β-casein gene probes. However, numerous rearrangements of the α- and β-casein genes were observed in the EcoRI-digested DNAs, e.g., note Figure 7, lane 12, compared with thymus DNA in lane 16. Thus, tumor DNA may not be static and undergo mutation only by single base changes. Instead, it is possible that transpositions, rearrangements, deletions, and inversions may occur following transformation by chemical and viral gents. In the latter case, it is intriguing to

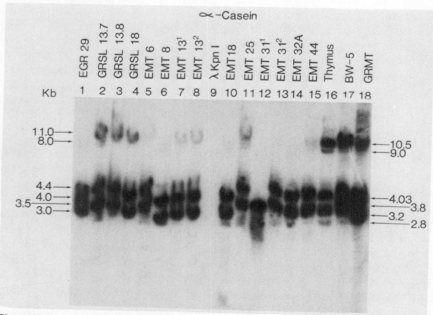

Figure 7

Rearrangement of the α-casein gene in mammary tumor DNA. Somatic cell hybrid clones were derived from primary cultures of GR mammary tumors and the E-36 hamster cell line. Here, 15 μg of EcoRI-digested DNAs were electrophoresed in each tract as described in the legend to Fig. 3. The mouse parental lines are shown in lanes 2-4 and different GR mouse tissue DNAs shown in lanes 16-18. Hybrid lines are shown in lanes 1, 5-8, and 10-15. Lane 9 was an internal λ DNA standard cut with KpnI.

note that casein gene amplication has been observed in several MMTV-induced mouse mammary tumors (Jones et al. 1980). Furthermore, analysis of the structure of MMTV DNA indicates the presence of short, inverted repeats and long, direct repeats at the ends of viral DNA, features that are analogous to those of transposable elements in DNA (Majora and Varmus 1981). It is likely, therefore, that further analysis of the structure of specific genes in tumor DNAs may be useful in understanding the etiology of the tumors, and more importantly, the loss of, or altered expression of certain genes in transformed cells. Such changes may occur at the level of DNA modification or rearrangement, or both.

EXPRESSION OF UNIQUE SINGLE-COPY DNA SEQUENCES IN DMBA-INDUCED MAMMARY TUMORS

In our previous studies (Supowit and Rosen 1980), the analysis of total poly(A^+) RNA from DMBA-induced mammary tumors and 14-day-midpregnant mammary gland by molecular hybridization and cell-free translation indicated that there were quantitative rather than qualitative differences between the two RNA populations. In these studies, two different types of hybridization experiments were performed: Homologous and heterologous cDNA complexity analyses and saturation hybridization to single-copy [^{3}H]DNA. Based upon the cDNA complexity experiments, it was concluded that most of the mRNA sequences that code for maintenance or housekeeping functions are shared between the neoplastic and normal mammary tissues. Furthermore, changes in the frequencies of the tissue-specific abundant and moderately abundant mRNAs may provide one mechanism by which the concentrations of specific proteins and ultimately the expression of the transformed phenotype may be regulated. In particular, the abundant milk protein mRNAs are present at 50-100-fold lower concentrations in the tumor compared to the normal mammary gland as previously described.

Saturation hybridization to single copy [^{3}H]DNA using tumor and midpregnant poly(A^+) RNA populations both individually and additively was also employed as a more sensitive method of examining scarce mRNA sequences. The majority of the infrequent or scarce mRNA sequences also appeared to be held in common between the two tissues. Thus, most of the mRNA sequences in the transformed and normal cells are held in common. A significant expression or depression of a large number of genes was, therefore, not evident in the DMBA-induced mammary tumors.

A more accurate method of detecting qualitative differences between two total RNA populations involves isolating single-copy DNA from DNA-RNA hybrids and then reacting this fractionated probe with homologous and heterologous RNAs (Ernst et al. 1979; Kamaley and Goldberg 1980). Recently, we have performed similar experiments to determine if there is a distinct set of high-complexity RNA sequences, presumably of nuclear origin, that are unique to the DMBA-induced tumor.

As we have shown previously by saturation hybridization with [³H]DNA that there are no detectable qualitative differences between the total poly(A⁺) RNAs from DMBA-induced tumor and midpregnant mammary glands, we prepared a sensitive probe for those sequences absent from the midpregnant RNA. This was done by two cycles of hybridization of single-copy DNA with midpregnant RNA. The DNA that remained single-stranded is termed the midpregnant null mDNA. This probe hybridized with midpregnant RNA to a saturation value of approximately 3.0% (Table 2) compared with 8.7% hybridization observed initially. It appears that the presence of midpregnant RNA complementary sequences in the null tracer is due to a failure to bind all of the RNA-DNA hybrids during the HAP fractionation. Assuming that these residual sequences are representative of the entire set of midpregnant RNAs, the presence of these sequences should not preclude use of this tracer to detect nonmidpregnant sequences. Reaction of the null mDNA with tumor poly(A⁺) RNA gave a saturation value of 7.5%, which is 2.5 times higher than the reaction of the null tracer with midpregnant RNA (Table 2). Reaction of the probe with identical RNA samples, hydrolyzed first with alkali to monitor potential DNA contamination, showed virtually no hybridization. This demonstrates that the DNAase treatment of the RNA samples effectively removed all of the contaminating DNA.

The 4.5% difference between the saturation values obtained with tumor and midpregnant RNAs when reacted with the null mDNA probes represents a complexity of 6.7×10^7 nucleotides (assuming asymmetric transcription). This is equivalent to 9500 different 7-kb genes that are expressed in the tumor, but not in the normal mammary gland. (An average gene size of 7 kb was employed in these calculations.) Therefore, this experiment suggests that the tumor poly(A⁺) RNA contains a set of sequences that are absent in midpregnant RNA.

The reciprocal experiment involved the hybridization of a [³H]DNA probe, which was complementary to the RNAs expressed in the midpregnant gland (midpregnant mDNA), with homologous and heterologous RNA populations. The data from these experiments is shown in Figure 8. At saturation, the mDNA reacted with midpregnant RNA to an extent of 80%. In contrast, there was a decrease in the saturation value to roughly 50% when tumor RNA is reacted with the mDNA. The data in Table 2 revealed that there are approximately 12,800 sequences in the midpregnant mDNA that do not react with the tumor RNA. This implies that there are some DNA sequences expressed in the midpregnant mammary gland, but not in the tumor. Although it appears that the hybridization of the mDNA with its homologous RNA has reached saturation, it is probable that this has not occurred for the heterologous reaction. It is possible that the actual difference is less than that observed if the heterologous reaction has not gone to completion. However, these results indicate that there are detectable qualitative differences in the total poly(A⁺) RNA populations in the normal and neoplastic tissues.

Table 2
Summary of mDNA and Null mDNA Hybridization Reactions

RNA	Null mDNA reactions			mDNA reactions		
	percent of null [3H]mDNA[a] hybridized	complexity[b] (nucleotides $\times 10^7$)	number of 7-kb genes[d] not shared with midpregnant	percent of [3H]mDNA[a] hybridized	complexity[c] (nucleotides $\times 10^8$)	number of 7-kb genes[e] not shared with tumor
Midpregnant	3.0	4.5	—	80.0	2.6	12,800
Tumor	7.5	11.0	9500	50.0	1.7	—

[a] Represents the terminal values obtained from the hybridization data presented as shown in Fig. 8. These values were normalized to 100% of their reactivity.

[b] Rat single-copy DNA has a complexity of 1.9×10^9 nucleotide pairs. The null mDNA complexity equals that of total-copy DNA (1.0×10^9) less the complexity of midpregnant mDNA (3.3×10^8 nucleotide pairs assuming asymmetric transcription), or 1.5×10^9 nucleotide pairs. Hence complexity = (% of null [3H]DNA hybridized) $\times$ (1.5×10^9).

[c] Complexity of midpregnant mDNA (3.3×10^8 nucleotide pairs) is equal to $1.9 \times 10^9 \times 0.087$ (% of hybridized [3H]mDNA $\times$ 2 (this value corrects for asymmetric transcription).

[d] This value = (complexity of null mDNA) $\times (0.045) \div 7 \times 10^3$.

[e] This value = complexity of midpregnant RNA hybridized to probe (2.6×10^8) less the complexity of tumor RNA reacted with the same probe (1.7×10^8). This value (9×10^7) was then divided by 7×10^3.

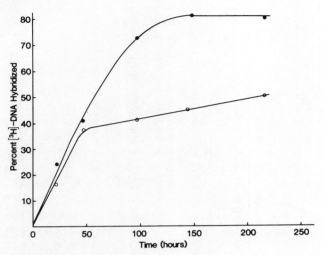

Figure 8
Hybridization of midpregnant [^{3}H]mDNA probe to RNA. Single-copy [^{3}H]DNA that was complementary to midpregnant poly(A$^+$) RNA was hybridized to midpregnant (O) and tumor (●) poly(A$^+$) RNAs. The concentration of the RNA samples was 17.2 mg/ml. All values were corrected for 100% probe reactivity.

Thus, use of fractionated probes revealed the presence of distinct sets of high-complexity RNAs, presumably of nuclear origin, that were unique to either the neoplastic or normal tissue. It is not known, at present, if these RNAs represent distinct sets of structural genes that are transcribed in only one tissue and then are processed and transported to the cytoplasm of the cell as functional mRNAs. Even though these qualitative changes have been found in sets of RNAs isolated from DMBA-induced mammary tumors and midpregnant mammary tissue, overall, it can be concluded from our hybridization experiments that the regulation of the abundancies of abundant and moderately abundant RNAs plays an important role in the expression of both the normal and transformed phenotype. It is likely that the mRNAs that code for housekeeping and maintenance functions are shared between the neoplastic and normal mammary tissue. Thus, changes in the frequencies of tissue-specific, abundant and moderately abundant mRNAs may provide one mechanism by which the concentration of specific proteins and ultimately the expression of the normal or transformed phenotype may be regulated. The regulation of mRNA frequency in the abundant and moderately abundant RNA classes may, in large part, be due to some type of posttranscriptional regulatory mechanism (Guyette et al. 1979; Jacobs and Birnie 1980; Supowit and Rosen 1980). It is possible that the regulatory proteins necessary for the expression of a specific phenotype are coded for by scarce mRNAs. Thus, the differences we observed between DMBA-tumors and midpregnant mammary tissue may be brought about by a relatively small number of specific RNAs in conjunction with the regulation of the abundancies of sequences that are held in common between the two tissues.

CONCLUSION

In this presentation, I reviewed our recent studies concerning the hormonal regulation of specific gene expression in the mammary gland. The complex regulatory mechanisms present in both normal and neoplastic tissue make the elucidation of the precise role of hormones in controlling gene expression quite difficult. However, by applying the latest techniques of molecular biology, we have obtained some insight into these processes. Future studies designed to investigate the mechanisms of posttranscriptional regulation of mRNA accumulation, the role of methylation in gene expression, and the higher-order structure of the milk protein gene domain currently are in progress in our laboratory. These approaches may help explain the regulation of differentiated function in the normal mammary gland and how these regulatory mechanisms have deviated in hormone-dependent breast cancer.

ACKNOWLEDGMENTS

The authors wish to acknowledge the excellent technical assistance of Mr. Donald Kessler. This work was supported by a National Institutes of Health (NIH) Postdoctoral Fellowship, CA-06645 (L.Y.), an NIH Career Development Award, CA-00154 (J.M.R.), and NIH grant CA-16303.

REFERENCES

Bolander, F.F., Jr. and Y.J. Topper. 1980. Loss of differentiative potential of the mammary gland in ovariectomized mice: Prevention and reversibility of the defect. *Endocrinology* **107**:1281.
Bolander, F.F., Jr., K.R. Nicholas, and Y.J. Topper. 1979. Retention of glucocorticoid by isolated mammary tissue may complicate interpretation of results from in vitro experiments. *Biochem. Biophys. Res. Commun.* **91**: 247.
Crick, F. 1979. Split genes and RNA splicing. *Science* **204**:264.
Elias, J.J. 1957. Cultivation of adult mouse mammary gland in hormone enriched synthetic medium. *Science* **126**:842.
Ernst, S.G., R.J. Britten, and E.H. Davidson. 1979. Distinct single-copy sequence sets in sea urchin nuclear RNAs. *Proc. Natl. Acad. Sci.* **76**:2209.
Fritsch, E.F., R.M. Lawn, and T. Maniatis. 1980. Molecular cloning and characterization of the human β-like globin gene cluster. *Cell* **19**:959.
Ganguly, R., N. Ganguly, N.M. Mehta, and M.R. Banerjee. 1980. Absolute requirement of glucocorticoid for expression of the casein gene in the presence of prolactin. *Proc. Natl. Acad. Sci.* **77**:6003.

Gullino, P.M., H.M. Pettigrew, and G.H. Grantham. 1975. N-Nitrosomethylurea as a mammary gland carcinogen in rats. *J. Natl. Cancer Inst.* 54:401.

Gupta, P., A.A. Hobbs, D.E. Blackburn, P. D'Eustachio, F.H. Ruddle, J. Hilgers, A. Sonnenberg, and J.M. Rosen. 1981. Characterization of the murine casein family: Evolution and chromosomal localization. *FEBS Proc. Meet.* (in press).

Guyette, W.A., R.J. Matusik, and J.M. Rosen. 1979. Prolactin mediated transcriptional and post-transcriptional control of casein gene expression. *Cell* 17:1013.

Jacobs, H. and G.D. Birnie. 1980. Post-transcriptional regulation of messenger RNA abundance in rat liver and hepatoma. *Nucleic Acids Research* 8: 3087.

Jones, R.F., W.A. Prass, and C.M. McGrath. 1980. Changes in casein sequence abundance in DNA of mouse mammary tumors. *Biochem. Biophys. Res. Commun.* 97:1241.

Kamalay, J.C. and R.B. Goldberg. 1980. Regulation of structural gene expression in tobacco. *Cell* 19:935.

Leder, P., D.A. Konkel, Y. Nishioka, A. Leder, D.H. Hamer, and M. Kaehler. 1980. The organization and evolution of cloned globin genes. *Recent Prog. Horm. Res.* 36:241.

Majors, J.E. and H.E. Varmus. 1981. Nucleotide sequences at host-proviral junctions for mouse mammary tumor virus. *Nature* 289:253.

Maniatis, T., R.C. Hardison, E. Lacy, J. Laver, C. O'Connell, D. Quon, G.K. Sim, and A. Efstratiatis. 1978. The isolation of structural genes from libraries of eucaryotic DNA. *Cell* 15:687.

Matusik, R.J. and J.M. Rosen. 1978. Prolactin induction of casein mRNA in organ culture. *J. Biol. Chem.* 253:2343.

Meo, T., J. Johnson, C.V. Beechey, S.J. Andrews, J. Peters, and A.G. Searle. 1980. Linkage analyses of murine immunoglobin heavy chain and serum prealbumin genes establish their location on chromosome 12 proximal to the T (5; 12) 31 H breakpoint in band 12F1. *Proc. Natl. Acad. Sci.* 77: 550.

Nakhasi, H.L. and P.K. Qasba. 1979. Quantitation of milk proteins and their mRNAs in rat mammary gland at various stage of gestation and lactation. *J. Biol. Chem.* 254:6016.

Ono, M. and T. Oka. 1980. α-Lactalbumin-casein induction in virgin mouse mammary explants: Dose-dependent differential action of cortisol. *Science* 207:1367.

Qasba, P.K. and P.M. Gullino. 1977. α-Lactalbumin content of rat mammary carcinomas and the effect of pituitary stimulation. *Cancer Res.* 37:3792.

Razin, A. and A.D. Riggs. 1980. DNA methylation and gene function. *Science* 210:604.

Richards, D.A., D.E. Blackburn, and J.M. Rosen. 1981a. Restriction enzyme mapping and heteroduplex analysis of the rat milk protein cDNA clones. *J. Biol. Chem.* 256:533.

Richards, D.A., J.R. Rodgers, S.C. Supowit, and J.M. Rosen. 1981b. Construction and preliminary characterization of the rat casein and α-lactalbumin cDNA clones. *J. Biol. Chem.* 256:526.

Rodgers, J.R., D.A. Richards, and J.M. Rosen. 1980. Rat milk protein mRNAs have unique, multiple high molecular weight processing intermediates. *Fed. Proc.* **39**:1653A.

Rosen, J.M. and S.W. Barker. 1976. Quantitation of casein messenger RNA sequences using a specific complementary DNA hybridization probe. *Biochemistry* **15**:5272.

Rosen, J.M. and S.H. Socher. 1977. Detection of casein mRNA in hormone-dependent mammary cancer by molecular hybridization. *Nature* **269**:83.

Rosen, J.M. and D. Shields. 1980. Post-translational modifications of the rat mammary gland caseins: In vitro synthesis, processing and segregation. In *Testicular development, structure and function* (ed. A. Steinberger and E. Steinberger), p. 343. Raven Press, New York.

Sibley, C.H. and G.M. Tomkins. 1974. Mechanisms of steroid resistance. *Cell* **2**:221.

Supowit, S.C. and J.M. Rosen. 1980. Gene expression in normal and neoplastic mammary tissue. *Biochemistry* **15**:3452.

Supowit, S.C., B.B. Asch, and J.M. Rosen. 1981. Casein gene expression in normal and neoplastic mammary tissue. In *Cell biology of breast cancer* (ed. C. McGrath, M. Brennon, and M. Rich). Academic Press, New York.

Swan, D., P. D'Eustachio, L. Leinwand, J. Seidman, D. Keithley, and F.H. Ruddle. 1979. Chromosomal assignment of the mouse κ light chain genes. *Proc. Natl. Acad. Sci.* **76**:2735.

Taborsky, G. 1974. Phosphoproteins. *Adv. Protein Chem.* **28**:1.

Teyssot, B. and L.-M. Houdebine. 1980. Role of prolactin in the transcription of β-casein and 28S ribosomal genes in rabbit mammary gland. *Eur. J. Biochem.* **110**:263.

Topper, Y.J. 1970. Multiple hormone interaction in development of mammary gland in vitro. *Recent Prog. Horm. Res.* **26**:287.

NOTE ADDED IN PROOF

The rat and mouse clones designated in this chapter as coding for α-lactalbumin and used in the studies described in Figures 1-3 have been sequenced recently in our laboratory and shown not to code for α-lactalbumin. Instead, they code for an unidentified hormone-regulated abundant mammary gland mRNA of unknown function.

COMMENTS

DAO: Jeff [Rosen], I am not very current on the subject of the heterogeneity of the cells and so forth. Really, you are looking at a picture of loss of casein mRNA in the neoplasm measurement. Probably, in the majority of tumors, you are not finding casein synthesis at all. We did some experiments, for example, with mammary tumor and DMBA and did not see any casein at all. I think that you might see occasionally some small amounts of the synthesis of casein, but this seems to have nothing to do with endocrine sensitivity of the tumor.

ROSEN: I think, Tom [Dao], that depends on the assay sensitivity. There is a very low level being expressed in all these tumors, and your assay really wasn't capable of picking that up.

DAO: I agree with you.

ROSEN: And if a sensitive cDNA hybridization assay is used, we have found that 70% of the hormone-dependent tumors do show detectable casein mRNA levels (Rosen and Socher 1977). However, I really think that it is a very small percentage of the cells, as I have shown, that are actually capable of synthesizing casein. You are right, the majority of cells have lost that capability.

    The critical question is this relation between hormone-dependent growth and hormone-dependent differentiation. Can you reactivate the cells to synthesize casein, for example? There are several ways to inhibit methylation, such as using the drug 5-azacytidine. There are several nice studies that have been done in other systems with, for example, temperature-sensitive viruses and myogenic or chondrogenic cells. These studies have shown that if you grow infected cells at a permissive temperature, they are transformed and do not express differentiated functions; if you grow them at the nonpermissive temperature, where the cells are not transformed, then they can express the differentiated functions. In some cases, you can switch back and forth.

    We are now trying to separate these two cell populations cleanly, put them in culture on a collagen-gel matrix, similar to what Dr. Nandi has described, and see if we can reactivate expression under conditions where they should maintain hormonal responsiveness.

DAO: You see, my idea is contrary to this. I think that loss of casein mRNA is an expression of neoplastic transformation.

ROSEN: I don't think it has anything to do necessarily with casein mRNA as a good marker for hormone-dependent breast cancer. I think it is important to understand the relationship between hormonal regulation of growth and hormonal regulation of differentiated function.

TOPP: Did the treatment with prolactin alter the splicing pattern?

ROSEN: No. Hormones may influence the accumulation of mRNAs by affecting their processing, which is something we are studying actively. If you look in the literature, there is no known effect of hormones as a rate-limiting event, on the processing of mRNA at the present time. Right now, processing is probably not a rate-limiting step. We are trying to see if there are any hormonal effects at the level of RNA processing.

TOPP: But you don't, in fact, see lots of transcript that is not properly spliced and rapidly degrading.

ROSEN: We have identified a whole series of putative primary transcripts in nuclear RNA at steady state and we are now looking at their processing, using intervening and structural gene probes to study the effects of hormones on precursor RNA processing and exporting out of the nucleus. But, right now, I think most of the hormonal effect we have observed is actually on the stabilization of the mRNA in the cytoplasm and not on processing.

HILF: You have only looked at DMBA-induced tumors in the pregnant animal under the hormonal milieu effects. Is that correct?

ROSEN: We have performed studies on one other group of NMU-induced tumors, the data from which I didn't have time to show. Paul Kelly at the University of Laval was nice enough to send some tumors that were taken either from rats treated with thioproperazine to elevate serum prolactin, a control group, or a group of ovariectomized animals. We observed that tumors from thioproperazine-treated animals displayed a 2-fold induction over the control group and that the ovariectomized group displayed a 2-fold reduction in casein mRNA levels in NMU tumors. We haven't done immunocytochemistry on those tumors, but we have performed some DNA blots which indicate that the methylation patterns are similar both in the NMU and the DMBA-induced tumors.

HILF: I asked that question because in 1960, Huggins showed in methylcholanthrene-induced tumors that estrogen treatment gave a very delightful secretory response, a milk-like response. Doug Reese did it with DMBA tumors a little later. We have done it with the R3230AC tumor. I just wonder whether you are going to look at such a possible alteration to see if you can suit this up a little bit more before eliminating the fact that only a few cells might be doing something.

ROSEN: Actually, I reviewed those studies in several chapters that I have written previously (Rosen 1978); several laboratories have observed this milk-like response. This response is usually seen in older tumors. We usually remove tumors in the first month or two after carcinogen administration. Some of the earlier work on DMBA tumors showed an apparent estrogen-induced secretion in tumors that appeared after 6 months (Archer 1969).

What we are really interested in studying is separating the different cell populations and not going back to the numerous in vivo models. I think the more we have heard at this meeting, the more it is apparent that there are problems in interpretation if you are going to work in the whole animal system to try to really look at the molecular mechanisms of hormone action in tumors.

What we are attempting to do is to take a given primary tumor, dissociate it so that we can, hopefully, obtain clean cell populations, and study gene expression in these populations in primary culture.

HILF: Lots of luck with clean cell populations when you try to separate them.

References

Archer, F.L. 1969. Fine structure of spontaneous and estrogen-induced secretion in breast tumor in the rat induced by 7,12-dimethylbenz[a]anthracene. *J. Natl. Cancer Inst.* 42:347.

Rosen, J.M. 1978. Experimental biology. In *Breast cancer: Advances in research and treatment* (ed. W.L. McGuire), vol. 2, p. 337. Plenum Press, New York.

Rosen, J.M. and S.H. Socher. 1977. Detection of casein messenger RNA in hormone-dependent mammary cancer by molecular hybridization. *Nature* 26:83.

New Concepts in Control of Estrogen-responsive Tumor Growth

DAVID A. SIRBASKU
Department of Biochemistry and Molecular Biology
The University of Texas Medical School at Houston
Houston, Texas 77025

The resolution of the problems of how estrogens promote mammary, pituitary, kidney, and uterine tumor cell growth in vivo has occupied our laboratory for some time. Our first efforts in this field were to attempt, by all means available, to demonstrate that estrogens were directly mitogenic for long-term tissue culture cell lines developed from estrogen-responsive rodent tumors. These efforts were largely without reward, and resulted in our statement in 1976 (Kirkland et al. 1976; Sirbasku and Kirkland 1976) that we believed that in the cases of two rodent tumor cell lines, the GH3/C14 rat pituitary (Kirkland et al. 1976) and the H-301 hamster kidney (Kirkland et al. 1976), the role of estrogens in vivo may be indirect. Our data suggested that estrogens in vivo may have an as yet unrecognized role in tumor growth, namely, that of induction of specific polypeptide growth factors, which then act as the primary mitogens for estrogen-responsive mammary, pituitary, and kidney tumor growth in vivo. We have reviewed previously (Sirbasku and Benson 1979; Sirbasku 1980; Sirbasku and Benson 1980) our reasons for proposing this new model of estrogen-responsive growth in vivo, and these are not described in detail here. However, it is important to emphasize that our original proposal of a new mechanism for estrogen-responsive growth in vivo was essentially consistent with classical endocrinology. Estrogens are well known to cause induction and secretion of blood-borne hormones (Meites et al. 1972) and secretory proteins (O'Malley and Means 1974; Meglioli 1976; Skipper and Hamilton 1977). We proposed that estrogens interact with target tissues, causing the synthesis and (or) secretion of polypeptide growth factors, and that these factors enter the general circulation and promote the growth of distant hormone-responsive tumor cells at whatever their location in the body. In rodents, we had found that two possible source tissues for this type of growth factor are rat uterus and rat kidney, both of which show estrogen-elevated growth factor activities (Sirbasku 1978a) for cell lines that form estrogen-responsive tumors in host rats and hamsters. For human mammary tumor cell lines, such as the MCF-7, that form estrogen-responsive tumors in nude mice (Shafie 1980), we have shown that growth factors from human blood platelets (Eastment and Sirbasku 1980) and from rat uterine extracts (Sirbasku and Benson 1980) are capable of supporting growth of these cells in serum-free medium. Up until the current report, our indirect estrogen action hypothesis has been that of a classical "endocrine" control that would be expected to be similar to that of the estrogen control of other polypeptide hormones. A summary of this model is shown in the left panel of Figure 1.

Nevertheless, as we progressed through our studies of estrogen-inducible growth factors, we made the observation (Benson et al. 1980; Sirbasku 1980; Sirbasku and Benson 1980) that MTW9/PL mammary tumors grown in vivo in response to estrogen stimulation (and possibly pituitary and kidney tumors as well) have a high specific activity growth factor associated with them. When such tumors are removed from the host animal and extracts prepared, 50 µg extract protein added per milliliter of culture medium are able to support sustained growth of the homologous MTW9/PL mammary tumor cell line in culture. One possible interpretation of these data is that this activity is growth factor made in other tissues and subsequently concentrated in the tumor. Two other possibilities are that the epithelial origin tumor cells are producing their own growth factor or that other elements of the tumor (presumably stromal or myoepithelial elements) are producing growth factor for the epithelial cells. Both of these last two mechanisms would represent a local production of growth factor that would not necessarily require the presence or secretion of the mitogen into the general circulation. If the stromal elements of a tumor could produce growth factors for epithelial cells, this would represent a "paracrine control," shown in the middle panel of Figure 1. If the epithelial cells produce

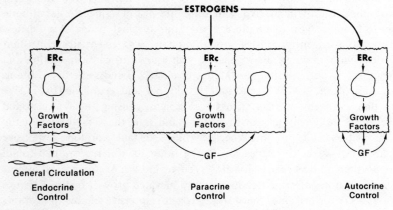

Figure 1
Three new models for estrogen-responsive tumor growth in vivo

growth factors that, after release, act back on specific receptors on the epithelial cells that produced the growth factor, this would represent an "autocrine control" of the tumor cell growth (Fig. 1, right panel). The role of estrogens in both of these mechanisms would be to induce production and (or) secretion of the factors by the appropriate cells.

Along these lines, Sporn and Todaro (1980) have reported most recently a very interesting new approach to promotion of growth tumors in vivo. They have data that supports the hypothesis that tumor growth could be promoted by endocrine, paracrine, or autocrine mechanisms. In this paper, we apply these observations to the problem of estrogen-dependent tumor growth in vivo, and we discuss the various data from our laboratory that support the possibility of all three of these mechanisms being important components of the growth of estrogen-dependent tumors in vivo.

In considering these models, it is very important to note that they probably are not separate or mutually exclusive processes but rather may be operating in concert to result in the experimentally seen continuous growth of the tumors in vivo. In view of the most current data about growth of cells in serum-free defined medium culture (Sato and Reid 1978; Bottenstein et al. 1979), it appears that several types of polypeptide hormone and growth factors are required for optimal growth rates. Hence, could it be possible that in vivo several factors may be essential for tumor growth?

The experiments described in this paper summarize the most current evidence supporting the estrogen endocrine control model. Herein we also review our reasons for believing that paracrine and (or) autocrine control may well be functioning in vivo as well.

EXPERIMENTAL PROCEDURES

Animal Studies

The rats used in this study were 150 g to 200 g outbred Sprague-Dawley animals purchased from Texas Inbred Mice Co. Surgery and estrogen pellet treatment were conducted as described before (Sorrentino et al. 1976; Sirbasku 1978b), and normal uterine and mammary tumor tissue extracts were prepared and sterilized exactly as described before (Sirbasku 1978a). The preparation of uterine luminal fluid (ULF) was described elsewhere (Sirbasku and Benson 1979).

Cell Line and Growth Conditions

The conditions for growth and passage of the MTW9/PL rat mammary tumor cells (Sirbasku 1978b) were as described in those papers cited above. When assays of the mitogenic effects of uterine organ extract, mammary tumor extracts, or ULF protein were performed, MTW9/PL cells were inoculated into 35×10-mm petri dishes at densities of 3 to 4×10^4 per dish in 3.0 ml Dulbecco's modified Eagle's medium (DMEM) containing 10% (v/v) fetal calf serum (FCS). After 24 hr, to allow cell attachment, the serum-containing medium was removed and replaced with medium containing the designated protein concentrations of the test samples. Control plates contained either 10% FCS or DMEM without serum. The cell population doublings occurring in the next 6 days were calculated from the cell number present at the time of change of medium to serum-free conditions.

Chromatography Methods

The samples of rat uterine extracts, ULF, and MTW9/PL tumor extract were submitted to various chromatographic separation procedures. Samples were submitted to ion exchange chromatography on carboxymethyl cellulose (CMC) equilibrated with 10 mM sodium phosphate buffer (pH 7.0) or on DEAE-cellulose chromatography at the same pH in the 10 mM sodium phosphate buffer. Affinity chromatography was conducted on Affi-Gel Blue resin (Bio-Rad) at pH 7.0 in 10 mM sodium phosphate buffer. Separation by apparent molecular weight was done by Sephadex S-100 or Sephacryl S-200 chromatography in standard phosphate-buffered saline (PBS) at pH 7.2.

RESULTS

Estrogen Induction of Uterine Growth Factor Activity

Our previous studies (Sirbasku 1978a) have shown that estrogen treatment of ovariectomized rats caused a 13.5-fold induction of a mammary-pituitary tumor cell growth factor activity in extracts of rat uterus. Further studies (Leland et al., unpubl.) have shown that this induction process is variable, depending on the relative presence of bacteria that originate from the vagina and migrate into the uterus during estrogen stimulation. The data in Figure 2 show a typical experiment, in which the uteri of the estrogen-treated animals showed moderate infection and which shows clearly that estrogen treatment causes only an approximate fourfold rise (half maximal growth) in apparent growth factor activity in uteri from these animals, as compared with uteri from animals that were only ovariectomized. Also, Figure 2 presents evidence that the ULF prepared from 10-day estrogen-treated ovariectomized rats contains low amounts of MTW9/PL cell growth factor, although this fluid activity does not appear as potent as that present in the tissue extract.

One of the first questions brought out by the data presented in Figure 2 is: What are the biochemical properties of this growth factor activity? Is it a lipid, steroid hormone, or polypeptide-protein? Table 1 describes the biochemical properties of the uterine-tissue-derived mammary growth factor activity. From the information summarized in Table 1, it is reasonable to conclude that the uterine-derived mitogen does have properties consistent with a high-molecular-weight protein. No evidence was obtained supporting the possibility that the activity was either a lipid or a steroid hormone. Furthermore, from the summary

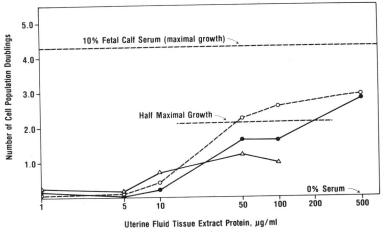

Figure 2

Growth of MTW9/PL rat mammary tumor cells in serum-free DMEM supplemented with the designated concentrations of protein from extracts of estrogen-treated ovariectomized rats (○), ovariectomized rats (●), and ULF collected from the estrogen-treated, ovariectomized females (△).

Table 1

Summary of the Properties of the Uterine-derived MTW9/PL Cell Growth Factor Activity

Property tested	Growth factor activity
Heat stability	90% labile at 80°C for 10 min
Dialysis	no dialysis over 8 days at 4°C at pH 7.2
Sephadex G-100 m.w.	70K
Trypsin treatment	100% labile in 4-6 hr at 37°C
Ammonium sulfate precipitation	33-67% saturation
Isoelectric focusing	pI 4.8-5.2
Charcoal extraction at 56°C	100% stable
Chloroform/methanol extraction	not in lipid soluble fraction
50% ethanol, acetone, or isopropanol treatment	50-70% denatured
6 M guanidine or 8 M urea at 37°C	50-70% denatured
pH 2.0 treatment	90-100% labile
pH 12.0 treatment	80% labile
Repeated slow freeze-thaw cycles	gradually labile
Augmentation of uterine factor growth promotion by added estrogen	no effect with estradiol added at 10^{-11}-10^{-8} M

presented in Table 1, it is clear that steroid hormones (or steroid hormone conjugates) are not necessary cofactors for the mammary cell mitogen, because exhaustive dialysis removes the conjugates, and the use of charcoal extraction to remove protein-associated steroids did not change the activity of the uterine growth factor.

Partial Purification of the Uterine Extract Mitogenic Activity

On the basis of our conclusion that the uterine-derived activity was probably a protein, our next course of action was to begin development of a purification procedure. As shown in Figure 3, a four-step partial purification scheme has

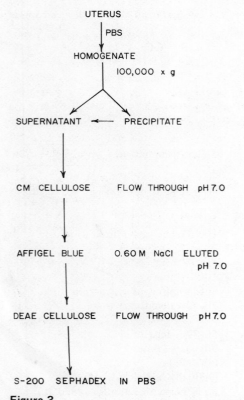

Figure 3

Partial purification scheme for the uterine-derived growth factor for the MTW9/PL rat mammary tumor cell

been developed, with the intent of applying at least four different criteria for separation of the mitogenic activity from other components in the crude extract. These criteria were chromatographed on a cation exchange (CMC) resin, an anion exchange (DEAE) resin, affinity chromatography, and molecular weight estimation. Each of these procedures separates components of the crude extract by different biochemical and physical properties.

The uterus (25 g wet weight) is homogenized initially in PBS (pH 7.2) containing 0.1% EDTA, and the broken cell debris removed by centrifugation at 100,000g. The supernatant is stored at 0°C, the pellet reextracted with 25 ml of the above buffer, and the supernatant from this extraction combined with the first supernatant. This crude solution is then applied directly to a 100 ml bed volume CMC column equilibrated as described in Experimental Procedures. The fraction that flows through the column contains 90-95% of the total protein and all of the activity. This flow-through fraction is then applied directly to the 50-ml bed volume Affi-Gel Blue column, and the fraction eluted with 0.6 M sodium chloride containing 40% of the total protein and 80-90% of the total activity. This fraction is then dialyzed against 10 mM sodium phosphate (pH 7.0) and applied directly to a 100-ml bed volume DEAE column equilibrated as described in Experimental Procedures. The flow-through fraction from this column contained 5-10% of the total protein, and 30-40% of the growth factor activity. When the DEAE column was eluted subsequently with steps of 0.15 M and 1.0 M sodium chloride in running buffer, no further activity could be found, although 40-50% of the total protein was accounted for. The reasons for the low yield of mitogenic activity from the DEAE chromatography have now been traced to two problems. First, a low amount of protein loaded on the 100-ml bed volume column causes a dramatic loss of the amount of total protein recovered from the column. Second, an inhibitory activity elutes with the main activity in the DEAE flow-through fraction.

The flow-through fraction of the DEAE was dilute and required vacuum concentration against PBS (pH 7.2). Volumes of 100–150 ml were reduced to 3–4 ml in 24 hr at 4°C. This concentrated sample was then applied to a 1 × 100-cm column of Sephacryl S = 200 and eluted with standard PBS (pH 7.2) at 4°C. The activity fraction eluted around the position of rat serum albumin (67K daltons).

Table 2 summarizes the purification achieved by these four steps. The fold purification achieved by these steps was approximately eightfold, which because of the co-purification of an inhibitor is not great, but which does define how the uterine-derived factor fractionates under four different sets of conditions. This should allow later comparison of this activity to activities extracted from mammary tumors and uterine luminal fluid.

What is the In Vivo Role of the Uterine-derived Growth Factor Activity?

Two of the critical questions concerning the identification of the uterine-derived mitogen are: (1) Is this mitogen the promoter of normal uterine growth, meaning that our isolation from this tissue simply represents the amount of growth

Table 2

Partial Purification of the Uterine-extract-derived and the ULF-derived
Mammary Cell Growth Factors

Fractions assayed	Amount protein added/ml culture medium to give standard growth response
Uterine-extract preparations	
Crude uterine extract	50 μg/ml[a]
Affi-Gel Blue, 0.6 M NaCl eluted	20 μg/ml
DEAE flow-through fraction	6 μg/ml
Sephacryl 200 (pooled fractions)	6 μg/ml
ULF preparations	
Crude ULF	200 μg/ml[b]
Affi-Gel Bue, 0.6 M NaCl eluted	23 μg/ml
DEAE flow-through fraction	0.8 μg/ml
Sephacryl 200 (pooled fractions)	1.0 μg/ml

[a]This amount of protein was added to serum-free DMEM to give 2.0 cell population doublings of MTW9/PL cells in 6 days.

[b]This amount of protein was added to serum-free DMEM to give 1.0 cell population doublings of MTW9/PL cells in 6 days.

factor found in the rapidly multiplying estrogen-stimulated uterus? and (2) Is the growth factor formed in the uterus and subsequently secreted into the general circulation, where it then can exert primary action on other estrogen target tissues, such as mammary and pituitary gland? The answer to the first of these two questions is now under study, since we have succeeded very recently in developing a smooth muscle cell line from the myometrium of the hamster uterus and another cell line from the endometrium of hamster uterus. Now we will be able to test whether the extracts of estrogen-primed uteri are able to promote growth of either or both of these permanent cell lines. If this proves to be the case, it may well indicate that the uterine extract activity is a primary mitogen for the uterus. However, these data would still not exclude the possibility that the uterine mitogen could act not only on uterus but also on both mammary and pituitary cell growth in vivo during estrogen stimulation. Previously, we have shown (Sirbasku and Benson 1979) that uterus, mammary, and pituitary tissues grow in concert in the rat when estrogen stimulation is present. Thus, the uterine-derived activity could have broader biological implications than we now recognize. These questions remain open, but surely they represent an interesting hypothesis for further experimental testing.

Nevertheless, we have approached the second question stated above: Does the uterine-tissue-derived activity appear in the extracellular fluids of the uterus? Ever since the observations of Shih et al. (1940), it has been recognized that estrogen treatment of castrated female rats results in the accumulation of large volumes of ULF. We have observed this phenomenon as well (Sirbasku and Benson 1979) and have identified in this fluid potent mammary and pituitary tumor cell mitogens (Leland et al., unpubl.). This activity, or activities (Leland et al., unpubl.), appears to be masked by inhibitors generated by the vaginally originated bacteria that invade the uterus. These organisms invade the uterus within 2 days after start of estrogen treatment and continue to multiply, killing the rat within 30 days. Although within 8 days after initiating estrogen treatment many bacterial forms were isolated from ULF (Leland et al., unpubl.), the two most common were *Psuedomonas aeruginosa* and *Proteus mirabilis*. *Pseudomonas* appears to produce the most toxic material present in ULF that we have identified, in part as the well-known exotoxin A (Liu 1966). This cytotoxin is known to be cytolytic to a great many mammary cell lines (Middlebrook and Dorland 1977a,b). It is now apparent that the low growth factor activity found in crude ULF (Fig. 2) is due probably to the presence of bacterial origin inhibitors. We have shown (Fig. 4 and Table 2) that Affi-Gel Blue chromatography is an effective first step in purification for uterine extract, and when it is applied to the ULF (data, Table 2) it is just as effective. It is readily apparent that the ULF fraction eluted from the Affi-Gel Blue with 0.6 M NaCl contains a potent mammary cell mitogen, comparable to that found in the uterine tissue extracts. To characterize the activities further, we compared the heat stabilities of the ULF mammary mitogen (Fig. 5) and the uterine extract mitogen (Fig. 6) and

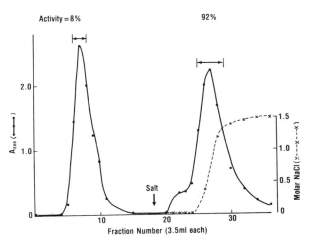

Figure 4
Affi-Gel Blue chromatography of uterine extract. Chromatography was conducted as described in Experimental Procedures. The flow-through fractions and the 1.5 M NaCl eluted fractions (after dialysis against PBS) were assayed at 20, 50, and 100 μg/ml DMEM.

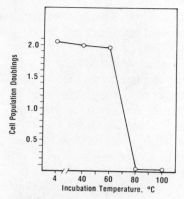

Figure 5

The 1.4 M NaCl eluted Affi-Gel Blue fractions (Fig. 4) of ULF (2.0 mg/ml) were sterilized by passage through 0.22-μm pore diameter filters and 1.0 ml transferred to sterile glass ampuls, sealed, and heated for 10 min at the designated temperatures. After this period, the ampuls were cooled to 0°C, opened, and the contents diluted with 9 ml of DMEM for assay with MTW9/PL cells.

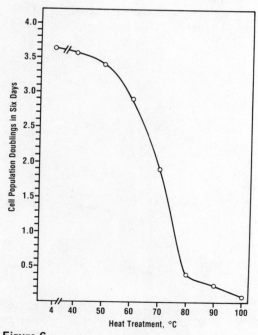

Figure 6

Heat stability of the uterine extract activity was conducted without prior Affi-Gel Blue chromatography, at 2.5 mg/ml in sealed glass ampuls exactly as described in the legend of Fig. 5.

434

demonstrated that both activities essentially were lost after 80°C incubation. The pH stabilities were, likewise, compared with the ULF mammary cell mitogen showing lability at pH 2.0 or pH 12.0 (Fig. 7), which was comparable to that seen with the uterine extract activity (Fig. 8). Further confirmation of the similar properties of the uterine tissue extract activity and the ULF activity was carried out by conducting the partial purification shown in Figure 3 with ULF. The results, summarized in Table 2, indicate that the ULF activity co-purified with that extracted from uterine tissue.

Although these data do not necessarily prove that the activities in the ULF and uterine extract are identical, they are consistent with this possibility, and they offer encouragement that the form of mammary-pituitary cell mitogen found in the uterine extract may be secreted in response to estrogens into the ULF or plasma. This last point about secretion into plasma raises another interesting question. Could the growth factor activity found in the ULF actually reach the plasma and, therefore, become a blood-borne agent? This process, and the experimental approach to test this possibility, are summarized in Figure 9.

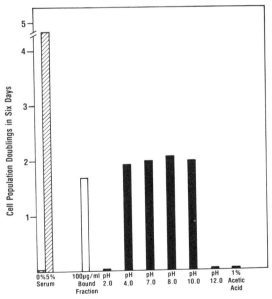

Figure 7
The 1.4 M NaCl eluted fraction of Affi-Gel Blue chromatography (Fig. 4) of ULF was used to determine the pH stability of the MTW9/PL cell growth activity. The samples were dialyzed for 18 hr at 4°C against 100 volumes of phosphate buffers adjusted to the designated pH values, after which the individual dialysis bags were transferred to PBS (pH 7.2) for 24 hr to return the pH to neutral. The contents of the bags were then assayed for residual cell growth.

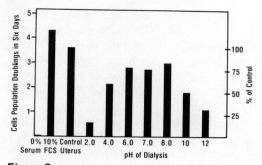

Figure 8
The pH stability of the uterine tissue extract was tested under the same conditions as the ULF (described in the legend of Fig. 7), except that the Affi-Gel Blue chromatography step was omitted.

To test whether proteins of apparent molecular weight 70K could reach the plasma from the ULF, we prepared ^{125}I-labeled rat serum albumin (^{125}I-RSA) and microinjected this protein into the ULF of a group of estrogen-treated, ovariectomized rats. The horns of the uterus were filled with small (1-2 ml) volumes of fluid at the time of injection. After 24 hr, serum samples were prepared from these rats and the serum analyzed for the presence of intact, high molecular weight ^{125}I-RSA monomers (m.w. 67K) and ^{125}I-RSA dimers. Both of these proteins were found in the serum of the ULF injected animals, confirming that between 5% and 10% of the total intact ^{125}I-RSA injected into ULF finds its way undegraded into the serum. We thus felt that the evidence was consistent with the conclusion that uterine tissue could secrete a mammary-

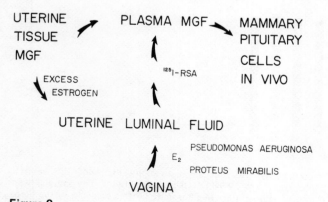

Figure 9
Diagrams of possible routes of entry of uterine-tissue-derived estromedins into plasma and the pathway for the estrogen-induced invasion of bacteria into the ULF.

pituitary growth factor into ULF and that this growth factor could pass into the serum by a mechanism not yet established.

Beyond these studies, we have sought to establish the presence of an estrogen-inducible growth factor in the serum from estrogen-treated rats. These experiments have met with difficulties owing to the presence of platelet-derived growth factor (Sirbasku and Benson 1979; Eastment and Sirbasku 1980). These problems have been discussed elsewhere (Sirbasku and Benson 1979) and will not be reiterated here.

Nevertheless, our most recent approach to the question of circulation was suggested by preliminary studies reported by our laboratory during the past year (Benson et al. 1980; Sirbasku 1980; Sirbasku and Benson 1980). We have found that extracts prepared from MTW9/PL rat mammary tumors growing in estrogen-treated, ovariectomized females contain a potent growth factor for the homologous MTW9/PL cells in culture. This growth factor activity in the extracts could be added back to cultures of MTW9/PL cells in serum-free DMEM: As little as 10 μg/ml gives significant growth (Fig. 10) and addition of 200 μg/ml gives nearly complete replacement of the serum requirement of MTW9/PL cells in culture.

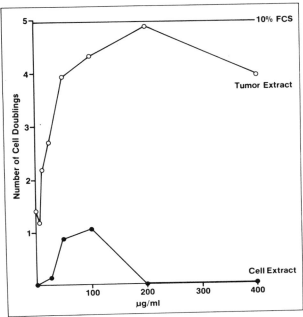

Figure 10
Growth of MTW9/PL rat mammary tumor cells in response to crude extracts of MTW9/PL tumors growing is estrogen-treated ovariectomized rats (O) and in response to extracts of MTW9/PL cells growing in culture (●).

The next obvious question is whether the growth factor in the MTW9/PL tumor extracts is the same as that in the uterus or ULF. Table 3 shows a comparison of the properties of the two activities. Notable differences in heat stability, trypsin sensitivity, acetone inactivation, and pH 2.0 inactivation show that by these several criteria, the tumor-derived and the uterine-tissue-derived activities are quite different, at least in the crude extract state.

Another striking difference is the character of the fractionation of the MTW9/PL tumor extract in Affi-Gel Blue resin (Table 4). The tumor activity shows an almost equal separation between the amount (and specific activity) of mitogen that bypasses the resin and the amount that is eluted with the high-salt step. This is clearly not the case with uterine extract, because greater than 90% of the activity in the normal tissue extract associates with the Affi-Gel Blue resin. These data suggested to us that the model of indirect estrogen control designated "endocrine control" (Fig. 1) could not necessarily explain the presence of the growth factor in mammary tumor extracts. In view of the fact that tumor cells are well known to produce growth factors in vitro (De Larco and Todaro 1978; Roberts et al. 1980), we considered the possibility that the MTW9/PL cells could be producing growth factors in vivo by either a paracrine or an autocrine mechanism as shown in Figure 1. We have grown the MTW9/PL cells in serum-free DMEM supplemented with the hormones prolactin, thyroxine, insulin, and estradiol, harvested the cells after 48 hr, prepared cell extracts, and asked whether these extracts could now support the growth of MTW9/PL cells in culture. As shown in Figure 10, the culture-grown cells supported minimal growth at low-protein concentrations, but they were ineffective at higher protein concentrations. These data suggest, but do not as yet conclusively

Table 3

Comparison of the Properties of the MTW9/PL Solid Tumor Growth Activity and Those of the Uterine-derived Mitogen

Treatments	MTW9/PL tumor extracts	Rat uterus extracts
Dialysis	nondialyzable	nondialyzable
100°C for 10 min	20-30% inactivation	100% inactivation
m.w. by Sephadex G-100 gel filtration	50K-80K	70K
Trypsin at 37°C	~30% loss	100% loss
Chromatography on Affi-Gel Blue resin at pH 7.2	50-70% flow-through and 30-50% bound (eluted with 1.4 M NaCl)	10% flow-through and 90% bound (eluted with 1.4 M NaCl)
1 N acetic acid at 4°C for 18 hr	100% inactivation	100% inactivation
Acetone (50%) at 37°C	no inactivation	50-70% inactivation
pH 2.0-4°C for 30 min	no inactivation	100% inactivation

Table 4
MTW9/PL Growth in MTW9/PL Tumor Homogenate from Affi-Gel Blue
Chromatography

Fraction	Cell number	Cell population doublings over control
Flow-through[a]		
10 μg/ml	6.16	0
50 μg/ml	27.8	1.92
100 μg/ml	29.2	1.99
Bound[b]		
10 μg/ml	5.29	0
50 μg/ml	28	1.93
100 μg/ml	28	1.93
Control		
10% FCS	137.8	4.23
0%	4.05	0

[a]The flow-through fraction contained 40-50% of the total protein.
[b]Eluted with 1.4 M NaCl in running buffer. This fraction contained 50% of the
original amount of protein applied to the column.

demonstrate, that the MTW9/PL cells could produce their own growth factor, although the data offers no clear distinction between a possible paracrine or an autocrine mechanism, especially since even with repeated cloning, this population of cells contains several morphologically different members. These matters may come to a resolution when purified factor is available to conduct immuno-fluorescent labeling of cells to determine which members of the MTW9/PL population possess receptors to the fluorescent-labeled factor.

DISCUSSION

In this paper, we have described the experimental results that suggest that the estrogen-dependent growth of mammary tumors in vivo may well involve more complex controls than previously recognized. We have proposed three new mechanisms by which estrogen may promote the growth of mammary tumors in vivo, and have presented evidence that these mechanisms are all possible in vivo. Our data is most extensive for the endocrine control mechanism (Fig. 1), which we have described previously (Sirbasku 1978a; Sirbasku 1980; Sirbasku and Benson 1980). Although we have studied extensively the properties of the uterine-derived mammary-pituitary tumor cell growth activity, we have not as yet resolved whether a single factor from the uterus is responsible for growth of both cell types or whether there are two separate but related factors for

MTW9/PL and GH3/C14 cells. This problem should be resolved by purification of the factor(s) to homogeneity.

Another unresolved question, which is equally important to the models presented in Figure 1, is whether the kidney-derived growth factor is the same as the uterine-derived mitogen(s). We have shown elsewhere (Sirbasku 1978 a) that rat kidney extracts contain an estrogen-inducible (twofold) growth factor activity for both the MTW9/PL mammary (Sirbasku 1978 a) and the GH3/C14 pituitary (Sirbasku 1978 a) cell lines in culture. Jefferson Officer of our laboratory has begun a partial purification of this kidney activity; within the near future, he should establish whether the kidney and uterine activity are the same and whether the kidney mitogen for GH3/C14 cells is the same as that which promotes MTW9/PL cell growth. If one considers the various possibilities, it may be that there is only one "estromedin" activity found in both the uterus and the kidney that promotes the growth of the two cell lines or that there are as many as four separate activities.

Beyond these studies, the presence in the MTW9/PL tumor growing in vivo of a mitogen that has very different properties from that seen in the uterine extract suggests a more complex control of mammary tumor cell growth than has been recognized previously. We believe pursuit of our studies into paracrine and autocrine control should result in a new conceptual basis for understanding mammary tumor growth and should further expand the possible role of the estromedin mechanism.

ACKNOWLEDGMENTS

The work presented in this report was supported by an American Cancer Society grant BC-255B and a National Institutes of Health grant 1-R01-CA26617. The author is a recipient of a Faculty Research Award (FRA-212) from the American Cancer Society. Many colleagues have discussed with me the various aspects of these new models; they have offered invaluable comment and criticism, especially Dr. Gordon Sato of the University of California in La Jolla, Mrs. Frances Leland of the University of Texas Medical School, and Dr. Judson Van Wyk of the University of North Carolina. The author also acknowledges the experiments performed by Dr. Caroline Eastment, who first showed that the MTW9/PL tumor extracts contained a potent growth factor activity for MTW9/PL tumor cells in culture. I wish also to express my very deep appreciation to Donna M. Sirbasku, M.D., who often discussed this research with me and encouraged me to pursue these new areas.

REFERENCES

Benson, R.H., C.T. Eastment, and D.A. Sirbasku. 1980. Properties of mammary growth factor(s) extracted from estrogen-responsive mammary tumors growing in rats. *Endocrinology* 106 (suppl.):273.

Bottenstein, J., I. Hayashi, S. Hutchings, S. Masui, J. Mather, D.B. McClure, S. Ohasa, A. Rizzino, G. Sato, G. Serrero, R. Wolf, and R. Wu. 1979. The growth of cells in serum-free hormone supplemented media. *Methods Enzymol.* 58:94.

De Larco, J.E. and G.J. Todaro. 1978. Growth factors from murine sarcoma virus-transformed cells. *Proc. Natl. Acad. Sci.* 75:4001.

Eastment, C.T. and D.A. Sirbasku. 1980. Human platelet lysate contains growth factor activities for established cell lines derived from various tissues of several species. *In Vitro* 16:694.

Kirkland, W.L., J.M. Sorrentino, and D.A. Sirbasku. 1976. Control of cell growth. III. Direct mitogenic effect of thyroid hormones on an estrogen-dependent rat pituitary tumor cell line. *J. Natl. Cancer Inst.* 56:1159.

Liu, P.V. 1966. The roles of various fractions of *Pseudomonas aeruginosa*. II. Concentration, purification and characterization of exotoxin A. *J. Infect. Dis.* 128:514.

Meglioli, G. 1976. Oestrogenic sensitivity of rat uterine secretion. *J. Reprod. Fertil.* 46:395.

Meites, J., K.H. Lu, W. Wuttke, C.W. Welsch, N. Nagasawa, and S.K. Quadri. 1972. Recent studies in functions and control of prolactin secretion in rats. *Recent Prog. Horm. Res.* 28:471.

Middlebrook, J.L. and R.B. Dorland. 1977a. Serum effects on the response of mammalian cells to the exotoxins of *Pseudomonas aeruginosa* and *Corynebacterium diphtheria*. *Can. J. Microbiol.* 23:175.

_____. 1977b. Response of cultured mammalian cells to the exotoxins of *Pseudomonas aeruginosa* and *Corynebacterium diphtheria*: Differential cytotoxicity. *Can. J. Microbiol.* 23:183.

O'Malley, B.W. and A.R. Means. 1974. Female steroid hormones and target cell nuclei. *Science* 183:610.

Roberts, A.B., L.C. Lamb, D.L. Newton, M.B. Sporn, J.E. De Largo, and G.J. Todaro. 1980. Transforming growth factors: Isolation of polypeptides from virally and chemically transformed cells by acid/ethanol extraction. *Proc. Natl. Acad. Sci.* 77:3494.

Sato, G. and L. Reid. 1978. Replacement of serum in cell culture by hormones. In *Biochemistry and mode of actions of hormones* II (ed. H.V. Rickenberg), vol. 2, p. 219. University Park Press, Baltimore, Maryland.

Shafie, S.M. 1980. Estrogen and the growth of breast cancer: New evidence suggests indirect action. *Science* 209:701.

Shih, H.E., J. Kennedy, and C. Huggins. 1940. Chemical composition of uterine secretions. *Am. J. Physiol.* 130:287.

Sirbasku, D.A. 1978a. Estrogen-induction of growth factors specific for hormone responsive mammary, pituitary and kidney tumor cells. *Proc. Natl. Acad. Sci.* 75:3786.

_____. 1978b. Hormone-responsive growth in vivo of a tissue culture cell line established from the MT-W9A rat mammary tumor. *Cancer Res.* 38:1154.

_____. 1980. Estromedins: Uterine derived growth factors for estrogen-responsive tumor cells. In *Control mechanisms in animals cells: Specific growth factors* (ed. L.J. De Asua et al.), p. 293. Raven Press, New York.

Sirbasku, D.A. and W.L. Kirkland. 1976. Control of cell growth. IV. Growth properties of a new cell line established from an estrogen-dependent kidney tumor of the syrian hamster. *Endocrinology* 98:1260.

Sirbasku, D.A. and R.H. Benson. 1979. Estrogen-inducible growth factors that may act as mediators (estromedins) of estrogen-promoted tumor cell growth. *Cold Spring Harbor Conf. Cell Proliferation* 6:477.

_____. 1980. Proposal of an indirect (estromedin) mechanism of estrogen-induced mammary tumor cell growth. In *Cell biology of breast cancer* (ed. C. McGrath and M. Rich). Academic Press, New York. (In press)

Skipper, J.K. and T.H. Hamilton. 1977. Regulation by estrogen of the vitellogenesis gene. *Proc. Natl. Acad. Sci.* 74:2384.

Sorrentino, J.M., W.L. Kirkland, and D.A. Sirbasku. 1976. Control of cell growth. I. Estrogen-dependent growth in vivo of a rat pituitary tumor cell line. *J. Natl. Cancer Inst.* 56:1149.

Sporn, M.B. and G.J. Todaro. 1980. Autocrine secretion and malignant transformation of cells. *N. Engl. J. Med.* 303:878.

COMMENTS

TOPP: Dr. Sirbasku, if you believe that the estrogens are acting at a site other than in the mammary tissue to cause the production of another growth factor, is there some way, surgically, that one could prevent that from happening so that the relationship between estrogen and mammary tumor growth is short-circuited?

SIRBASKU: Yes. We short-circuited it so well that we killed about 96 rats in 76 hr. If you remove the kidneys and the uterus from an animal and administer estrogen, the animals are all dead within 72 hr. So you have a real problem with that experiment.

HILF: David [Sirbasku], you showed a series of growth curves in which, as the amount of extract or factor that you added increased, the growth curve increased, seemed to come to a peak, and then come flopping down at the other end of that. Would you like to comment regarding what that flopping down phenomenon is?

SIRBASKU: Sure. In the case of the uterus, if you are not extraordinarily careful when you make your uterine extracts, there is a gross error that is made. When you administer even twice the normal physiological level of estrogen to a rat, the cervical plug is released and vaginal organisms invade. The vaginal organisms can be cultured. The organisms here are everything from Staphylococcus aureus, which has been implicated in toxic shock syndrome, to *Pseudomonas aeruginosa. P. aeruginosa* makes exotoxin A, 66K m.w., and we have purified it from our preparations. So when you add uterine extract, you may see something like that (bell-shaped curves), indicating that you have got inhibitors and activators in the same preparations.

All tissue extracts suffer from inhibitors. I am sure you are all aware of the chalone theory, which states that there are growth inhibitors in all tissues.

Role of Hormones in Mammogenesis and Carcinogenesis

SATYABRATA NANDI, JASON YANG, JAMES RICHARDS,
AND RAPHAEL GUZMAN
Department of Zoology and Cancer Research Laboratory
University of California
Berkeley, California 94720

It is not a debatable question whether hormones play a role in carcinogenesis of their target tissues, including mammary tissues (Huseby 1965; Clifton and Sridharan 1975; Furth 1975; Noble 1977; Welsch and Nagasawa 1977; Nandi 1978; Rivera and Bern 1980). The question is: What is their role and how do they act? Although hormones have many effects on mammary tissues, one of their principal in vivo effects on carcinogenesis appears to be their growth-promoting actions on these cells. Studies during the last quarter of a century have clearly demonstrated and delineated the roles of different ovarian, adreno-cortical, and hypophysial hormones in the growth of mammary tissues in vivo (Forsyth and Hayden 1977; Topper and Freeman 1980). The hallmark of in vivo hormonal studies has been the basic finding that mammary tissues regress following removal of specific endocrine glands and that growth can be restored and even stimulated in these regressed tissues by supplying the hosts with specific hormones from these same endocrine glands. For example, in mice, hormones such as estrogens, progesterone, prolactin, growth hormone (GH), and placental lactogen have been shown to have sustained mammary growth-promoting activity when given singly or in combinations depending on the endocrine status of the host (see Topper and Freeman 1980). Yet, none of these hormones, alone or in combination, have been shown consistently to be growth-promoting in vitro for unprimed or regressed mammary tissues. The only hormone that consistently has been found to be mitogenic in vitro for mouse mammary tissues has been insulin, and even this particular hormone has never been shown to cause more than a few rounds of DNA synthesis (Banerjee 1976; Topper and Freeman 1980). Thus, there is a paradox between in vivo and in vitro findings, and at this time the specific nature of hormonal influences on mammary growth remains unresolved. It follows, therefore, that it would be difficult (if not impossible) to determine the role of hormones in mammary carcinogenesis until more is known about their role in the growth of normal mammary cells. During the last 2 years, we have been attempting to develop cell culture systems to analyze the role of hormones, growth factors, and other agents in the growth, differentiation, and transformation of mammary cells. We are still far from achieving these goals, but our preliminary studies with mouse and human mammary cells, employing our recently developed culture system (Yang et al. 1979), agree with previous in vitro findings and have failed to show any appreciable growth-promoting effects of the so-called in vivo mammogenic hormones. How can these results be reconciled with the existing overwhelming evidence that hormones do promote the growth of mammary cells in vivo? This will be the subject matter of our discussion. In our presentation, based on our recent studies (Yang et al. 1979, 1980a,b,c; Nandi et al. 1980), we first describe the development of a collagen gel system for growing mammary cells in vitro; this is followed by the elaboration of our studies on the effects of hormones and growth factors on mouse and human normal mammary cells. Finally, we speculate briefly as to what might be the significance of these in vitro results in terms of the in vivo growth promotional effects of hormones.

Because of time and space limitations, we make no attempt to review the existing literature in this area, except to cite only the most pertinent literature. The readers are directed to the following recent reviews on the role of hormones in growth and carcinogenesis: Jimenez de Asua et al. (1979); Stiles et al. (1979); Elias (1980); Rivera and Bern (1980); Sonnenschein and Soto (1980); Topper and Freeman (1980).

MATERIALS AND METHODS

Collagen Gel Technique for Cultivation of Mammary Cells

Essentially, the culture method used by us is a modification of the method used by Michalopoulos and Pitot (1975). The procedures for the dissociation and for Percoll gradient enrichment of epithelial cells from virgin and midpregnant mouse mammary gland and from normal human breast tissues derived from reduction mammoplasties, and areas away from primary lesions in mastectomies, have been described previously (Yang et al. 1980a,b,c). Normal cells were also obtained from human colostrum samples by centrifugation in Hanks' balanced salt solution (HBSS). These cell pellets were dispersed and embedded directly inside collagen gels without further enzyme treatment or Percoll gradient centrifugation.

Collagen solution and gel were prepared as originally described (Michalopoulos and Pitot 1975). Briefly, rat tail collagen fibers (1 g) were sterilized in alcohol overnight and dissolved in 1:1000 acetic acid (300 ml) in sterile distilled water; the supernatant after centrifugation at $10,000g$ for 30 min was the stock collagen solution. Eight volumes of stock solution were mixed with 2 volumes of a 2:1 mixture of 10X-concentrated Waymouth's medium and 0.34 N NaOH and kept on ice to prevent immediate gelation. Appropriate numbers of cells ($2-10 \times 10^4$ cells/ml) were added to cold gelation mixture, and 0.5 ml of this mixture was added on top of 0.3 ml of previously gelled collagen in each well of Falcon multiwell plates and allowed to gel at room temperature. After this layer had gelled, cultures were fed with 0.5 ml of Ham's F-12 medium (Grand Island Biological Co.) containing 12.5% horse serum (HS) (Sterile Systems and Flow Laboratories), 2.5% fetal bovine serum (FBS) (Sterile Systems), 100 units/ml penicillin, 100 μg/ml streptomycin, 2.5 μg/ml amphotericin B, and various additives. The cultures were fed with fresh medium every 2 days.

For cell number estimates at the end of the experiment, each gel was transferred into a 10 X 75-mm test tube and 0.1 ml of 1% stock collagenase made up in HBSS was added and the mixture incubated on a gyratory water bath shaker for 30-60 min at 37°C. After digestion of collagen gel, cells inside the gel were recovered by centrifugation at 100g for 5 min. Samples were stored frozen until the time of DNA assay. The DNA content was determined by a fluorometric assay (Heingardner 1971) utilizing Babl/cfC3H mammary cells, counted in a hemocytometer, as a standard.

The procedures for tissue, organ, and urine extracts were as follows: Tissues and organs were excised from mice and homogenized with a Polytron (Brinkman, Switzerland) in 3 volumes of distilled water per gram of tissue. The homogenates were centrifuged at 10,000g for 30 min and the supernatant placed in dialysis tubing with a molecular cut-off of 3,500 daltons. Urine was placed directly in dialysis tubing. After dialysis against water for 2-3 days at 4°C, the volume was concentrated by absorption with polyethylene glycol 6000 (J.T. Baker Chemical Co.). The concentrated extract was centrifuged at 105,000g for 1 hr and the supernatant sterilized by Millipore filtration. The protein content was determined by the Bio-Rad protein assay.

RESULTS

General Aspects of Growth of Mammary Cells Inside Collagen Gel Matrix

A major difficulty in the cultivation of mammary cells has been the contamination with fibroblasts, which will overgrow the culture if not removed. In our procedure, there has been a virtual elimination of fibroblast overgrowth even after long-time cultivation because of our use of Percoll density-gradient-enriched epithelial cell fractions and the addition of 0.01 μg (mouse cells) or 0.1 μg (human cells) cholera toxin (CT)/ml to the basal medium, which inhibits fibroblast growth. Additionally, cholera toxin appears to have a growth-stimulatory effect on mammary epithelial cells.

In general, primary cultures of normal and neoplastic mouse and human mammary epithelial cells grow well when cultured within a collagen gel matrix. Proliferation of cells within the collagen gel is greater compared with cells that are grown on top of a collagen layer or on plastic. Normal mammary cells of mice fail to grow whem embedded in soft agar. However, cells grow in soft agar if they can attach to collagen fibers embedded in it (J. Richards, unpublished), indicating that both the embedded state and the attachment to collagen fibers were necessary for maximal growth.

Growth of mammary cells inside the collagen gel matrix is three-dimensional in nature. Mouse mammary cells produce outgrowths that frequently have ductlike projections, whereas human cells produce a variety of outgrowths. In general, human mammary cell outgrowths ranged in morphology from a ductlike appearance to a spherical mass.

Growth of Normal Mouse Mammary Epithelial Cells Inside a Collagen Gel Matrix: Effect of Hormones and Growth Factors

In initial studies, mammary cells were cultured for 13 days in basal medium containing .01 μg CT/ml with various concentrations of HS and FBS. Inclusion of serum in the medium was essential for the growth of mammary cells in culture. The extent of growth was dependent on the concentration of HS and the maximum growth was attained at 50%. A serum concentration of 12.5% HS and 2.5% FBS, along with CT, allowed maintenance without any appreciable increase in cell number during the experimental period of 2 weeks. This maintenance medium (containing Ham's F-12 medium with 12.5% HS, 2.5% FBS, 0.01 μg/ml CT, and antibiotics) was used in subsequent experiments to determine the effects of steroids, protein hormones, growth factors, and organ extracts on the proliferation of mammary cells in culture. The following is a summary of the results obtained from our studies of normal mammary epithelial cells (midpregnant and nonpregnant) in primary culture (Yang et al. 1980a,b):

1. Protein hormones—insulin (I), prolactin (PRL), and the steroid hormones estradiol (E), progesterone (P), cortisol (F), d-aldosterone (A), and testosterone (T)—singly at various dose levels showed little if any proliferative effect on midpregnant mammary cells in cultures. Similarly, no proliferative effects were observed on these cells when they were exposed to various combinations of these steroid and protein hormones (IE, IP, IF, IEP, IEPF, IEPA, IPRL, IPRLA, IPRLEP, IPRLAF, IPRLEPF). Recent studies also have failed to show any proliferative effects of steroid and protein hormones in collagen gel cultures of normal mammary epithelial cells from nonpregnant mice.

2. In contrast to the lack of effects of the classical steroid and protein hormones described above, epidermal growth factor (EGF), in conjunction with CT, stimulated as great a proliferative response on nonpregnant mammary cells as that obtained with 50% HS plus CT. The synergistic effects of EGF and CT were found to be less in normal cells from pregnant mice, suggesting that the cells may be less responsive to EGF during pregnancy.

3. Inclusion of optimal concentrations of various crude tissue (kidney, brain, spleen, uterus) and urine extracts to the maintenance medium resulted in proliferative response of midpregnant cells as great as, or greater than, that obtained by 50% HS plus CT. As kidney extract was found to be a rich source of stimulatory activity, such extracts were then prepared from mice at different physiological states (midpregnant, adult virgin, adult virgin with

pituitary isografts for 1-2 months). However, the level of stimulatory activity in the kidney extract did not seem to be affected by the hormonal status of the donor.

4. Recent unpublished observations from our laboratory indicate that insulin alone in the presence of low serum concentration (3% swine) is able to cause a six- to eightfold increase in the number of midpregnant mammary epithelial cells during a culture period of 1 week. Although insulin stimulated growth when the serum concentration was low, this effect was either abolished or greatly reduced when the basal serum concentration was increased.

Growth of Normal Human Mammary Epithelial Cells Inside a Collagen Gel Matrix: Effects of Hormones and Tissue Extracts

Initial studies with human mammary epithelial cells were directed toward finding an optimal culture condition that would allow maximal growth of these cells. We needed to be able to generate sufficient numbers of cells from one source for use in our studies to determine the effects of hormones on the growth of human mammary cells. The results from these studies (Yang et al. 1980c) are summarized below.

1. Sustained growth leading to an increase of 10-30-fold in cell number over the initial value can be attained in 2-3 weeks in primary culture in Ham's F-12 medium containing 12.5% HS, 2.5% FBS, 0.1 μg CT/ml, human male urine extract (6 μg protein/ml), and a hormone combination of 10 μg insulin/ml, 1 μg d-aldosterone/ml or (.005 μg/ml estradiol plus 0.5 μg/ml progesterone), 0.5 μg cortisol/ml, and 10 μg human placental lactogen/ml. Similar growth was also achieved in secondary culture after 1 : 8 split.

2. The maintenance medium used for hormonal studies consisted of Ham's F-12 containing 12.5% HS, 2.5% FBS, and 0.1 μg CT/ml. Inclusion of serum into the maintenance medium was essential for the maintenance of cells without any proliferation in culture.

3. Addition of either urine extract or hormones alone to the maintenance medium did not result in significant proliferation of mammary cells in culture. However, the addition of extract and hormone combinations (ILAF or ILEPF) together resulted in considerable proliferation of human mammary epithelial cells. In a few cases, primary cultures grew in response to the addition of hormone combinations alone to the maintenance medium. However, growth was not sustained when the same cells were treated identically in secondary culture.

4. Urine extracts were replaceable with extracts prepared from human kidney and brain as well as with EGF.

5. Studies were done to determine which of the hormones used in the combination was essential for growth. When hormones were added individually to urine extract in maintenance media, only cortisol was found to be essential.

DISCUSSION

Speculations of the Reasons for Differential In Vivo and In Vitro Effects of Hormones on the Proliferation of Mammary Epithelial Cells

The in vitro results on hormonal effects on mammary cell proliferation (described herein) are radically different from what is known with regard to the role of hormones in vivo in mammogenesis. Hormones such as estrogens, progestins, prolactin, and placental lactogen have been shown to induce mammary cell proliferation in vivo (Bern and Nandi 1961; Forsyth and Hayden 1977; Topper and Freeman 1980). Yet none of these hormones singly or in combinations were capable of stimulating mammary epithelial cell proliferation in our culture conditions. Although current studies have demonstrated the possible mitogenic effects of insulin and cortisol on mammary cells in vitro, these hormones are not considered major mammary cell mitogens in vivo. Contrary to in vivo findings, in vitro studies demonstrated the necessity for tissue extracts or growth factors alone or through their synergistic actions with hormones (exogenously added or those present in sera) in the promotion of sustained proliferation of mammary epithelial cells. Therefore, the chief question requiring analysis at this time is: What is reason for this discrepancy between in vivo and in vitro proliferative effects of hormones on mammary cells? The simplest explanation would be that either the current in vitro findings are artefacts of the cell culture system or that the so-called in vivo mammogenic hormones may not be directly mitogenic for mammary cells. The in vitro system used by us is by no means identical to the in vivo environment and a clear explanation of our results is difficult because of the presence of contaminating hormones and unknown growth factors in our sera-containing culture media. Therefore, at present, we have no way to ascertain unequivocally whether our culture conditions allow us to generate physiologically significant results. However, the finding that mammary cells in vivo and in vitro respond to the same hormone combinations with regard to casein production (Emerman et al. 1977) suggests that such culture systems may be suitable for analyzing hormonal effects on target cells.

Assuming that culture studies provide "physiologically" significant results as to the role of hormones, several explanations can be provided for the discrepancy between in vivo and in vitro results. As one explanation, Sirbasku (1978) has suggested that growth-promoting effects of estrogens in vivo on several sensitive mammary tumor lines may be due to an estrogen-induced factor from certain tissues. We have felt that an explanation of the in vivo-in vitro discrepancy of the hormonal effects on target cells (Nandi et al. 1980) must take into account the explanation for the presence of specific hormone receptors in these cells as well as their growth responsiveness to the same hormones in vivo. The following is a summary of our current notions in this area.

At this time, we think that the explanation for the observation that so-called mammogenic hormones are growth-promoting in vivo lies in the fact that hormone-induced growth of a tissue or organ in vivo is a complicated phenomenon encompassing a number of biological events at the tissue level, including cell division. Thus, to be growth-promoting, hormones do not have to be directly mitogenic on the target cells. Unfortunately, there has been a tendency to ascribe hormone-induced growth of target cells only to cell division. Yet it has been known that growth of target tissue such as mammary tissue in vivo is associated with the occurrence of a series of hormone-induced events such as (1) alteration of the epithelial cell shape, e.g., squamous to cuboidal and columnar (see Richardson 1947); (2) induction of hormone receptors (see Forsyth and Hayden 1977); (3) probable production of angiogenic factor (Soemarwoto and Bern 1958)—angiogenesis being necessary for nourishment and waste product removal by the growing tissue; and (4) a spreading factor (Elliot and Turner 1951) for the penetration of the mammary epithelial cells into the stromal component of the fat pad. Thus, it is a possibility that the mammogenic hormones do not have to be mitogenic at the target cell level to be effective in growth promotion. They can still affect target cells directly (justifying the presence of specific hormone receptors) and initiate a cascade of events, e.g., receptor modulation or cell shape alteration, essential for the ultimate growth of the organ.

Our current thinking is that mitogenic growth factors are ubiquitous and evolutionarily more primitive than classical hormones—and that they act on cells only after they have been prepared (appropriate modulation of cell shape, receptor content, angiogenic factor, etc.) by the classical hormones. Thus, hormones might be the ultimate regulators of tissue growth, although they are not directly mitogenic. Growth, regeneration, and repair are fundamental to the survival of multicellular organisms, and it is likely that evolution to multicellularity necessitated a continuous presence of the mitogenic growth factors, whereas hormones evolved later on as modulators of growth.

Finally, although our results are preliminary and will undoubtedly require reevaluation as techniques improve, it is obvious from our studies that a clear understanding of the role of hormones in normal growth and differentiation will be a prerequisite to understanding the hormonal role in mammary carcinogenesis.

ACKNOWLEDGMENTS

This investigation was supported by grants CA05388 and CA09041, awarded by the National Cancer Institute.

REFERENCES

Banerjee, M.R. 1976. Response of mammary cells to hormones. *Int. Rev. Cytol.* 47:1.

Bern, H.A. and S. Nandi. 1961. Recent studies of the hormonal influence in mouse mammary tumorigenesis. *Prog. Exp. Tumor Res.* 2:90.

Clifton, K.H. and B.N. Sridharan. 1975. Endocrine factors and tumor growth. In *Cancer, a comprehensive treatise* (ed. F.F. Becker), vol. 3, p. 249. Plenum Press, New York.

Elias, J.J. 1980. The role of prolactin in normal mammary gland growth and function. *Hormonal Proteins and Peptides* 8:37.

Elliot, J.R. and C.W. Turner. 1951. Some hormones involved in elaboration or activation of the mammary spreading factor. *Proc. Soc. Exp. Biol. Med.* 77:320.

Emerman, J.R., J. Enami, D.R. Pitelka, and S. Nandi. 1977. Hormonal effects on intracellular and secreted casein in cultures of mouse mammary epithelial cells on floating collagen membranes. *Proc. Natl. Acad. Sci.* 74: 4466.

Forsyth, I.A. and T.J. Hayden. 1977. Comparative endocrinology of mammary growth and lactation. *Symp. Zool. Soc. Lond.* 41:135.

Furth, J. 1975. Hormones as etiological agents in neoplasia. In *Cancer, a comprehensive treatise* (ed. F.F. Becker), vol. 1, p. 75. Plenum Press, New York.

Heingardner, R.T. 1971. An improved fluorometric assay for DNA. *Anal. Biochem.* 39:197.

Huseby, R.A. 1965. Steroids and tumorigenesis in experimental animals. In *Methods in hormone research* (ed. R.I. Dorfman), vol. 5, p. 123. Academic Press, New York.

Jimenez de Asua, L., K.M.V. Richmond, A.M. Otto, A.M. Kubler, M.K. O'Farrell, and P.S. Rudland. 1979. Growth factors and hormones interact in a series of temporal steps to regulate the rate of initiation of DNA synthesis in mouse fibroblasts. *Cold Spring Harbor Conf. Cell Proliferation* 6:403.

Michalopoulos, G. and H.C. Pitot. 1975. Primary culture of parenchymal liver cells on collagen membrane. *Exp. Cell Res.* 94:70.

Nandi, S. 1978. Role of hormones in mammary neoplasia. *Cancer Res.* 38:4046.

Nandi, S., J. Yang, J. Richards, R. Guzman, R. Rodriguez, and W. Imagawa. 1980. Role of growth factors and classical hormones in the control of growth and function of mammary tissues. In *Hormones, adaptation and evolution* (ed. S. Ishi et al.), p. 145. Japan Scientific Press, Tokyo, and Springer-Verlag, Berlin.

Noble, R.L. 1977. Hormonal control of growth and progression in tumors of Nb rats. *Cancer Res.* 37:82.

Richardson, K.C. 1947. Some structural features of the mammary tissues. *Br. Med Bull.* 5:123.

Rivera, E.M. and H.A. Bern. 1980. Hormones and cancer. In *Hormones in development and aging* (ed. A. Vernadakis and P.S. Timiras). Spectrum, New York. (In press)

Sirbasku, D.A. 1978. Estrogen induction of growth factors specific for hormone-responsive mammary, pituitary, and kidney tumor cells. *Proc. Natl. Acad. Sci.* 75:3786.

Soemarwoto, I.N. and H.A. Bern. 1958. The effect of hormones on the vascular pattern of the mouse mammary gland. *Am. J. Anat.* 103:403.

Sonnenschein, C. and A.M. Soto. 1980. But .... are estrogens per se growth promoting hormones? *J. Natl. Cancer Inst.* 64:211.

Stiles, C.D., W.J. Pledger, J.J. Van Wyk, H. Antonides, and C.D. Scher. 1979. Hormonal control of early events in the BALB/c-3T3 cell cycle: Commitment to DNA synthesis. *Cold Spring Harbor Conf. Cell Proliferation* 6:425.

Topper, Y.J. and C.S. Freeman. 1980. Multiple hormone interactions in the developmental biology of the mammary gland. *Physiol. Rev.* **60**:1049.

Welsch, C.W. and H. Nagasawa. 1977. Prolactin and murine mammary tumorigenesis. *Cancer Res.* **37**:951.

Yang, J., J. Richards, P. Bowman, R. Guzman, J. Enami, K. McCormick, S. Hamamoto, D. Pitelka, and S. Nandi. 1979. Sustained growth and three-dimensional organization of primary mammary tumor epithelial cells embedded in collagen gels. *Proc. Natl. Acad. Sci.* **76**:3401.

Yang, J., J. Richards, R. Guzman, W. Imagawa, and S. Nandi. 1980a. Sustained growth in primary culture of normal mammary epithelial cells embedded in collagen gels. *Proc. Natl. Acad. Sci.* **77**:2088.

Yang, J., R. Guzman, J. Richards, W. Imagawa, K. McCormick, and S. Nandi. 1980b. Growth factor- and cyclic nucleotide-induced proliferation of normal and malignant mammary epithelial cells in primary cultures. *Endocrinology* **107**:35.

Yang, J., R. Guzman, J. Richards, V. Jentoft, M.R. DeVault, S.R. Wellings, and S. Nandi. 1980c. Primary culture of human mammary epithelial cells embedded in collagen gels. *J. Natl. Cancer Inst.* **65**:337.

COMMENTS

SHELLABARGER: Dr. Nandi, can you get transformation in the mouse cells?

NANDI: So far we have not been able to induce transformation in vitro. One of the major problems here is to identify the transformants because there is no in vitro assay for that. So that is where we are spending much time right now.

SHELLABARGER: Are these virus-free?

NANDI: In the mouse that we are using, they don't express the virus.

SHELLABARGER: Are you talking about nondispersed cells or are you dealing with clumps?

NANDI: These are clumps of 10–20 cells. It is virtually impossible to use monodispersed cells, because 90% of the cells will be dead or will not be growing.

ROSEN: You make a distinction, which is sort of interesting, between primed and unprimed animals. As you know, all of the other earlier work always was done with estrogen-progesterone-primed animals in which the gland was removed and subsequent hormonal effects were studied in culture. In these studies, a marginal effect on growth of hormones was observed when they were added in culture.

NANDI: Of course they do. We did it first with the primed cell. You can take a regressed mammary gland from a hypophysectomized-ovariectomized animal and, by giving estrogen, progesterone, and prolactin, and so on, you can stimulate complete mammary growth. That should be the model. One ought to be able to repeat this in vivo phenomenon in the culture system. However, nobody has been able to do it yet. So nobody really knows what priming does.

There is a tremendous carryover of hormones and other agents which somehow modify the hormonal effects in vitro. We know that with human cells we can at times show excellent effects of hormones alone, if we use primary cultures. But as soon as the same cells are taken to secondary culture, they are no longer responsive to hormones alone. Now, if you add hormones and extract together, they will take off and grow, indicating that there is some kind of synergistic effect.

ROSEN: It suggests, though, that these growth factors have a fairly long half-life, because if you treat for 6-9 days with estrogen and progesterone and then remove the gland, obviously there is something that has been induced over that period that can be maintained for at least a short period in culture.

NANDI: As you know, in his latest work Sam Soroff has caused regression of mammary cells in organ culture. Then, by adding not mammogenic hormones alone but EGF plus hormones, he has been able to restore growth of these cells.

SIRBASKU: I think, along those lines, Dr. Nandi, the most important papers right now that fit that kind of model are coming from Chuck Stiles and Jack Pledger. They are saying that the cell cycle is divided into two portions. Cells that are arrested in G_0, which an unprimed mammary gland would be, would require something called competence factors, and these competence factors could bring a cell from G_0 into the G_1 period, meaning they have now entered in the cycle.

I think that what I am looking at—and I have been working along the same lines as Jack Pledger for a year now—are not the competence factors, but factors involved in the second phase of the cell cycle. You must have factors to go from G_1 into S, after commitment, and those are called progression factors. I think that I am looking at progression factors. I still don't think I ever arrived at what the competence factors were. That is my interpretation of my data.

ROSEN: Have you ever used a pituitary extract? I noticed that seemed to be missing from all the various extracts. That seems to be a logical extract.

NANDI: Have you ever used a mouse pituitary?

ROSEN: I know they are small, I agree. I realize that.

SIITERI: I want to draw attention to a very recent paper by Henri Rochefort in which he showed that the ordinary charcoal extraction procedures which remove free steroids do not remove sulfated hormones. Furthermore, he showed that estrogen sulfates are active in his culture systems. This has probably caused a lot of confusion in the past. It is easy to solve the problem, but most people have not addressed it.

SIRBASKU: It is an excellent paper. You have to treat the serum with aryl sulfatase. Also, you have to assay your cells for aryl sulfatase, which is a trivial assay, because you can use the ether-soluble layer as your count measure and just mix with the radioactive glucuronide or sulfate, allow it to stand 30 min, add ether, separate the layers, and count the ether-soluble fraction.

SIITERI: Dr. Nandi, I don't understand the collagen gel system, but, you know, steroids love to stick to proteins. Are steroid hormones, particularly progesterone, available to the cell in your gel?

NANDI: We haven't measured whether they are available to cells or not. But we do know that if we put the cells on the top of the collagen gel, the gel is floating, and then we add hormones. We can show a direct response to corticoids and prolactin in terms of casein synthesis by these cells. So the steroids are effective, but I don't know how much binding of progesterone or estrogen with cells has taken place.

KORENMAN: We are doing some studies on the interaction of various hormones on the cell surface. Dr. Nandi, your presentation brought to mind a couple of relevant matters.

CT is a chronic stimulator of cAMP through permanent ADP ribosylation of the coupling protein of the adenyl cyclase. Recently, it has been demonstrated that this coupling protein is found in the cytosol of many cells and also that this coupling protein normally will enter the cell membrane of the cell that you expose it to. It is quite conceivable to me that the cell extract, a potent element of the cell extract, is something like coupling protein and that what you may be seeing is a release of inhibition of cell division, which you are producing by AMP activation.

Now, you said that you use CT to prevent fibroblast overgrowth. But after several generations, that may not be such a problem. Have you studied these cells at all without CT?

NANDI: Yes, we have. It is possible to induce growth. For example, with CT, we might get a 15-fold increase in 2 weeks. Without CT, we will get maybe 7-fold growth within that period. So the growth is reduced. However, we can obtain growth in the absence of CT.

Name Index

Subject Index